Strong State, Weak Links

Strong State, Weak Links
Eugenics and the Southern Politics of Welfare

ANNA L. KROME-LUKENS

The University of North Carolina Press
Chapel Hill

This book was published with the assistance of the H. Eugene and Lillian Lehman Fund of the University of North Carolina Press.

© 2026 Anna L. Krome-Lukens
All rights reserved
Set in Minion Pro by Westchester Publishing Services

Library of Congress Cataloging-in-Publication Data
Names: Krome-Lukens, Anna L. author
Title: Strong state, weak links : eugenics and the southern politics of welfare / Anna L. Krome-Lukens.
Description: Chapel Hill : University of North Carolina Press, 2026. | Includes bibliographical references and index.
Identifiers: LCCN 2025045119 | ISBN 9781469693668 cloth | ISBN 9781469693675 paperback | ISBN 9781469693682 epub | ISBN 9781469693699 pdf
Subjects: LCSH: Eugenics—North Carolina—History—20th century | Eugenics—Government policy—North Carolina | People with mental disabilities—North Carolina—Social policy | Involuntary sterilization—North Carolina—History—20th century | Public welfare—North Carolina—History—20th century | African American women—North Carolina—Social policy | Poor women—North Carolina—Social policy | BISAC: POLITICAL SCIENCE / Public Policy / Social Policy | SOCIAL SCIENCE / Discrimination
Classification: LCC HQ755.5.U5 K76 2026
LC record available at https://lccn.loc.gov/2025045119

Cover art: *Biennial Report of the North Carolina State Board of Charities and Public Welfare, 1922–1924*, p. 87. North Carolina Collection, Louis Round Wilson Special Collections Library, University of North Carolina at Chapel Hill.

For product safety concerns under the European Union's General Product Safety Regulation (EU GPSR), please contact gpsr@mare-nostrum.co.uk or write to the University of North Carolina Press and Mare Nostrum Group B.V., Doelen 72, 4831 GR Breda, The Netherlands.

Contents

List of Illustrations, vii

Introduction, 1

Chapter 1 The Social Pulse of North Carolina, 16
  The Emergence of Progressive Reform Networks

Chapter 2 Constant Care and Anxiety, 41
  Institutional Segregation and the Eugenics Debate in the 1910s

Chapter 3 Save the Feeble-Minded Girl, 68
  The Limits of Institutions and the Logic of Sterilization

Chapter 4 The Root of Social Problems, 90
  Eugenics and the Training of Social Workers

Chapter 5 The Burden of the Socially Useless, 123
  Eugenics Research and the Campaign for Sterilization Laws in the 1920s

Chapter 6 Brewer v. Valk, 158
  Legal Strategies in Addressing Female Delinquency and Feeblemindedness

Chapter 7 The Human Element in the Modern Welfare State, 184

Epilogue, 214

Acknowledgments, 221
Notes, 223
Bibliography, 299
Index, 321

Illustrations

Figures

2.1 Caswell dormitory, 52
2.2 "Where Four Important Measures Are Taken," 64
4.1 Kate Burr Johnson, 94
4.2 Two families, 113
4.3 "County Homes Breeding Places for the Feebleminded," 116
4.4 "North Carolina's Best Crop—Her Children," 117
4.5 "Cross Roads Through Mothers' Aid," 119
5.1A Text introducing the report on a family in Swamp Island, 132
5.1B Fannie Wilks and her sister, 132
5.2 The Wake family, 135
5.3 Nancy Fehler Rode, 136
5.4 Don Fehler and his family, 138
5.5 Lina Fehler Eck, 139
5.6 Fehler family chart, 140
5.7 "Which One Would You Choose for the Brightest?," 145
5.8 Operating room, State Hospital at Raleigh, 148
6.1 1929 sterilization form, 161
6.2 "$100 Now," 163
6.3 Samarcand cottage, 166
6.4 John S. Bradway, 176
6.5 Duke Law class of 1933, 179
7.1 1933 sterilization form, 204

Map

7.1 Noninstitutional sterilization petition rates by county, 1934–44, 202

Tables

6.1 Sterilization operations by year, location, and type of operation, 1929–32, 164

7.1 Sterilization operations by year and type of operation, 1929–44, 197

7.2 Sterilization operations performed before and after the creation of the Eugenics Board, by origin of petition, 198

7.3 Noninstitutional sterilization petition rates in selected North Carolina counties, 1934–44, 200

Strong State, Weak Links

Introduction

In January 1919, North Carolina Governor Thomas Bickett addressed the state legislature to urge a sweeping range of reforms, including better roads, tax reform, and a law to prevent the reproduction of "idiots and imbeciles." This final goal was realized two months later when he signed the South's first statewide eugenic sterilization law. North Carolina had also been the first state in the South to open an institution to contain people who were "feebleminded"—a catchall category denoting low intelligence—during their reproductive years. To Bickett and other reformers, these eugenics programs were part of a suite of changes that would modernize North Carolina and make the Anglo-Saxon race "hardier and holier . . . not unlike the giants that walked the earth when the sons of God mated with the daughters of men."[1]

At the time, many leaders agreed with Bickett's sentiments. In the first half of the twentieth century, a majority of states in the United States had eugenics programs, which their proponents hoped would encourage "fit" people to procreate together and *dis*courage "unfit" people from reproducing. Like many other states, North Carolina passed restrictive marriage laws and institutionalized thousands of supposedly delinquent or defective people. In other ways, however, North Carolina's eugenics programs were among the most aggressive. Officials in the state surgically sterilized more people per capita than any other state: around 5,700 people, mostly women, between 1929 and 1974.[2] Unlike most other states, North Carolina sterilized people beyond the confines of custodial institutions, so eugenics programs had greater potential to touch the lives of average North Carolina citizens. Decades after the sterilization programs ended, in 2014, North Carolina also became the first state to offer financial compensation to sterilization victims.

This book focuses on the early twentieth century, when North Carolina created eugenics policies and programs that shaped the modern welfare state for years to come. Between 1900 and 1940, white leaders in the state engaged with eugenics ideology as part of broader state-building efforts. Reformers and officials built a policy framework that reflected their vision for the region: a society with a diversified economy and government programs to meet white citizens' basic needs, but one that enshrined inequality. In particular, reformers used eugenics-inspired metaphors to rationalize the unequal distribution of welfare services, giving new and supposedly scientific authority to long-standing prejudices about the undeserving poor. Social workers learned to see "feeblemindedness" as the "root of social problems." In their minds, moreover, feeblemindedness was inextricably linked to lower-class white people and African Americans. White reformers believed that eugenics programs could prevent "unfit" white people from passing on their supposed inferiority, thus strengthening the so-called Anglo-Saxon race and reinforcing the notion of white superiority. This conviction explains a phenomenon that surprises many people today: the state's eugenics programs initially targeted poor and allegedly sexually promiscuous white women. Only in the 1950s did officials shift their focus to Black women, who were then gaining greater access to social service programs, as part of the broader backlash in the South to civil rights victories.[3] Although the 1950s and 1960s were by far the most active years of the eugenic sterilization program, in this book I focus on the critical preceding years, during which eugenics ideology became cemented in policy. By focusing on the intertwined histories of welfare and eugenics in the early twentieth century, I show how welfare programs have been racialized in different ways across time.

This book is about the people who inscribed eugenics policies into the modern state, their reasons for doing so, and the consequences of their actions. These people included academics interested in studying the problems of the New South, newly trained welfare officials genuinely eager to uplift the poor, white middle-class businessmen and clubwomen dedicated to urban reform and rural revitalization, medical doctors concerned about rampant disease, and legislators and other elected officials. I examine how these white reformers' beliefs, influenced by both their upbringing in Lost Cause ideology and their interactions with reformers across the region and the nation, shaped the ways they presented problems of poverty and mental defects to the public. Their unwillingness to acknowledge the exploitative nature of the South's economic and political systems, I show, defined the policy solutions they saw as possible and necessary. Finally, I demonstrate how the policy choices they enshrined in law engendered ongoing inequality and perpetuated their beliefs.

It is important to note that few of these reformers would have considered themselves "eugenicists," in that their pro-eugenics activism was driven more by personal or political motivations than by dedication to any particular scientific theories. Because they did not proclaim themselves as eugenicists, I do not use that label. Nevertheless, many of the reformers in this book agreed with the core principle of eugenics: that by influencing who did and did not reproduce, they could improve the human race, particularly the Anglo-Saxon race. Eugenics ideology had a profound impact on their thinking and, in turn, on the institutions and policies they built. Importantly, while I focus on their interest in eugenics, many other principles shaped their beliefs. At the same time they lobbied for eugenics policies, they participated in numerous other reform campaigns, including campaigns about child labor, female suffrage, education, and public health, to name just a few. These reformers embody the widespread internalization of eugenics ideology among the Southern middle class as part of broader social reform efforts.[4]

The reformers at the heart of this book matter because they were also the architects of the modern state. I focus on mid-level policy actors, who often fall in a chasm between the traditions of political history and social history. Although not always formal agents of the state, they wielded power at a defining moment in the creation of strong-state liberalism. If we seek to understand both the promise and the shortcomings of our modern state, we must understand these actors' assumptions, their goals, and their methods. I document the process by which they built consensus, transformed ideology into social policy, and put policy into practice. Their efforts underscore the ways that public policy is implemented through the accretion of actions of many individuals, each with complex belief systems whose tenets shape their daily decisions.[5]

These reformers' assumptions about heredity, mental defects, and inherent racial potential shaped the creation of welfare programs at a critical stage in their development. Reformers' ideas thus also informed emerging conceptions of the ideal citizen of a modern nation-state. Anglo-American poor laws had long reflected the idea that only some people were worthy of financial beneficence, while other people's moral failings excluded them. Eugenics ideology carried that dichotomy between the deserving and undeserving poor into the modern era, using rhetoric of rationality, scientific expertise, and bureaucratic efficiency to justify continued discrimination. At this critical moment of state development, reformers reinscribed into the modern welfare state definitions of fitness for both parenthood and citizenship that were dependent on class and race biases.[6]

Beginning in the late nineteenth century, the "Southern problem" drew national attention. Many critics, both within and outside of the South, saw the region as backward and its people as not yet ready to be incorporated into the modern American nation. They lamented the region's "race problem" and its pervasive poverty and disease. Others saw hope in a "New South" where industrial growth, taking advantage of the region's natural resources and cheap labor, would bring the region into the fold of the nation. As Natalie Ring argues, the "Problem South" and "New South" were two sides of the same coin, a framing of the region that generated an extraordinary impulse for reform. The coalition of reformers who both lamented and attacked the South's problems included Southern and Northern liberals and Progressives, philanthropists, and federal agencies.[7]

Crucial to the solution of the Southern problem was building a citizenry capable of laboring in the modern industrial economy and participating in the democratic process. Critics saw the South's population, both Black and white, as too poor, sickly, and uneducated to do either. Their reforms consequently tackled the South's poverty, health, and education, using the tools of social science to define and address the problems. Poor white people in the South drew particular interest from white reformers, many of whom saw them as evidence of possible racial degeneration and as a sign that the South might not ever be fully integrated into the nation-state. Fundamentally, poor white people posed a challenge to the ideology of white supremacy.[8]

Like other Southern states, North Carolina faced a tangle of challenges at the turn of the century: rural poverty, a fast-hardening racial caste system, and a model of limited government that allowed for pockets of business growth but provided little economic opportunity for the majority of its citizens. North Carolina's economy was predominantly agricultural, and the last three decades of the nineteenth century were marked by falling commodity prices, high costs of supplies and high interest rates, and economic depressions. Life remained difficult for many North Carolinians. Small farmers and sharecroppers had a particularly hard life, working long days in all seasons. As industrialization took hold, more rural dwellers left their farms to find jobs in new mills or factories. Yet even in 1900, nine out of ten North Carolinians still lived in rural areas, and the state's per capita income was barely a third of the national average.[9]

Meanwhile, white elites fostered anti-Black racial animosity among poor white people and systematically removed political rights and economic opportunity for Black people. Bare-knuckled violence and rhetoric pandering to white supremacy—which reached its peak in the Wilmington coup of 1898—allowed the state's Democratic Party to consolidate its hold on the state for the next half century. White elites in North Carolina and other Southern states also began using legal tactics to maintain racial divides and minimize political threats. Under Jim Crow, they instituted a racial hierarchy that relied on disfranchisement, legalized segregation augmented by an elaborate code of social interaction, and the omnipresent threat of violence. In cementing their hold on political power, white elites also maintained their economic dominance. With a Democratic stranglehold and a strong tradition of local government, white political leaders hewed to a low-tax, low-service model of government. State legislators made only cursory attempts to provide a social safety net, leaving local officials to support the poor, elderly, and disabled with whatever money they judged they could spare from tiny tax revenues.

In response to these challenges, a coalition of reformers emerged in North Carolina in the first two decades of the century. Many of these reformers considered themselves to be part of the Progressive movement, which arose in the late nineteenth century to address the challenges of a modern, urban, industrialized society. The movement had myriad strands—indeed, so many that some scholars have claimed it was too divided for a coherent movement to have existed. But North Carolina's reformers, like Progressives elsewhere, saw themselves as unified around common values and goals, namely the principles that democratically elected governments should intervene for the common good using expert knowledge. Their campaigns in the United States included child labor reforms, public health, the Australian ballot, settlement houses, Americanization of immigrants, good roads, tax reform, and trust-busting. North Carolina's reformers took up many of these campaigns themselves, albeit within the context of a largely rural economy, an extreme racial hierarchy, and the restrictions born of a political economy predicated on maintaining cheap labor and low taxes.[10]

Thus, while North Carolina's white reformers took pride in being Progressive and shared ideologies with Progressives elsewhere, they also adhered closely to traditional power structures and operated under political constraints particularly evident in the South. Like reformers in other Southern states, they were engaged in constant battles with small-government conservatives, which forced them to rationalize every dollar they spent. At every turn they confronted skepticism about the need for government intervention. These patterns pulled their reform efforts in a more conservative direction. Rather than pushing for a more generous, universal social safety net, they created a welfare framework that met only the most basic needs of the people whom they and their political opponents agreed were most worthy. At the same time, reformers' failure to argue for more radical alternatives was often due to lack of imagination more than pragmatism. Their vision of an ideal society, like that of Progressive-Era reformers elsewhere, was limited by their own economic interests. Progressives were almost by definition people with ample resources that allowed them time to engage in reform. Their economic interests led toward maintaining the status quo. Although some Progressives were enticed by a social democratic vision, in the South that brand of politics invoked the specters of communism and racial equality.[11]

Southern white Progressives were constrained by their racial beliefs and the constant imperative to keep economic and political power in the hands of white elites. In many ways, their beliefs about racial differences mirrored those of white Americans across the nation. Many middle- and upper-class native-born white Americans assumed they were morally and intellectually superior to Black people, Indigenous people, Asian and European immigrants, and most other racial and ethnic groups. Progressive white reformers believed their campaigns to protect the white race from miscegenation and degeneration were, in fact, much-needed reforms. In the South, however, the stakes were higher. White power and social practices in the South were premised on racial capitalism, in which white people reaped the benefits from a subaltern labor force marked by Blackness. The architects of Jim Crow in the South—including many Progressive reformers—continually faced challenges to the stark logic of white supremacy. Despite common white rhetoric to the contrary, racial boundaries were neither simple nor self-evident. Racial mixing had occurred for generations, in situations ranging from partnerships of genuine affection and respect to white slaveholders raping enslaved Black women. Many Southerners with some Black ancestors could "pass" as white. Setting and policing the boundaries between white and Black was thus no easy task. White policymakers also had to decide how to interact with Indigenous groups, including North Carolina's Lumbee and the Eastern Band of Cherokee Indians, who complicated the dichotomous assumptions of Jim Crow. In this context, many Southern white reformers found eugenics ideology appealing as well as politically useful.[12]

Of course, eugenics was not merely a Southern phenomenon. Its principles appealed to many early twentieth-century leaders as a reform strategy that promised to remake the very essence of humanity. Prominent thinkers brought eugenic ideas from their birthplace in Britain to the United States shortly after the turn of the twentieth century. They argued that principles of animal breeding could be applied to the human race to produce stronger, more intelligent, even more moral human beings. Eugenicists' tools fell into two categories: positive eugenics approaches encouraged the reproduction of desirable or "fit" people, and negative eugenics mechanisms discouraged or prohibited the reproduction of "unfit" people. Positive eugenics efforts tended to be less coercive and usually were tailored to people with social and political capital. Negative eugenics focused on populations that were almost always poor, immigrants, or otherwise socially and politically disadvantaged. The principal tactics were sterilization operations and "segregation," the physical sequestration of target populations in sex-segregated institutions during years of reproductive potential. Some states also passed marriage laws intended to prevent people with mental illness, venereal disease, or other undesirable traits from marrying each other. Many eugenicists added immigration restrictions to their list of desired policies. Beginning in the 1930s, German fascists took negative eugenics to what they saw as the logical extreme, killing Jewish, Romani, and gay people, as well as other people they believed were unfit.[13]

American eugenicists of the early twentieth century believed the principles of eugenics led toward a better future. They argued that by selectively promoting or opposing the reproduction of various groups, they could eradicate poverty, crime, mental illness, and other social problems. Because of their only rudimentary understanding of genetics and their zeal for social engineering, they believed that a whole host of traits were heritable and that eugenics-based interventions would produce meaningful results. In addition to attributes that modern science has confirmed as having some hereditary component, such as vision, eugenicists fixated on character traits such as laziness and criminality, or on temperamental qualities such as "constructive imagination" and "prevailing mood." Many advocates assumed that character traits in their entirety were passed on, and they believed that poverty and other social problems were hereditary. They labeled undesirable heritable traits as "cacogenic."[14]

Their most common concern was "feeblemindedness," a term that is understandably offensive to modern ears. I have chosen to use this term throughout the book because it has no precise modern equivalent. Experts in the early twentieth century believed feeblemindedness encompassed a range of degrees of intellectual disability, often paired with physical disability. They sorted feebleminded people into "high grade" and "low grade," sometimes using results of intelligence tests to further divide their subjects into "imbeciles," "idiots," and "morons." (I use these terms in the text as well, when they are important in understanding how historical actors categorized people.) Yet to most Americans in the early twentieth century, feeblemindedness was defined as much by social class and sexual behavior as by intelligence. According to the accepted knowledge of the day, feebleminded parents were almost certain to have "defective" offspring. Eugenics experts were often unclear about the relative influence of genetics versus environmental conditions, but they argued that both could contribute to the problem—either feeblemindedness was a hereditary trait or feebleminded people were incapable of providing adequate parenting to raise "normal" children. Long-term solutions thus hinged on preventing feebleminded people from having children. Eugenicists claimed that sufficient dedication to eugenic principles would eradicate a range of undesirable traits within years or decades. Despite the now-apparent scientific futility of their project, eugenicists believed that their failures were due simply to insufficient dedication to eugenic principles: if feeblemindedness still existed, it was only because laws and social institutions did not go far enough in realizing negative eugenic principles.[15]

Progressive-Era proponents of eugenics formed elaborate institutions and networks to promote its spread. Much of this activity centered in the Northeast and Midwest. The American Breeders Association (later the American Genetic Association), founded in 1903, held its first annual meeting in St. Louis, Missouri; the Eugenics Record Office was founded in 1907 in Cold Spring

Harbor, New York; and the Race Betterment Foundation was founded in 1914 in Michigan. For people tied in to social reform networks, exposure to eugenics principles was almost inevitable. The general public also learned about eugenics as its promoters spread its gospel in newspapers and periodicals. People across the nation formed their own opinions as they read these publications or books about eugenics, such as Arthur Estabrook's influential family study, *The Jukes in 1915*. Although eugenics was inherently elitist and lacked true grassroots appeal, its principles were nonetheless common intellectual currency in the first decades of the twentieth century. Eugenics appealed to some middle-class white Americans because it offered a hint of personal control or validation: by choosing the proper spouse they could equip their children with a better inheritance and thus a brighter future. To others, eugenics helped justify privileged social positions. Its appeal was evidenced in popular movies, prescriptive literature, "better baby" contests at state fairs, and many other popular cultural productions. Its very malleability is what made eugenics so popular. While its claims to being scientific lent it credibility, eugenics rested equally on unscientific assumptions that anyone could adopt and manipulate.[16]

Eugenics policy in the United States took shape at the state level and varied by region.[17] The Northeast, Midwest, and West were the earliest to adopt eugenics programs, creating institutions to house feebleminded people in the late nineteenth century. Southern states built similar institutions a decade or two later. Similar patterns hold for the passage of sterilization laws, which thirty-two states passed at some point in the twentieth century. Indiana passed the first sterilization law in 1907 and eighteen other states followed suit by 1922. Southern states passed sterilization laws slightly later. In addition to chronological differences, states' programs varied in emphasis, depending on local concerns. But eugenics everywhere went hand in hand with concerns about the sanctity of particular races, and all states focused on some permutation of anxiety about racial purity or fitness. In Virginia, for example, pro-eugenics reformers were concerned with maintaining the "integrity" of the white race; in Vermont they were driven by pride in white self-reliance; and in California they focused on regulating white female sexuality and morality to prevent what they saw as racial degeneration. In Northeastern cities, the explosion of "new immigrants" from Southern and Eastern Europe lent urgency to policing immigration and the boundaries of whiteness. In the Jim Crow South, immigration was not a significant concern, but racial segregation and discrimination framed conversations about fitness and feeblemindedness.[18]

In the first half of the twentieth century, white leaders in North Carolina used the supposedly scientific authority of eugenics to prop up white supremacy, part of the long, contested process of creating a Jim Crow state.[19] For these reformers, poor white people challenged the logic of innate white superiority because their very existence presented alarming evidence of possible white degeneracy. Eugenics ideology posited both a social analysis and a solution: in white people, poverty and other social problems were most frequently the result of feeblemindedness or other mental defects. By reducing the frequency of these problems, they believed, eugenics programs could strengthen the so-called Anglo-Saxon race. "Anglo-Saxon" was a term white reformers used for rhetorical purposes. It denoted the purest and most noble strain of whiteness, inherited from the original white settlers of the state. In their minds, Anglo-Saxon racial purity was also linked to cultural superiority and the foremost achievements of modern government and civilization. Many white reformers and state welfare leaders adopted this analysis. Rather than addressing the economic and political system that caused widespread poverty, they taught social workers to identify where hereditary mental defects lurked in white families and to prevent these people from passing on their supposed inferiority. Eugenics principles, they claimed, were the "consummation of the true ideals of betterment of the race by elimination of the unfit." Policies such as sterilization and "suitable matings" were a "great constructive, scientific agency for promoting the welfare, the happiness and the general well-being of mankind." White reformers and welfare officials believed that mental defects were far more common among Black people, so their goals for Black people were merely to reduce what they believed were criminal and antisocial tendencies.[20]

Facing strong traditions against even rudimentary social services, North Carolina's reformers promised that, in the long run, eugenics programs would curb the costs of aid to the poor and disabled. They created a welfare system that relied on going only halfway: providing relief but attaching stigma; requiring means testing; and carrying forward the dichotomy of deserving and undeserving poor, couched in a newer, supposedly scientific language of eugenic fitness. In essence, they agreed upon a compromise in which public money would be spent in moderation so the deserving poor could create wholesome environments where "fit" children would not be tainted, while money would not be wasted on "unfit" people except to suppress their reproduction. Their efforts to shape the behavior of North Carolinians were partly symbolic, as they tried to educate the public about what a "fit" person looked like. Their decisions, however, also carried real and sometimes damning consequences for people who were sterilized, institutionalized, or denied welfare benefits.[21]

Working at a critical moment in the development of welfare, these reformers helped to define ideas of citizenship and belonging in the modern state.

The early twentieth century was a moment of many transitions in Americans' understanding of their relationship with the state—what they could expect the state both to provide and to demand.[22] We now see citizenship as a package of rights and responsibilities to be gained through either birth or naturalization. In the early twentieth century, that package was ill-defined, and answers were still evolving to the questions of who could be a citizen and what rights and duties citizenship entailed. For much of American history, legal citizenship was an option only for white men, thanks to the myopia of the Constitution's framers and restrictions such as the Chinese Exclusion Act, and despite the protections of the Fourteenth Amendment. Sustained efforts to disenfranchise Black and poor white people drastically shrank the electorate in North Carolina and other Southern states in the 1890s and 1910s. White women then gained the vote with the ratification of the Nineteenth Amendment in 1920. As crucial as these changes were in maintaining the balance of power in the Jim Crow South, citizenship was about more than the vote. By the late twentieth century, a mix of federal legislation and court cases extended the option of citizenship to most adults, and citizenship came to carry more extensive benefits, such as the legal ability to work, protection from deportation, and eligibility for social welfare benefits.

In this book, I use the word "citizenship" to mean more than the legal right to vote or to live in the United States. Instead, the term signifies questions about who belongs in American society and why. I examine citizenship as an identity, considering both who had access to that identity and how citizens were supposed to behave in social, political, and economic terms. In doing so, I recognize that although citizenship in the United States is a binary category—either one is a citizen or one is not—in practice, "citizenship can be delivered in different degrees of permanence or strength," as Nancy Cott has phrased it.[23] The reformers I highlight usually did not consciously set out to define the terms of citizenship. Yet the decisions they made had lasting consequences for our understanding of citizenship.[24]

Like many people today, reformers in the early twentieth century were concerned with the American body politic. They built a modern state that defined membership in that body politic—the citizenry. To reformers invested in improving the efficiency and power of the state, eugenics offered a seemingly logical mechanism to improve the individual citizens who comprised that body politic. To some reformers, the very quality of the social fabric depended on a sound racial heritage, and neglecting eugenics would cause "racial, and consequently social, degeneration." A dedication to eugenics, on the other hand, would eliminate the feebleminded, with the resulting "splendid feature" of a "noteworthy decrease in crime and the resultant betterment of citizenship in the state."[25]

Reformers also had to decide the privileges that accompanied citizenship status. As both federal and state governments created more services during the Progressive Era and New Deal, policymakers had to decide who was eligible for these services, including welfare benefits.[26] Defining rights of citizenship was a greater challenge in a rural environment. North Carolina's reformers aimed, like the federal government at the time, to expand the modern state into rural areas.[27] In many of their decisions about welfare, North Carolina's reformers and officials relied on eugenics ideology. They divided the "fit" from the "unfit," undermining the idea that social welfare provisions are a basic right, in favor of a welfare model that grants only certain individuals the full rights of citizenship. Moreover, reformers' definitions of both fitness and citizenship were racialized and gendered, with the pinnacles of both categories reserved for white men.

Reformers used the language of "citizen" when they wanted to emphasize people's rights to get a benefit or their potential to contribute to society. In this framing, citizens were white people who could contribute their labor in a capitalist system or behave in a noncriminal way. Citizenship included the abilities to care for one's family and to "think straight," as well as to "act honestly . . . to work industriously, to live thriftly." When welfare officials wanted to justify their work, they talked about the potential of benefit recipients to behave as citizens *with* the support of social workers and their interventions. In contrast, reformers and welfare officials rarely used the language of citizens when they referred to "defective" people. Although they believed a small group of "unfortunates" could be trained in self-care and become "productive citizens," some reformers singled out other "defective" people as unfit for citizenship.[28] The best that could be done for these people, they believed, was preventive work, including eugenics programs. One reformer wrote that eugenic sterilization should be "regarded as an integral part of a broad system of protection and supervision of those unable to meet unaided the responsibilities of citizenship in a highly competitive society." These reformers thus viewed citizenship as dependent on both body and mind, on one's current ability and future potential to be self-supporting and to comply with law and social norms.[29]

The first half of the twentieth century was a period of significant change for North Carolina. While North Carolina in 1900 was a poor and predominantly agricultural state, by the eve of World War II the state—and its government—were transformed in many ways. By the 1920s North Carolina led the South in industrial development, with textile, tobacco, and furniture factories providing wages for workers and enormous profits for their owners. Railroads connected small towns to national markets and allowed the greater movement of people and goods. In response to these changes, Progressive reformers expanded the state's stake in education, health, welfare, roads, and economic development. These changes continued in the 1930s: not only did the federal response to the Great Depression rapidly expand the state's welfare system, but the state took control of many local operations, including roads and school funding, and instituted the first state sales tax. By 1940, although the state's residents were still relatively poor and predominantly rural, North Carolina had the administrative apparatus of a modern state, and its strong industrial sector meant it was poised for postwar economic and population growth.[30]

The creation of this modern state was a moment of opportunity for potential redefinition of citizenship. White reformers' reliance on eugenics ideology and rhetoric—as a seemingly scientific approach that simultaneously reinforced their racial prejudice—helped them build into the modern state an exclusive rather than an expansive version of citizenship. In the crucible of attention to Southern problems, reformers used eugenics ideology to justify their decisions about welfare and citizenship, and they implemented eugenics programs to address concerns about white degeneracy.

This book is organized into seven mostly chronological chapters. The first chapter focuses primarily on welfare, the next two focus primarily on eugenics, and the final four chapters show how eugenics and welfare became intertwined. At the heart of each chapter are complex individuals: white welfare officials and well-connected reformers who fought simultaneously for eugenics programs and expanded social welfare provisions. I take up the story of these reformers at the turn of the twentieth century, when North Carolina elites were building a framework of racial capitalism that supported their economic power. I follow them through the height of Progressivism in the 1910s, the strife of World War I, the challenges of modernity in the 1920s, and the crisis of the Great Depression. Their beliefs and their choices show the profound impact of eugenics ideology on their activism and on the institutions and policies they created.

In chapter 1, I introduce the network of reformers who began to apply methods of the Progressive movement to rural problems. They developed a shared vision of social progress that relied on state and expert intervention to ameliorate a host of problems, including poverty, poor education, child labor, juvenile delinquency, and poor public health and sanitation. White poverty was a particular concern for these reformers. A network of middle-class and elite white men and women began to discuss new responses to the state's endemic poverty. In 1912, they coalesced in a statewide group called the North Carolina Conference for Social Service that championed a greater role for government in addressing the causes and consequences of rural poverty. As the "social pulse of North Carolina," the Conference was a potent political force in the next two decades.

In the 1910s, reformers began to pass laws and build institutions that supported their social vision, often using eugenic ideas of "fitness" to express broader concerns about maintaining the social order. Chapter 2 traces the growing interest in eugenic ideas in the 1910s by focusing on Caswell Training School, the brainchild of physician Ira M. Hardy. Following Northern models, reformers envisioned Caswell as an institution that would both train feebleminded children to be self-sufficient and serve the purpose of eugenic segregation, rendering the inmates unable to procreate. In the process of institution-building, medical and social welfare professionals educated other North Carolinians about eugenic principles. Although they faced some opposition, these leaders linked eugenic ideas of fitness to fears about poverty and race relations—ideas that resonated among middle-class white reformers who hoped to improve social services and prevent future social problems.

Within a few years it was apparent that neither was Caswell's physical space sufficient to house all the state's feebleminded white children, nor could institutional officials control residents' behavior. With the public fascinated by the repeated escape attempts of a deviant and supposedly feebleminded white teenager named Lydia Spruill, politicians and reformers reopened the question of Caswell's efficacy. Chapter 3 follows the resulting policy shifts in the 1910s. As wartime concerns about prostitution and mental defects mounted, reformers began to consider more drastic eugenic measures of sterilization and even euthanasia. Although the latter option never gained traction, doctors and reformers passed a sterilization law in 1919, with much of the public discussion highlighting fears about white womanhood.

While reformers were building institutions and passing laws to address the problem of the "feebleminded," they were also creating the bureaucratic infrastructure for expanded social welfare programs. Chapter 4 analyzes that work, beginning with a landmark welfare bill in 1917, which made North Carolina the first state to create a "county-unit" system to serve rural areas and attracted attention from welfare experts around the nation. With this legal framework in place, the new welfare commissioner, Kate Burr Johnson, filled out her staff in partnership with philanthropies and academic institutions. By the end of the 1920s, their county-unit welfare system reached even the most isolated parts of the state and provided the nation's first state bureau to coordinate Black social work. The new welfare board, although far from meeting poor families' needs, did provide centralized oversight and training of all social workers. This structural feature both standardized the distribution of relief and laid the groundwork for eugenic sterilization. Crucially, state officials taught homegrown social workers to see feeblemindedness—which they associated with lower-class white people and African Americans—as "the root of social problems." They were particularly concerned about the menace of "mental defectiveness . . . as a factor in race deterioration."[31]

During the 1920s, state welfare officials conducted eugenics education campaigns that resulted in a push for a new sterilization law. Chapter 5 examines welfare officials' extensive mental testing regime, their studies of deviant families, and their publicity efforts. In 1929, after multiple attempts, reformers succeeded in passing a new sterilization law that gave officials more power with less oversight. Many white leaders were now convinced that sterilization served dual goals of minimizing spending on welfare and creating a "pure bred stock." The champions of the bill in the statehouse made arguments in the language reformers had been using for years, highlighting the supposed social benefits of eugenics programs.[32]

When the Great Depression arrived, North Carolina's welfare officials were just beginning to implement sterilization programs. Despite the magnitude of the economic crisis and the structural forces demonstrably responsible for widespread hunger and unemployment, social workers continued to associate some kinds of white poverty with feeblemindedness. Even as the state raced to provide some measure of relief to the "worthy," state officials promoted sterilization and "eugenical social work" for the "socially useless."[33] Chapter 6 analyzes a little-explored but important case, *Brewer v. Valk et al.* (1932), which emerged in this context. The case centered on Mary Brewer, a poor white woman from Winston-Salem nominated for sterilization. The reformers who brought the case to the North Carolina Supreme Court intended to strike down only a narrow section of the 1929 sterilization law and pave the way for a new law. Within days after the court's decision in *Brewer*, the same activists who had brought the case on Brewer's behalf *and* argued on behalf of the state were drafting a new bill. The resulting 1933 law created a state Eugenics Board, which had authority over sterilizations for the next four decades. Their choice to embed the Eugenics Board within the welfare bureaucracy built an enduring link between eugenics and social welfare programs. Although the 1933 law and the Eugenics Board ostensibly provided greater due process protections for its targets, the reformers' real aim was to protect the state from legal challenges to sterilization—an echo of the collusion behind Virginia's infamous *Buck v. Bell* (1927) and an indication of the weaknesses in democratic policymaking structures at this critical moment in the development of the modern welfare state.

Chapter 7 examines the lasting effects of eugenics on welfare policies during and after the New Deal, as the state recommitted to sterilization. By the time the New Deal infused federal funds into social welfare work, North

Carolina had built a surprisingly effective, homegrown network of welfare offices filled with trained social workers. Although federal programs imposed new regulations on existing agencies, federal funds often flowed through established state channels. From 1935 onward the state welfare board administered federal funds, including for Social Security programs. With these funds, local welfare departments grew in number and size, fulfilling earlier reformers' vision of a strong network of county departments with centralized supervision. Moreover, state welfare officials continued to train local administrators of federal funds, and eugenics principles remained an important part of the state's welfare programs and professional training. As part of the scrutiny they applied to recipients of relief programs, state officials taught social workers to differentiate between "normal" and "abnormal" poverty. As the budgetary constraints of the Great Depression created additional financial incentives to sterilize recipients of welfare benefits, a state commission called in 1937 for expanding the existing sterilization program.

The state did, in fact, expand sterilization programs in subsequent years. For nearly four decades, with encouragement from state welfare officials, social workers actively used sterilization as a tool that they thought would reduce poverty, with a notable increase in the mid-1950s in the proportion of sterilizations targeting people living outside of institutions. Simultaneous fears about growing welfare costs, which many white people blamed on Black single mothers, led North Carolina and several other states to expand the scope of their sterilization programs while shifting their racial focus. In the early years of North Carolina's eugenics program, Black people had been sterilized at lower rates than white people, but by the mid-1950s, they were sterilized at higher rates, with Black women targeted in particular. From 1957 onward, the majority of people sterilized were African Americans.[34] North Carolina's eugenic sterilization program continued until 1974, by which time the state had sterilized around 5,700 people, mostly women. For the duration of the program, social workers looked at people in poverty and often saw feeblemindedness.[35]

Chapter 1

The Social Pulse of North Carolina

The Emergence of Progressive Reform Networks

In the late summer heat of 1905, a forty-one-year-old woman named Daisy Denson stepped off a train in Raleigh, North Carolina. She was returning from New York, where she had attended the New York School of Philanthropy's summer course for social workers. There, she had spent several weeks absorbing experts' lectures, visiting model institutions, and chatting with classmates from other states. Now Denson, the sole employee of the state's welfare bureau, was returning to North Carolina to tackle the problems she saw there.[1]

As the state capital, Raleigh was growing quickly, exemplifying the promise of the "New South." In this vision of the region, business and civic leaders aimed to build an economy that melded new industry with the South's abundant natural resources, while taking advantage of cheap labor. Industrialists in the Piedmont region had fared particularly well in recent decades. The American Tobacco Company in nearby Durham now dominated the nation's growing cigarette market, and High Point, to the west of Raleigh, had rapidly become a major furniture manufacturer. Thousands of miles of new railroads connected these industries to the rest of the nation.[2]

As Denson made her way home from the train station to her mother's house a few blocks north of the capitol building, she saw reminders of the major improvements since she had moved to Raleigh two decades earlier: streetcars, streetlights, telephone lines, and municipal water and sewer systems had been added during the 1880s and 1890s, as in North Carolina's other cities. Downtown, workers built dozens of new stores and office buildings. Yet Raleigh, with a population around 14,000, must have struck Denson as quiet compared to the bustle of New York City's millions of residents. Despite the recent proliferation of small towns and cities in North Carolina, the state lacked a metropolis comparable in scale to other Southern cities, let alone Northern ones. Wilmington, the state's largest urban center, had just over 20,000 people, roughly half the size of Birmingham or Little Rock, and less than a quarter the size of Atlanta or Richmond. Only four other cities in the state had a population over 10,000: Asheville, Charlotte, Greensboro, and Winston.[3]

Nearby Pittsboro, where Denson had spent her childhood, represented another side of the New South. As the Chatham County seat, Pittsboro was also a business depot for local farmers. The roads leading there were unpaved, but in 1886 a new railroad to Raleigh, thirty miles east, became an artery to outside markets. The surrounding countryside was dotted with new factories and textile mills. These light industries mushroomed as the challenges of farming drove many North Carolinians to seek steady wages and as the prospect of cheap Southern labor drew Northern investments in bigger factories. By 1900 the state had 177 cotton mills, almost all in the Piedmont, with company towns huddled next to them. As farm families moved to mill villages, they tried to maintain some of the communal values they brought from rural life, while dealing with paternalistic mill owners. Children worked alongside their parents; in 1900 a quarter to a third of mill workers were boys and girls under sixteen. Many white textile mill owners chose to segregate the work force, offering poor white families "racial exclusion as an employee benefit" and relegating African Americans to the worst and dirtiest of the jobs.[4]

Beyond mill towns lay farmland. This rural landscape was the least familiar to Denson, but over 90 percent of the state's roughly 1.9 million people still lived in rural areas. Most made their living from the soil. Although Denson's ancestors were slaveholders who owned large farms, the typical farmer in 1900 worked land about the third the size of antebellum farms. Many of these farmers owned their land, growing cash crops such as cotton or tobacco in addition to subsistence gardening that helped keep food on the table. Over a third, however, were tenants or sharecroppers, renting land at the bidding of the landowner and often falling further into debt each year. African American farmers were even more likely to be tenants or sharecroppers. Whether they owned land or not, small farmers often struggled with falling commodity prices, high costs of supplies, and high interest rates, as well as economic depressions in the 1870s and 1890s. For all these farmers, survival meant long days of hard work in all seasons.[5]

From her perch in Raleigh, Denson led a phalanx of men and women who set about addressing North Carolina's social problems, including widespread poverty, health problems, child labor, and poor education. North Carolina's reformers mirrored other Progressives in their underlying beliefs and in many of their strategies, but they also adapted ideas circulating among Progressives in urban areas to suit North Carolina's rural landscape, political traditions, and racial hierarchy. North Carolina became known as the "Wisconsin of the South" for its advances in education, health, and social welfare. The state's network of dedicated reformers expands our notions of the reach and significance of reform in the Progressive Era.[6]

This chapter introduces the middle-class and elite North Carolinians who began to respond in a coordinated way to the problems of the New South, developing along the way a shared vision of social progress—albeit one hamstrung by their prejudices. Linked through organizations such as the North Carolina Conference for Social Service, a generation of reformers learned about conditions in North Carolina and about Progressive policies elsewhere. White reformers developed a foundation of shared beliefs about the causes and consequences of rural poverty. Like other Progressives, they came to believe that they needed to do more to prevent social problems, and that doing so would require strong government intervention. They pushed for measures to improve the standards of living for North Carolinians, particularly for the neediest white people. They were interested in child labor, education, public health, and juvenile delinquency, but a campaign for improved social welfare united many of their concerns. The state's welfare bureau, the Board of Public Charities, became one center of activity. Although the Board was constrained by a tiny budget and lack of formal powers to intervene in local institutions, its leader Daisy Denson built an effective network of volunteers who reported on undesirable conditions and established some political impetus for change.

Beneficent Provision for the Poor

At the turn of the century, the railroads and factories of the New South were reshaping North Carolina's landscape and daily life for many people. The economic windfall of the New South, however, accrued to only a few. In 1900, North Carolina's per capita income was only 36 percent of the national average. Sharecroppers, factory workers, and other common laborers lived a tenuous existence, with a single failed crop or bout of illness spelling debt, hunger, or worse. African American farmers and laborers faced additional perils, including racial prejudice, legalized racial discrimination, and extralegal violence, all of which restricted their economic opportunities and punished them for challenging social and economic hierarchies. With lower rates of landownership and blocked out of the highest-paying jobs in the mills and factories, they were more likely to be poor.[7]

White or Black, poverty in the South's rural agricultural areas differed from the urban poverty that prevailed in the Northeast. To be sure, for poor people everywhere, adequate shelter and clothing could be hard to come by. Living in the country had some advantages, though. Poor people in rural areas avoided the rampant disease of crowded northeastern slums. And farming families, even those with little cash, could avoid the worst ravages of hunger if they grew some food alongside their cotton, or better yet, maintained some chickens or other livestock. As families moved to mill villages, some continued this subsistence gardening. Many poor rural or mill village families nevertheless suffered from nutritional deficiencies that led to pellagra (a chronic disease that produced skin problems and diarrhea but could also lead to insanity and death). Parasitic hookworm affected almost 40 percent of the population.[8]

Public support for the needy was minimal. Historically, local Southern communities cared for their own poor, while state governments offered more centralized support for orphans, the insane, and people with mental disabilities. After the Civil War, several Southern states created statewide boards to oversee charitable poverty-relief efforts. North Carolina was the first. During Reconstruction, its Republican-led legislature established a Board of Public Charities as part of larger efforts to establish basic rights for all citizens. In the state's "forward-looking" 1868 constitution, the legislature entrusted to the Board "the management of all charitable and penal State institutions," arguing that "beneficent provision for the poor, the unfortunate and orphan [is] one of the first duties of a civilized and christian State."[9]

The Board's broad constitutional mandate did not translate readily into action. The Board was charged with investigating and supervising all institutions, which included state-run mental hospitals, homes for veterans, and orphanages; county homes and jails; and dozens of private institutions. It was also instructed to study social problems such as insanity, crime, and vagrancy, and to recommend changes to the legislature. In its early years, however, the Board was "practically inactive," hindered by a lack of funding and legislative interest. The Board received a new jolt of life only when a state investigation of the State Hospital at Raleigh in the late 1880s made the governor aware of the stagnant Board. In 1889, the state appointed a new five-member Board, and in 1891 the Board began to receive some state funding and paid a secretary to conduct some of its work. Still, the Board's purview did not extend to providing services or financial relief to the state's indigent population. That task fell mostly to individual counties.[10]

Most counties had a poor home or workhouse, usually for the aged or infirm. Conditions at county homes were often far from desirable; the Board reported in 1901 that conditions there were often worse than in jails. One visitor to the county home in mountainous Cherokee County described it as "utterly destitute of all means of comfort. The houses are old log structures, and the logs are rotten. . . . There is not a shade tree in 100 yards, and it is one of the most horrid places I ever saw used for the purpose. It will be impossible to live comfortably in the house in the winter." Residents of the county homes lived under the watchful eye of superintendents, who might confine or punish them for disobedience. The able-bodied inmates were usually required to labor on county-owned farms to make the homes self-sustaining. Despite these limitations, county homes served a vital function by providing shelter and sustenance to the most desperately poverty-stricken people. At the turn of the century, county homes supported a statewide average total each year of 1,300 people, both Black and white.¹¹

County supervisors helped support other poor families through "outdoor relief," small monthly payments to help them purchase essentials while living on their own. Although counties generally allocated 10 percent of local tax revenues to support the poor, counties' provisions varied markedly. In 1903, while the commissioners of mountainous Transylvania County gave six dollars per month to ten families on outdoor relief, Iredell County, in the Piedmont, distributed one dollar per month to seventy-five families, and some counties distributed no outdoor relief at all. Most counties' spending fell between these extremes, with the average monthly payment in 1903 at $2.08. The Board estimated that 3,918 people received public funds each year between 1896 and 1901. The number of people receiving outdoor relief thus far exceeded the number residing in poor homes, perhaps because they preferred to maintain their independence or because of space constraints in county homes. Local officials, however, probably agreed with state board members that distributing poor funds without the supervision afforded by residence at poor homes could "encourage idleness and degeneracy."¹²

In towns and cities, private charity supplemented these meager public efforts but operated with no oversight or coordination, as did corporate welfare programs in mill villages.¹³ Associated Charities funded some rudimentary social services and provided food and clothing for the poor. Private groups, often with religious affiliations, ran orphanages. Other groups ran hospitals and sanitariums, some of which cared for the poor.

The state Board of Public Charities was charged with overseeing all these institutions but had limited funding and little power to sanction institutions for mismanagement. The state board did have power to license private hospitals caring for "inebriates," "drug habitués," or other mental patients, but not privately run orphanages, maternity homes, reformatories, or sanatoria. In addition, the Board's funding was restricted to office expenses and members' travel to meetings. Notably, the state did not provide funds for Board members' travel to inspect any of the institutions they purportedly managed. Perhaps in response to this quandary, the Board developed the idea of three-member county boards of visitors who would file reports about conditions in local institutions, including county poorhouses and jails. This informal arrangement helped the Board fulfill its obligation to report on conditions in institutions around the state.¹⁴

The Board's abysmal lack of funding and political authority was no accident, but rather was a logical extension of the ruling political ideology in North Carolina. As one welfare official later wrote, "this State is so strong for local self government, for state's rights, opposed to paternalism, in fact loves liberty[,] that it is a delicate thing to talk of 'inspectors.'"[15] The political tradition in North Carolina was one of localism and individualism, with one analyst noting that North Carolina in the nineteenth century "approached the political philosophers' concept of the 'minimal state.'" The state supreme court even explicitly took a low-tax stance in rulings in 1870 and 1885. In keeping with this tradition, at the turn of the century, state revenues were almost always less than combined county tax revenues, and a "good portion" of the state's spending on welfare actually went toward pensions for Confederate veterans. Both state and county spending increased gradually after 1870, as the government increased its stake in roads, education, hospitals, public health, and welfare, but state spending remained low until the 1920s.[16]

New Responses to Endemic Poverty

In the 1900s, North Carolina reformers began to address poverty and other social problems in an organized fashion. Like Progressive reformers nationwide, they were bolstered by their faith in expert knowledge, coordinated action, government intervention, and the efficacy of preventive measures where charitable responses had failed. They applied these principles to problems of the New South. White reformers focused on pushing the government to address persistent rural poverty, new forms of urban poverty, poor-quality schools, and malnutrition and other public health threats, while Black reformers tackled similar problems with little possibility of government support. Strong traditions of low-tax strategies and local political control often allowed only incremental change. At the state level, the concentration of political power in the hands of Democratic Party leaders required reformers to capitalize on personal connections and existing networks, including women's clubs and church organizations. A few well-positioned people connected various groups, creating overlapping networks of like-minded reformers.

Daisy Denson, the secretary of the Board of Public Charities from 1903 to 1917, was one of these key players. In many ways Denson was typical of her generation of reformers. She was a member of the white Raleigh Woman's Club, an Episcopalian, and a daughter of a Confederate soldier. Her vision of public welfare grew from her belief in Christian charity, her genuine concern for "the unfortunate and the weak," and her desire to maintain what she saw as the state's proud Anglo-Saxon heritage. Yet in other ways Denson stands apart from her peers. She was the first woman in North Carolina to hold an executive position at the state level and the first female state welfare executive in the nation.[17] She used her position to promote her vision of public welfare, which she refined through correspondence with Progressive reformers beyond state lines. Denson's career demonstrates the development of the state's systems of social welfare from the turn of the century through the First World War and the importance of a generation of female reformers who claimed responsibility for the public welfare.

Daisy Denson was born on December 1, 1863, amid the Civil War. Her mother Margaret Matilda Cowan Denson came from a prosperous North Carolina family that in 1860 enslaved eighty people on a large plantation near Wilmington. Her father Claude, born in Virginia, was a captain in the Confederate army, and after the war he opened a school in Pittsboro, North Carolina. The Densons established a comfortably middle-class life in Pittsboro, with Daisy the oldest of seven surviving children. The family had means enough to send her to the Leache-Wood School for Young Ladies, in Norfolk, Virginia, where she received a satisfactory, if unusual, education: among other courses, the school offered instruction in accounting and office management. In her early twenties she returned to Pittsboro to teach with her father. She later recalled that "when I grew up Southern girls were just beginning to venture out into the great world of business—teaching was about the only so-called 'respectable' opening for them."[18]

Denson's upbringing also included a heavy dose of Lost Cause mythology, including white supremacist ideology and nostalgia for antebellum social hierarchies. Her father served as the secretary of the North Carolina Confederate Veterans' Association. In 1887, the family moved to Raleigh for Claude to take a new teaching job, and soon Claude became a member of the organizing board of Raleigh's centennial celebration, which celebrated the city's ancestry as "pure English blood." The implicit theme of the weeklong event was reverence of the city's "Anglo-Saxon forefathers" and celebration of a mythic past in which white supremacy went unchallenged. Throngs at a parade "saluted with reverence" as eight Confederate veterans marched by. The Denson family also attended a more exclusive Centennial Ball, where the city's elite white youth danced "dressed in the quaint costumes of 'ye olden time'" while hundreds of less privileged spectators looked on "from outside of the ball netting."[19]

Unmarried at age thirty and residing at home with her parents, Daisy Denson filled some of her time with club and association work, a suitable occupation for a single Southern woman of means. After the family moved to Raleigh, she served as secretary for the Wake County Memorial Association and was for years an active member of the United Daughters of the Confederacy, spreading the Lost Cause creed she had been raised to venerate. She also joined the Monday Evening Club, a mixed-sex literary group whose intellectual discussions, according to a newspaper profile of Denson, "satisfied, in a measure, the intellectual cravings of the active brain which . . . longed to do more than was expected of the well bred Southern girl of that period." In

1904 Daisy and her sister Mary became founding members of the Woman's Club of Raleigh, which quickly became one of the largest member clubs in the white state Federation of Women's Clubs.

Denson had her first experience with "organized altruistic work" as a member of the Ministering Circle of the King's Daughters. Her altruism derived partly from her sense that social work was a Christian calling. The Densons attended Christ Church, Raleigh's oldest Protestant Episcopal church, where women worked on charitable efforts through various guilds and organizations. Because of her faith, Denson believed that there was no realm that social service could not reach and that "there would be no social work but for the life of Jesus and the influence of the church."[20]

Denson and many of her fellow reformers were part of a social movement with religious underpinnings called social Christianity or the social gospel. Although the social gospel had many variants, some core beliefs united its followers. These liberal Protestants believed that the moral teachings of Jesus called Christians to social service and reform. The central concept of the social gospel, as imagined by one of its foremost theologians, Walter Rauschenbusch, was the kingdom of God on earth—not a utopia, but a constant seeking of greater perfection. The social gospel movement was in many ways the religious analog of the secular Progressive movement, in that both movements embraced the potential of science to address the inequities of industrial society. Many religious leaders found inspiration in the social gospel message for their Progressive reforms. In the South, women in particular drew on religious justifications for their social service and reforming activities.[21]

In 1903, Daisy Denson's charitable work became her formal profession when she was appointed the secretary of the Board of Public Charities, succeeding her father, Claude Denson. Claude had been the board's first secretary, selected because of his political connections. Beginning in 1889 he conducted the Board's business from the family home in downtown Raleigh while still teaching at the Raleigh Male Academy. Daisy often helped him with the Board's work, particularly after his health began to decline in 1898, and she was named assistant secretary shortly before Claude's death on January 15, 1903. Daisy carried on in that role until July 1903, when she received word that Governor Aycock had approved her appointment as secretary. This decision made her the first woman appointed to public office in North Carolina.[22] By February 1904, Denson had persuaded the governor to give her office space in the west corner of the Senate gallery, "just under the roof." From her new office near the center of power, she was able personally to lobby senators and meet with other officials near their places of business. She gradually organized her work: she fixed regular office hours, "systematically arranged" all her records and "valuable books," and purchased a typewriter for her correspondence.[23]

Denson ran day-to-day Board affairs as she pleased. As she pointed out in 1912, she was the "only paid employee except the office janitor." Board members generally supported Denson and allowed her to work with minimal oversight. She sent monthly reports and requests for feedback about urgent issues to Chairman William A. Blair, a prominent banker and lawyer in Winston-Salem who headed the Board from 1904 until his death in 1948. She also submitted more formal reports to all five members of the Board at their quarterly meetings and occasionally consulted with Carey J. Hunter, the sole member of the Board who lived in Raleigh.[24]

Some people objected to having a woman in the job. Denson would never have been considered for the position without her father's recommendation. State law actually excluded women, as nonvoters, from public offices, although no one raised this issue with regard to Denson. But some observers wondered whether she was fit for the job, including one man who reported that he had got "hold of information which would not be given to you because you are a lady."[25] Such critics apparently believed that institutional staff would be shy about disclosing unpleasant details to Denson because of a woman's supposedly delicate sensibilities. It quickly became clear to Denson that in the male-dominated world of politics, professional credentials were one way to shore up her authority.

During the early twentieth century, charity workers nationwide began to receive professional training as social workers. Social work professionals absorbed and embodied the Progressive faith in expert knowledge. These new professionals sought to differentiate themselves from members of benevolent organizations and to claim control over growing welfare programs on the state and national level. They argued that charity was not sufficient; in fact, charity might even be counterproductive. Instead, they emphasized preventive measures that could stem public health problems or social problems of poverty, insanity, or deviance before they fully took hold.[26]

To enhance both her credibility and her effectiveness, Denson maintained connections with national social work organizations and experts in other states. Of primary importance was the National Conference of Charities and Correction (NCCC), founded in 1874. Upon her father's death, Denson took over as state corresponding secretary and faithfully attended the annual conferences to present North's Carolina report, even though she had to take unpaid leave and cover her own expenses. She also served on several NCCC committees. When Denson was not able to attend the national conference, she would have received a bound copy of the proceedings and could read the latest discussions of social welfare issues. She also attended other conferences, such as a 1910 meeting of the International Prison Congress in Washington, DC, which attracted delegates from thirty-nine countries. She sometimes toured institutions in other states, and she maintained an active correspondence with her counterparts elsewhere. From all these experiences, she culled recommendations that she saw as relevant to North Carolina and shared them with legislators in her annual reports.[27]

Denson also sought out training at the Summer School of Philanthropy in New York, which she attended in July 1905, again taking unpaid leave but receiving a scholarship from the Charity Organization Society of New York. As she wrote to the school's director, "I want to see and know! Then I shall speak with no uncertain voice of the needs of the state. I see these needs now, but I must be in position to offer not only an ideal but a practical plan." The summer school program included visits to model institutions and discussions with experts about current social welfare approaches. Denson traded on the school's cachet to gain respect in relationships with other professionals. In 1910, writing to an official at the Chicago School of Civics and Philanthropy, she referred to herself as "an old scholar of the New York school, summer, 1905," stretching the truth to her advantage. She kept in touch with her classmates even ten years later. Back in North Carolina, Denson's work reflected her professional training; her daily diary entries were terse accounts of facts uncovered and paperwork completed, while her correspondence referred to experts' opinions on how to approach the problems she faced.[28]

Yet professional training was little help in Denson's biggest challenge: singlehandedly overseeing dozens of institutions spread across more than 50,000 square miles, with a bare-bones budget and limited legal power to intervene when conditions were inadequate. Although the state considered it a misdemeanor for institutional officials to fail to report on conditions at the institutions, there was no such sanction for *tolerating* poor conditions such as housing mentally ill patients in county jails. Publishing the names of the delinquent counties was Denson's only real recourse. Her annual reports included descriptions of the conditions in state and local institutions, but the effect of these illustrations on the public was probably negligible.[29]

To accomplish her job of overseeing the state's institutions, Denson relied on a network of volunteers: untrained members of county boards of visitors, medical doctors who felt called to Christian charity, ministers who headed orphanages, and clubwomen imbued with the spirit of reform. Most of these volunteers shared Denson's sensibilities of Christian social service and a Progressive faith in preventive measures. They also shared similar social positions as members of the state's white, urban elite, endowing many of them with political connections. As Denson told a colleague from Minnesota, such local operatives were often "the direct cause" of a new county home because "these local men are often placed on important work for the State and are sometimes members of the Legislature, etc."[30]

Although Denson tapped into established networks, including the white Federation of Women's Clubs and religious groups, the goal of social welfare reform also transformed extant organizations and sparked the creation of new groups. As reformers sought each other out, they shared their knowledge and optimism about their reform efforts. Powerful people and organizations coalesced around the ambition of seeking Progressive solutions to a number of interconnected social problems. In the process, like Progressive reformers elsewhere, they became a political force, pushing North Carolina to take a more proactive, interventionist approach to endemic poverty, poor educational opportunities, and rampant public health problems.

Organized Womanhood

Women's clubs across the nation were important sites of Progressive reform, and North Carolina's women's clubs were no exception. In a patriarchal society that otherwise restricted elite and middle-class women to the domestic sphere, a woman's club served as an outlet for her energy, as well as a supportive social circle that recognized her abilities and nurtured her talents. For both white and Black women, clubs provided an important space to organize around issues of shared concern and to pool their political power. Even without the vote, women drew on their influence as mothers and as moral guardians to tackle a multitude of social ills, both through charitable efforts and by pushing Progressive reforms through the legislature. Their collective efforts expanded the state's responsibility for community welfare and were critical in placing North Carolina at the forefront of Progressivism in the New South.

Clubwomen's Progressive-Era social reform was an outgrowth of earlier charitable and reform efforts. Nationwide, such Progressive-Era reforms built on a robust tradition of women's political activism, including the temperance and abolition movements. In the antebellum South, the first women's clubs were religious organizations. By the late nineteenth century, some clubs were focused on temperance or philanthropic activities, and for white women patriotic and hereditary societies were popular. Building on women's status as caregivers, many clubs began to explore aspects of social welfare, including education, child welfare, prison conditions, and public health. For many middle-class women, charitable work with less fortunate North Carolinians opened their eyes to social problems and sparked their interest in substantive reform. For example, clubwomen who were distressed to find infrequent religious services at county homes might push county commissioners to provide new management for the homes. Many clubs' work focused on "practical things," such as providing books or clothing for schoolchildren, raising funds for nurses, and providing "travelers' aid" at railroad stations.[31]

At the turn of the century, Black and white clubwomen's reform efforts in the South were almost entirely segregated but sometimes ran in parallel streams. North Carolina had many types of women's clubs, but the white Federation of Women's Clubs (FWC) and the Black Federation of Colored Women's Clubs were statewide organizations that became the central arenas for women's social welfare work. After its organization in 1902, the white federation grew quickly in size and influence. The Black federation, founded in 1909, was a smaller group with considerably less influence with white power brokers; nevertheless, it was an important meeting ground for middle-class African American women. Other powerful club networks included the white United Daughters of the Confederacy and white and Black members of the Kings' Daughters and the Women's Christian Temperance Union.[32]

The white Federation of Women's Clubs facilitated reform efforts by educating members and disseminating information about club activities, with charitable work and social reform occurring under many names. From 1902 to 1914, for example, the FWC had departments focused on health, child study, state charities, social service, constructive philanthropy, and village improvement. To inform and inspire other clubs, the annual yearbook included accounts of member clubs' activities. The FWC collected papers written by women for their own clubs on a variety of subjects and lent them out to any clubs studying those subjects. Although many of the papers were on literary, cultural, or historical topics, others tackled areas related to social reform such as the "feeding of infants" and "the development of brain cells." The state FWC also provided materials for members to make presentations in their local communities. In 1912, the civics department provided stereopticon slides and an accompanying lecture on civics and health. Clubs that borrowed this set of materials could read the prepackaged lecture while showing the slides for an effective public presentation.[33]

To learn about the state's most pressing issues, club leaders invited experts as guest speakers. At the FWC's annual conventions, experts offered analysis of common social problems and sometimes influenced the direction of federation activity. At the 1910 convention, one expert spoke on hookworm and tuberculosis, and Dr. Watson Smith Rankin, the head of the state Board of Health, also made a "stirring address." After hearing these public health experts speak, delegates inaugurated a federation department of health. National leaders in social welfare, too, were invited guests at the Federation of Women's Clubs. In 1913, Julia Lathrop, the head of the Children's Bureau, spoke at the annual convention for thirty minutes, explaining "in a concise and illuminating way the methods of work and sphere of usefulness" of the bureau to a "spellbound" audience.[34]

The work of one dedicated chair of the health department demonstrates the FWC's approach to educating clubwomen. In 1911, Mrs. W. N. Hutt noted that one of her goals was "to encourage clubs to not scatter effort on several lines of work, but to concentrate on one definite line until results are reached." Her approach was first to send information about "health subjects" to all the clubs, asking that club members read them at meetings. Next, she had the hundreds of clubwomen in the state added to the mailing list of the state Board of Health "so that each one receives a monthly bulletin on health subjects." In a single year she gave almost two hundred lectures about health topics under the aegis of the Farmers' Institutes and the Board of Agriculture, targeting farm women who "need a knowledge of how to promote health in the home and in the locality." She also organized a statewide essay contest on topics of tuberculosis, hookworm, and general sanitation. As a result of her campaigns, Hutt reported that local clubs had organized for food safety, had educated other women about disease prevention and pest control, and were "instrumental . . . in the passing and enforcement of effective rules for town sanitation."[35]

As a clubwoman and a welfare professional with national connections, Daisy Denson was a crucial resource for many white clubs, helping to shape their reform platforms. She began this work in her home club, the Raleigh Woman's Club. As chair of its Social Service Department, her projects for the club in its inaugural year included a study of "child-saving" that examined the role of industrial schools and a discussion of "private charitable forces and public relief forces." Denson used her knowledge to help other clubs as well, with the chair of the state FWC's social service committee noting in 1913 that Denson's experience made her suggestions "most valuable in formulating our line of work." Clubwomen sometimes wrote to Denson asking for information about particular social issues. In 1912 one woman wrote on behalf of her club in Clayton as they took up the study of insanity. Denson sent her the latest report of the Board of Public Charities and lent her copies of two bulletins from the Indiana Board of State Charities. She described the state's current facilities, the latest developments in treatments for insanity, and her hopes for legislative appropriations for a psychopathic ward at a state hospital.[36]

In all her interactions, Denson strove to educate clubwomen about key principles of professional social work, particularly the necessity of prevention rather than ameliorative measures. As she noted to the clubwoman from Clayton, "on this subject, Insanity, as upon so many other subjects for social study and betterment[,] prevention is looming larger daily."[37] Many clubwomen were familiar with the importance of prevention in public health work, and the concept would have transferred easily to work in the closely related field of welfare.

Thanks to Denson, white clubwomen also became involved with the state's welfare system, where they extended Denson's influence and made lasting contributions through official oversight roles as members of county welfare boards. As late as 1894, there were no women on the county Boards of Visitors, although Claude Denson had trouble filling the seats and thought female involvement would be helpful. By the time Daisy Denson took office in 1903, many county boards had at least one female "Auxiliary Visitor" in addition to three male members. Denson pressed individual women to join county boards and worked with state FWC leaders to increase women's involvement in inspecting local jails and poor homes. Under her watch, women became strongly represented: in 1908, she began to list women's names with the men's as regular members of the county boards, and the next year forty-three of the ninety-three functioning county boards had least one woman among their members. Throughout the 1910s, the FWC's social service chairs pushed clubwomen to inspect local institutions and to join the official county boards.[38] Women's involvement with the welfare board reshaped both the state's power and their own understanding of welfare. Their increased presence gave Denson more insight into conditions at county institutions, ultimately affording her greater influence over counties' work and ammunition for more sweeping statewide reforms. It also gave women's local charitable efforts the weight of state authority. For many women, service on county welfare boards was also an important avenue of education and reform.

As they learned more about social problems and Progressive principles of social work, white clubwomen embraced a distinct role in social welfare reform. From Denson and other professional social workers, clubwomen learned that charity was not sufficient; in fact, charity might even be counterproductive because it could cause dependence. Instead, they learned, North Carolina needed trained social workers who were well versed in preventive measures that could stem social problems of poverty, insanity, or deviance before they fully took hold. But despite their eagerness to hear about emerging trends in the field of social reform, clubwomen's class status set them apart from the emerging profession of social work. Their role, instead, was to throw their political weight behind causes. When the Federation of Women's Clubs coordinated its efforts statewide, it massed the full force of thousands of white clubwomen. Their lobbying efforts included sending letters and petitions to legislators or voicing their opinions in person. They often relied on men sympathetic to their causes to speak on their behalf, but even so were essential in making governments take on social realms that had traditionally been the responsibility of families or communities.[39]

White clubwomen's purview was broad, the result of clubs' wide-ranging interest in personal and civic improvement. Sallie Southall Cotten, a founder of the Federation of Women's Clubs, recalled that "nothing was so occult as to intimidate the women of that day." A club could take up the study of insanity one month and Elizabeth Browning's poetry the next, and follow it with an exploration of environmental conservation. The result was a conception of "social welfare" that ignored the professional boundaries between education, public health, and social work. Instead, clubwomen integrated traditional areas of organized philanthropy with reforms in libraries, civic betterment, good government, and more. This approach recognized the intricate ties between many social problems, as when one department noted in 1912 that civics and health are "so closely allied."[40]

Yet while white clubwomen's treatment of the connections between branches of social reform was forward-thinking, in other ways their social vision was limited. Committed to maintaining the social order, they built their social reforms around middle-class ideals, strict gender roles, and racial segregation. Even as philanthropic efforts such as education of mill operatives highlighted the shortcomings of the New South economy, Southern white clubwomen's personal and economic ties to that economic system, as well as their faith in the race and class distinctions embedded in the New South's hierarchy, led them to abstain from real critique.[41]

Conversely, Black women could not claim "the privileges of ladyhood" and had a more difficult political task.[42] For Black women, organizing in clubs was an important means of providing for the community when the state shut them out. They began by transforming church missionary societies and other existing organizations into social service agencies. As Black clubwomen organized statewide and regional bodies such as the North Carolina Federation of Colored Women's Clubs, they also took up topics such as public school teaching, civic improvement, and public health campaigns.

Whereas white women focused on charity and were motivated by an abstract idea of Christian benevolence, Black women sought to provide services for African Americans without regard to class, reflecting the necessity of basic services in health and education. Perceived as less threatening politically than Black men (at least before the passage of the Nineteenth Amendment, which granted women the right to vote), Black women could safely "serve as emissaries to local governments" and organize institutions that supported Black communities, painting their reform activities as part of their duties as women rather than as part of a political agenda. Yet their work did have a political edge, even if they sometimes chose to hide it. By improving conditions for African Americans, promoting respectability and morality, and "uplifting" the race, Black women combated notions of Black inferiority.[43]

In campaigns to establish institutions or involvement with local welfare boards, North Carolina's reform-minded white and Black women repeatedly confronted and challenged ideas about women's capabilities and proper gender roles. As they drew on their gender and moral authority to justify their actions, they simultaneously expanded the bounds of acceptable female behavior. Still, their sex restricted their political options. Not yet enfranchised, these social crusaders had limited influence within the state. It was only with the support of like-minded male activists, officials, and legislators that North Carolina's women accomplished their goals. One pivotal organization where white men and women found common ground was the North Carolina Conference for Social Service.[44]

To "Save" and "Enrich Life": The North Carolina Conference for Social Service

The North Carolina Conference for Social Service, founded in 1912, became an important forum for reform-minded white men and women to learn about the latest developments in welfare and social service, as well as an avenue to coordinate political activities. Daisy Denson had long been convinced that North Carolina needed a state Conference of reformers to push legislative action, which some other states had. As early as 1903, she called for a "State Conference of Charities" that would advance "all movements for the benefit of the weak and unfortunate, [learn] each other's experience and educat[e] the masses to see these questions aright." But Denson could not create an organization singlehandedly.[45]

The North Carolina Conference coalesced after several of the state's leading reformers attended the May 1912 Southern Sociological Congress in Tennessee, where they found a new sense of purpose.[46] Four months later, seven influential North Carolinians convened at the Raleigh Chamber of Commerce to discuss the creation of a statewide social services Conference: Daisy Denson; Dr. Watson Smith Rankin, the head of the state Board of Health; Dr. Louis Burgin McBrayer, superintendent of the State Tuberculosis Sanatorium; Wiley Hampton Swift, former superintendent of Greensboro schools and a legal adviser of the National Child Labor Committee; Reverend M. L. Kesler, head of the Baptist Orphanage at Thomasville; Dr. James Yadkin Joyner, state superintendent of public instruction; and Clarence Poe, editor of the *Progressive Farmer*. After their meeting, they issued a call to "all social workers and all persons interested in the general uplift and betterment of the State" to attend a Conference in early 1913. Denson exulted to Rankin that "This is the greatest step taken for uplift in our history. It will flood the dark places with light" and awaken "the [moral] consciousness of the citizens."[47]

News about the Conference spread quickly as organizers recruited attendees. Progressive-leaning newspapers across the state published information about the upcoming Conference, highlighting its already large membership, including "many of the very prominent people of the state," and the eminence of invited speakers. Echoing press releases from Rankin, they also emphasized the breadth of the conference's reform goals, with topics ranging from illiteracy to taxation, human health, and the "negro problem." The Raleigh *News and Observer*, whose editor Josephus Daniels frequently sympathized with Progressive causes, encouraged attendance by those who shared the modern "progressive spirit": the idea that "it is not the few who are to be considered, but that it is the many whose interests are to be subserved."[48]

When the conference took place in February 1913, it was a resounding success. The 400 attendees from every part of the state far exceeded organizers' hopes of 150 attendees. The two-day event opened on a wintry Tuesday evening in February. Despite the "very bad weather," hundreds of people nearly filled Raleigh's First Baptist Church to hear speeches by luminaries, including a welcome by Governor Locke Craig. The featured speaker was Oklahoma Senator Robert L. Owen, a "militant progressive" and a crusader for a national public health bureau. The positive reaction to Owen, who had clear socialist leanings, indicates surprising political openness among North Carolina's Progressives. After Governor Craig introduced him as "a practical idealist," Owen gave an impassioned keynote speech about how "practically every evil" the conference hoped to address was attributable to poverty. The Raleigh *News and Observer* reported favorably on this opening session, praising Owen's "sanity" and knowledge."[49]

During the conference, attendees heard speakers on a range of topics, from "the dependent child" to legal reforms in criminal procedure. Some lively sessions took the full time allotted; at other moments, "the hush, born of deep interest, was tense" and there was a "feeling of earnestness and reverence." One evening, the state's legislative session adjourned to attend Conference addresses in the House chamber on "four of state's most pressing needs": taxation, public health, child labor, and public school attendance.[50]

For many listeners, one address on the first night encapsulated the Conference's aims: William L. Poteat's thoughts on the "correlation of social forces." Poteat was a professor of biology at Wake Forest University who became a Conference leader in the decades to follow. Poteat's speech summed up the need for cooperation among all those interested in "social amelioration." Like Denson a proponent of the social gospel, Poteat drew inspiration from the "practical aim of Jesus," which he said was "to extend the ministry of relief to human suffering and need." Unfortunately, he noted, the social forces of "the home, the school, religion, government, business" were working for the same goals but "independently of one another." He hoped to make each group aware of the others, "and by uniting them, multiply their efficiency."[51]

Poteat's listeners heard in his speech a "clear, convincing, ennobling" call to action. Instead of being daunted by the sheer variety and magnitude of the problems they faced, Conference members spied an opportunity in "allying the fighting forces" against problems with common roots of "poverty, ignorance, and crime." As speaker after speaker showed, the correlation of social forces would require government intervention. Broad social change required the state to supply "remedies for social evils," going beyond its traditional role of protecting life and property and administering justice.[52]

Conference members thus shared key beliefs that aligned them with other Progressives of the time, and the Conference claimed the notion of "progress" as central to their work. They acknowledged the deep-seated relationships among various social problems and felt a duty to address the roots of the problems. Moreover, they were optimistic that their efforts would not only "save life from disease, degeneracy, and poverty" but also "enrich life by a larger program of education, beauty, and maximum human development." Raised in traditions of charity and inspired by expert knowledge flowing from the burgeoning social sciences, they rarely questioned their conviction that they knew what was best for the poor, dependent, or delinquent. They revered social service as a sacred Christian duty, but they realized the need for concerted government action and hoped to change prevailing attitudes about the role of government. They believed that state spending on social programs, even when the state ran a deficit, indicated not "poverty of statesmanship but largeness of governmental heart."[53]

Conference members' vision of social "progress" was firmly rooted in beliefs about white supremacy and black inferiority—beliefs they shared with other members of North Carolina's white elite and professional classes and with white reformers elsewhere. Many reformers hoped to improve conditions for white people because of their pride in their racial heritage. For example, state Superintendent of Public Instruction James Y. Joyner framed his plea to the Conference for a six-month school term as necessary for "these children of yours, through whose veins courses the purest strain of Anglo-Saxon blood to be found on the earth."[54] When Conference members discussed the need for improving Black people's basic welfare or literacy, their goal was to polish the image of the New South. They sought to prevent the "negro problem" from dominating politics, to prevent Black resentment from cresting to violence, to prevent the intermingling of white and Black people that threatened the logic of the established racial order, and to stave off criticism about Southern poverty and backwardness.

The Conference was committed to maintaining strict hierarchies of race and expanding the state's system of legal racial segregation. Members feared that the continued presence of Black people in North Carolina—unfortunate but inevitable, in their view, given white elites' reliance on cheap Black labor—would "drag us down." One Conference leader called for "uplift[ing] the negroes" morally, socially, and economically, both "as a missionary enterprise . . . and also as a matter of self-protection." Despite calls for "an attitude of mutual helpfulness and respect," this endeavor was far from an equal partnership, based as it was in racist assumptions about Black inferiority. In its early years, the Conference passed resolutions to study the "negro problem" and favoring a law to criminalize cohabitation of the races.[55]

Occasionally the Conference discussed more drastic approaches to the presence of Black North Carolinians. Clarence Poe, a founder of the Conference and its president from 1913 to 1915, was perhaps the most ardent proponent of extending the logic of white supremacy and racial segregation. Poe's influential weekly *Progressive Farmer* voiced the concerns of farmers, and he headed a Conference committee dedicated to "improvement of country life," part of the nationwide Country Life movement. Inspired by a South African proponent of racial apartheid whom he met while traveling in Europe, Poe developed a vision of rural racial segregation for the American South. The Conference was receptive to Poe's argument that to improve country life, farmers needed not only more education and well-organized cooperatives, but also a "denser white population" to improve white "social life." Poe pushed further, however, arguing that "Negroes should buy land in communities to themselves" and trying to pass a constitutional amendment to this effect. His plan may have appealed to other Progressives as an extension of the ideals of efficiency and rationality—a chance to "redesign" rural North Carolina "by eliminating the potential for intermixing and conflict between blacks and whites." But Poe faced opposition from white planters and merchants who exploited cheap Black labor. Perhaps for this reason, the Conference stopped short of publicly backing Poe's plan, and Poe's effort ultimately failed.[56]

Conference leaders took pride in the organization's rapid growth and claimed that it was the "social pulse of North Carolina." Within three months of the first convention, the Conference had 542 members, including many well-connected elites. Subsequent conventions drew hundreds of attendees and invariably attracted newspaper coverage, not only in the host city but in other major cities. Each year's gathering centered on a new theme, but attendees could expect some regular program features: music, prayers, updates from committees, and visitors from national organizations. Within the Conference's first five years, attendees absorbed addresses from droves of state and national experts, women and men such as the president of the National

Congress of Mothers; the executive secretary of the National Organization for Public Health Nursing; Julia Lathrop, the director of the US Children's Bureau; the warden of Sing-Sing prison; a specialist on rural education from the US Bureau of Education; and the head of the National Committee on Provision for the Feeble-Minded. Attendees could also enjoy informal conversations with other reformers and social workers at lunch tables, after committee meetings, or at evening soirees. In between annual conventions, the Conference's quarterly publication, *Social Service Quarterly*, kept reformers linked.[57]

From the beginning, the Conference's leadership sought to make change, not merely to discuss problems. Conference members knew that their reforms would meet opposition, particularly in a state with strong local influence over politics and a single-party stranglehold on power. Their opponents included fiscal conservatives, proponents of individual rights, and business owners who feared that regulation would decrease profits. In response, Conference members planned from the beginning to "carry the fight to the enemy's corner." They planned annual Conference gatherings to coincide with legislative sessions, and the climax of each session was the endorsement of suggested legislation. At the first gathering, for example, attendees passed ambitious resolutions in favor of prohibition, restrictions on child labor, a vital statistics law, funding for the state Board of Health, parole and probation for prisoners, a longer school term, and compulsory school attendance.[58]

The Conference relied on the political connections of numerous members to make sure their proposals got a hearing in the legislature. A Conference pamphlet noted thirty years later that its presidents "have been the most prominent men and women of the State—an ex-Governor, legislators, university and college presidents and professors, newspaper editors, agricultural leaders, business men, lawyers, doctors, and social workers."[59] As members of the state's middle class and New South industrialists, Conference members did business with, attended church with, and had marriage or blood ties to Democratic Party insiders. North Carolina politics at the turn of the century remained a boys' club, an insular network of friends and political allies. Their leader was Furnifold M. Simmons, a lawyer who marshaled the state's white supremacist campaign in 1898 and ran the state's Democratic machine for the next three decades.

Conference members were closely linked to the Simmons machine. Conference President Clarence Poe, for example, was married to the daughter of the late Governor Charles B. Aycock (governor from 1901 to 1905), who was a close friend of Simmons. Aycock and Simmons were members of Raleigh's Watauga Club, along with Conference member Josephus Daniels, editor of the Raleigh *News and Observer*, and Thomas Dixon Jr., a former state legislator who wrote *The Clansman*, a novel that was adapted into the infamous film *The Birth of a Nation*. The Conference bestowed an "honorary presidency" on current Governor Locke T. Craige, a close friend of Aycock's while they were students at the University of North Carolina. Another Conference member in 1913 was Thomas Bickett, who chaired the committee on judicial reform and arbitration and was also the state's attorney general. In 1917 he was elected governor, and immediately after he finished his term he became president of the Conference, although he died before he could serve for long.[60]

Although the Conference included influential members such as Bickett and Poe, most members in its early years were laypeople with no professional training but with a personal or religious interest in social service. Most Conference members typified their generation of white social reformers: they were solidly middle-class people—ministers, lawyers, businessmen, or their wives—whose primary occupation usually reflected some interest in improving society. Ages of members ranged from twenty-four to eighty, but most, like Denson, were born in the decade after the Civil War and were now middle-aged.[61] They had the financial means to pay dues and to afford travel to conferences. Although these reformers lacked professional training, they educated themselves on the newest techniques of social science by reading publications and attending lectures and conferences.

The Conference for Social Service reflected the symbiotic ties between private citizens and official government agencies—a key factor in the success of nascent reform efforts in the South. From the first meeting of the Conference in 1913, members of the Board of Public Charities attended and even used the meeting as a chance to conduct Board business. Some of the Board members became dues-paying members of the Conference. The heads (and later the staff) of state agencies, too, were enthusiastic participants. Rankin and Denson, the heads of state public health and welfare agencies, relied on the support of sympathetic groups to push their needs before the legislature. Sometimes they lamented their isolation as the only full-time "professionals," surrounded by "a multitude of so-called charity workers" with "noble impulses" but "mistaken ideas of what is really needed to better the condition of the unfortunates around them."[62] Social work was a new profession, however, and in practice the lines were often blurred between professional social workers and laypeople interested in social reform. In this context, the Conference served as an important forum for bringing together officials, experts, politicians, and laypeople. Their shared beliefs and effective organizing strategies made the Conference both a potent political force and a clearinghouse for many of the Progressive social policies that took shape in the next two decades.

"Mothers of the Race": Gender and Social Service

Women played a notable role in the Conference for Social Service, as they did in other Progressive organizations in the state. For women whose hearts "overflowed with a great yearning to make this earth better," the conference was arguably the most exciting place to be. Its annual conventions offered reform-minded women from even the most isolated corners of the state chances to immerse themselves in discussions of social welfare from morning until late at night. Sallie Southall Cotten, one of the matriarchs of the white Federation of Women's Clubs, argued that the Conference mission, particularly its focus on children, naturally called to "every woman's heart." She hoped the Conference would awaken women "to the consciousness of their power and the need for their assistance."[63] When Cotten wrote in 1914, women constituted a quarter of the 726 Conference members. Among the more active members—the half of members who had joined a committee—married women were represented at about the same rate as men. Unmarried women, however, were more likely than men or married women to be active. Some of these women, such as Daisy Denson, worked in the field of social welfare or public health, while others were simply dedicated to the cause.[64]

Clara Swift Souther Lingle, a clubwoman and suffrage activist from Davidson, North Carolina, was one such woman. Born in Missouri in 1874, Clara Souther graduated from Mary Institute, a St. Louis girls' school with a Harvard-educated principal. The young Clara likely received an excellent education; students could take classes in higher-level math and natural sciences at nearby Washington University, and Clara studied modern languages, reputedly learning seven of them by the time she was thirty. In her early twenties, she went abroad to study violin at a conservatory in Leipzig, Germany. There she met Thomas Wilson Lingle, a North Carolina native three years her senior who was studying for a PhD. He soon completed his doctoral degree, followed by a degree from Princeton Theological Seminary. As a minister, he followed in the footsteps of his brother Walter Lingle, a Presbyterian minister whose sermons were already gaining him renown. After Clara and Thomas married they spent three years in São Paolo, Brazil, where Thomas taught philosophy and history at a college founded by a Presbyterian missionary. In 1904, they returned to the United States for Thomas to take a position as a philosophy professor and fundraiser for a small Presbyterian college in Illinois. The next year he was appointed president of the college.[65]

In 1908, Thomas got a job as a fundraiser at Davidson College, which he had attended and where his brother Walter was a trustee. The family, now including two children, moved to North Carolina—a return home for Thomas, who was born in nearby Rowan County, but a new place for Clara. The

Lingles quickly established themselves in the Davidson community, where they rented a house close to the college. Thomas completed his charge of raising $300,000 within two years and won a position as a member of the faculty in modern languages. Clara joined the Davidson Book Lovers' Club, becoming its president in 1912. She sometimes spent the summer with her children in the North Carolina mountains, and she took them on an extended trip to Switzerland while Thomas led a group of Davidson students on a bicycle tour of Europe.⁶⁶

Clara Lingle soon became a powerful figure among North Carolina's clubwomen. She was an ardent proponent of female suffrage, one of the members of the Equal Suffrage Association who appealed to the state legislature in 1915. She was elected to chair Federation of Women's Clubs' committees on civics and social service. She may have been influenced by her brother-in-law Walter, who was avidly reading works by Walter Rauschenbusch and other leading social gospel thinkers and trying to convince his fellow Presbyterians of the need for social action. Like Sallie Southall Cotten, Lingle viewed women as naturally attracted to and uniquely suited to social service, calling them "the original social service workers and agitators," because of their concern for "life and the care of human life."⁶⁷

In May 1915, Lingle was elected president of the North Carolina Federation of Women's Clubs, and she was determined to integrate the state's clubwomen more fully into the Conference for Social Service. According to one source, her "first official act" as president was to attend the Conference. Within three weeks of her election, she was sending material about clubwomen's social service efforts to Clarence Poe for publication in the Conference's quarterly journal, telling him that she had much more material, and asking how they could arrange to have the journal sent to all the state's clubwomen. Soon Lingle was elected first vice president of the Conference. She went on to serve as secretary and treasurer until at least 1922. She used her positions to coordinate the work of the two organizations, including having the FWC pass a 1916 resolution supporting the Conference's general aims.⁶⁸

While some of Lingle's appeals were intended to inspire clubwomen, at other times clubwomen aimed to justify women's participation to male Conference members. In 1914, Cotten argued that women deserved a place within the Conference for Social Service not only because they naturally wanted to mold their children's world, but also because they were stalwart allies. Men might sometimes lapse in their commitment to "the welfare of the next generation," but women—"as givers of life, as the mothers of humanity"—would not. She wrote, perhaps willing it to be true, that in reform efforts "men need and welcome the help of women." She continued, "Neither can accomplish much *alone*; together they must strive and overcome, together they must win or lose."⁶⁹

Male leaders of the Conference agreed to some extent but saw women as adjuncts rather than as necessary partners. When Lingle appealed to clubwomen to join the Conference, the official Conference response, likely penned by then-President Alexander W. McAlister, was that "no part of our active Social Service forces will be more welcome to become active helpers." His condescending choice of words betrays a sense that women were not equal partners in social welfare work. Similarly, several months after Lingle began to devote her enormous energies to the Conference, the *Quarterly* featured a photograph of her with a caption that described her as "a splendid helper in the planning of our Conference" and a "valued leader among the forward-looking women of North Carolina"—not a leader in her own right.[70]

These gender dynamics played out across all levels of the Conference. When Lingle became first vice president of the Conference in 1916, she served on an executive board whose other members were nine men. On the Conference's twelve committees in 1914, almost all the leadership positions were held by men. On most committees, membership was about a quarter female, in the same proportion of the larger body, but a few committees had skewed gender ratios, indicating the gendering of distinct areas. For example, women made up a disproportionately large number of the committee on temperance and moral conditions, and they constituted over half of the committee on insanity, eugenics, and mental hygiene. The only committee with entirely female membership (including a female chair and vice chair) was the standing committee on women and social service. One other committee was sex-segregated: the committee on the "negro problem" included only men.[71]

Lingle and the Conference's other female members thus had a complicated role within the organization. The Conference did both build on and further the goals of women's clubs, and the Conference often directed its amassed Progressive forces toward goals that had grown out of women's organizations. Yet while women's inclusion in the Conference spoke to their political capital, the rhetoric in Conference discussions of "what women can do for social service" suggested that women should focus their moral force and their maternal power in areas especially suited for women, such as child welfare and prison reform. Male leaders often sidelined women's concerns and dismissed their potential as leaders. As a single committee was devoted to "women and social service," so was their participation—addresses by women or issues supposedly of interest them—consolidated into one afternoon session during the first few annual gatherings. Despite women's significant contributions to the Conference's success, not until 1932 did a woman serve as president. Within the conference, as in many other arenas of early twentieth-century

North Carolina, women had certain forms of power, but the acknowledgment of their powers also was a restrictive embrace.[72]

As North Carolina joined the New South, changes in the South's political economy exacerbated persistent problems: poverty and associated diseases, poor education, child labor, and friction between Black and white people, to name a few. While the state's skeletal welfare bureaucracy produced only marginal successes, a growing number of reformers interested in social conditions found common cause. Reformers who tackled these problems shared social status, faith in their ability to intervene in complex social problems, and a commitment to government involvement where private charity had proved insufficient. Despite some efforts at interracial cooperation, reformers were divided along racial lines, with distinct strategies and ambitions.

Seeing opportunity in the midst of challenge, these reformers sought to educate themselves about Progressive social reform through both observation and participation. They asked trained professionals to address their women's clubs or the Conference for Social Service and followed expert opinions in publications. Many women and men also gained skills and experience through their work as volunteers, on institutional boards, or directing local philanthropic efforts. In the process, they imbibed the language and principles of Progressive reforms everywhere: the importance of efficiency, prevention, and expert knowledge. A growing number of reformers built their political efforts around a vision of "social service" that was founded on Christian duty, on reformers' elitist and unswerving conviction that they were correct, and—among white reformers—on their faith in the superiority of white over Black people. United by these principles, networks of reformers created a distinct brand of social reform that addressed conditions in a rural state while taking into account the state's political constraints.

With allies in the governor's office and legislative halls, reformers soon would have notable successes in improving the state's welfare and public health programs. At the same time, a clear vision of social progress based on Progressive principles was confined almost entirely to the state's elite and middle class. As late as 1922, one Progressive leader noted that "this stream of progress . . . does not seem to me to have the quality of permanence. . . . The so-called common people have not been taught to appreciate its significance."[73] Although white Progressives in North Carolina strove to improve the conditions of rural white people in poverty, their efforts were fundamentally paternalistic, as were most Progressive efforts across the country. Perhaps the most apt example of the divide between the concerns of middle-class reformers and the rest of the state can be found in the growing interest in eugenics.

Chapter 2

Constant Care and Anxiety

Institutional Segregation and the Eugenics Debate in the 1910s

On a summer morning in 1912, visitors from across the state converged on Kinston, a tobacco and cotton trading center in Eastern North Carolina. Newspapers had published an open invitation to attend a ceremony at the state's newly chartered school for feebleminded children, and officials had arranged for special reduced-fare train travel to Kinston that day. The visitors made their way to the school's lush campus, a mile outside of town, accompanied by the mayor and many other local residents. The crowd gathered in a field on a south-facing hill above the winding Neuse River and with a background of "living forest green" that wafted "the perfume of the pine and the cedar." They saw no buildings except for a farmhouse in a grove of "stately oaks," where the school's superintendent planned to live with his family, and an old tobacco barn that was being converted to office space.[1] The day's celebration was focused on the change to come: the laying of the cornerstone for the first building of an institution that its champions hoped would care for the state's feebleminded and, ultimately, erase the problem of feeblemindedness through eugenic segregation.

In the fanfare of the day—Masonic rites, an address by the lieutenant governor, musical performances by local church choirs and a military band—an address by Charles Laughinghouse stood out as particularly "brilliant." Laughinghouse, a doctor from nearby Greenville, laid out in his speech many of the medical profession's arguments for how segregation would gradually eliminate feeblemindedness, which he and other Progressive-minded reformers saw as the cause of many other social problems. His address mixed cautionary tales and optimism. Insanity, feeblemindedness, and crime, he warned, were increasing to the extent that "normal human beings will become extinct." Because these problems were primarily hereditary, "nothing but segregation, nothing but constant surveillance . . . will protect [feebleminded children] and protect society against their crime . . . and against their power to spoil future generations with hereditary taint." The school would "guide" feebleminded children to "self-support and happiness" while also preventing them from having offspring, assumed to be "more feebleminded and more dangerous than the parent." Segregation was "evolution's plan by which we will rid society to a large extent of its feeble-minded population" and gradually eliminate "social waste." The school trustees and the state board of public health so admired Laughinghouse's address that they printed copies and sent them to the legislature, judges, ministers, and other influential people.[2]

The establishment of this school, later called Caswell Training School, was a critical step in North Carolina's commitment to eugenic policies, transforming ideas into a brick-and-mortar institution. This chapter examines the creation of Caswell as part of the growing appeal of eugenics ideology to a circle of influential white North Carolinians during the 1910s, showing how the school became a touchstone for efforts to educate the public about eugenics principles. Reformers embraced eugenics ideology as part of their vision of a paternalistic white society, and they created institutions in line with both ideals. They envisioned Caswell as an institution that would both train feebleminded children to be self-supporting and serve the purpose of eugenic segregation, eliminating the possibility for "unfit" people to reproduce. For them, these dual goals of eugenic segregation and custodial care were not opposed. Chartered in 1911 and opened in 1914, Caswell became a physical manifestation of reformers' social vision, separating white children from Black, normal from deviant.

In the process of institution-building, medical and social welfare professionals—the earliest proponents of eugenics—educated many other North Carolinians about eugenic principles. Among these early experts were Ira Hardy, a doctor whose appeal for a training school for feebleminded children was based on both personal experience and medical expertise, and Sybil Hyatt, one of the first trained eugenics fieldworkers to be stationed in the South. In conversation with eugenics experts from national organizations, they helped establish Caswell Training School as an institution dedicated to principles of eugenic segregation and research to eliminate feeblemindedness. In practice, Caswell's mission was a matter of constant debate: Was its primary purpose to care for children or to protect society from the feebleminded? The process of creating the institution brought before the public these debates about eugenics and the role of the state in regulating reproduction, policing deviance, and defining disability.

Eugenics found a ready audience among white reformers interested in providing better social services and preventing future social problems.[3] Many of the same reformers who advocated for stronger social welfare measures in the Conference for Social Service or white women's clubs learned about eugenics through these organizations. Eugenics aligned well with key elements of their worldview, including their passion for Progressive principles of efficiency and prevention and social Christianity's emphasis on shaping humankind for God's kingdom on earth. North Carolina's reformers also found that eugenics spoke to the state's traditions and provided convenient language for their broader concerns about maintaining the social order. Reformers linked "the newest science, eugenics" to ideas that already had broad support among middle-class white people.[4] They used agricultural metaphors and religious rhetoric to frame the need to eliminate "bad stock," promote "fitness," and preserve a pure, white "North Carolina type"—all while saving the state money by preventing hereditary diseases that led to social problems. White women in particular were attracted to eugenic principles as a way to protect their children and fulfill their maternal duties to the Anglo-Saxon race.

The motivations of the school's most ardent supporters diverged from the public at large. While pro-eugenics reformers saw segregation as a way to contain social deviance, some families chose to send their children to Caswell because they sought help in caring for them. Other middle-class onlookers simply celebrated the school's role in housing the most pitiable children. Still, as Charles Laughinghouse's address shows, the school's founders were clear about their eugenic intent, and they met with few opponents. In discussing and institutionalizing eugenic principles, Progressive reformers reshaped the public's thinking about the relationship of the state to its least powerful citizens.[5]

The "Menace of the Feebleminded"

At the turn of the century, people around the country were warning of the "menace of the feebleminded." The concern about feeblemindedness was not new, although the definition of the term shifted over time in response to changing social conditions. In the 1880s and 1890s, influential thinkers linked feeblemindedness with social problems such as poverty, criminality, and immorality. They emphasized its heritability and high rates among the American population.[6] In the early twentieth century, feeblemindedness became increasingly visible in public discourse, particularly as experts during the 1910s began to insist that the feebleminded were not only associated with social problems but were in fact *responsible* for social problems. With this change, according to historian James Trent, the concern with feeblemindedness reached a "near hysterical pitch." A new idea of the "mental defective" permeated the American consciousness more than previous views of people with intellectual disabilities. Experts such as Henry H. Goddard, who headed research at the Vineland training school in New Jersey and published the influential pedigree study *The Kallikak Family* in 1912, estimated that only one in ten mentally defective people were in institutions. They claimed that enormous numbers of feebleminded people roamed unidentified, uncontrolled, and multiplying rapidly because of their supposed promiscuity.[7]

Discussions about the menace of the feebleminded dovetailed with conversations about eugenics. Indeed, feeblemindedness was the central concern of many eugenics experts. They promised that feeblemindedness could be controlled or eliminated if only society focused on preventing reproduction of the "unfit." One response was a call to contain more of the feebleminded, including higher-grade "morons," in institutions. Some institutions had been founded before the Civil War, but many were built during a surge in the late nineteenth century. Most followed the model of Massachusetts in taking people who presented a wide variety of cognitive disabilities and trying to train them for self-support or at least self-care. By 1910, twenty-eight states had at least one publicly supported institution for the feebleminded, and three more states had private institutions. States in the Northeast tended to have the most institutions: Massachusetts, Pennsylvania, New Jersey, and New York each had five or six, counting both public and private institutions.[8] Nearly every institution for the feebleminded was built on the colony model, which allowed officials to segregate inmates by type within the institution.[9] As concern about the feebleminded expanded, states in the South and West built new institutions, and existing institutions in the Northeast expanded their populations. The result was a growth in the institutionalized population of mental defectives from 14,347 in 1904, to 20,731 in 1910, to 32,727 in 1915. North Carolina's attention to the problem of the feebleminded, energetic discussions of eugenics, and the desire for institutional segregation were part of these larger patterns.[10]

Medical doctors were the first group to publicly discuss eugenics in North Carolina, a common pattern in the South. Their medical training predisposed them to seek a "scientific" rationale for feeblemindedness, as well as for social problems such as deviant behavior. Most were convinced that heredity played a large role in determining traits such as insanity, idiocy, alcoholism, and criminality. They believed that "defective" children were likely to pass on their own defects and, in the interim, become criminals, prostitutes, or vectors of disease. Like doctors and scientists elsewhere at the turn of the century, however, they did not understand how genes were passed from generation to generation, with some arguing that heredity was only "habit fixed by past environment." They disagreed about the relative influence of environment and heredity. Some argued that heredity determined as many as 95 percent of cases of feeblemindedness, while others claimed that "the particular kind" of feeblemindedness that "causes crime and poverty is mostly hereditary." Others looked to environmental causes; they argued that degeneration was due to "excess in the ancestor" or that exposure to American "civilization" and "freedom of thought" improved the bodies and brains of US-born children of immigrants.[11]

Religion, culture, and politics also influenced their views. More than one doctor backed up his argument that it takes four generations to breed a perfect man by quoting from the Bible that the "sins of the fathers shall be visited upon the children to the third and fourth generation." One believed that pursuing eugenics research would put reproduction "on the high moral plane which the Creator originally ordained." Some worried about "race suicide," echoing fearmongering by Teddy Roosevelt and others that the white race would be overtaken by hordes of inferior races. Citing research on fertility rates by British statistician Karl Pearson, they argued that while "pathological stocks" were increasing quickly, "the good old English stock in America" had a birth rate below replacement levels. To counter these trends, doctors argued that "race-regeneration" through eugenics would create a "purer and nobler race." Some even took heart from the "prospect of the extinction of the colored race" from venereal disease or other illnesses. Others extended the logic of eugenics far beyond the realm of heredity, as when one doctor argued that people should know the pedigree of their business partners.[12]

Doctors, as a group, favored certain eugenic measures. Their first concern was the care and treatment of the insane, and the state medical association called for increased and improved facilities for the insane. Doctors also discussed policies to prevent the spread of supposedly heritable traits, including insanity, epilepsy, and feeblemindedness. At the state medical society's annual meeting, they discussed some version of these policies almost every year from 1895 onward. They advocated marriage restrictions for a number of conditions, institutions to segregate the feebleminded, and teaching adolescent girls about "thoughtful marriage."[13]

Doctors also debated sterilization. In 1897 the medical society's president stopped short of endorsing a law to sterilize feebleminded, epileptics, and criminals, as one Western state was then debating, arguing that sterilization was doubtless effective but segregation could achieve the same ends. Some doctors questioned whether sterilization could improve the condition of individual insane or epileptic patients, one argument that eugenicists made in defense of the operation. On the other hand, others were in favor of sterilizing various populations, such as criminals, idiots, the insane, and even any alcoholic who had a child. Some doctors took more extreme positions, such as questioning whether criminals have a right to live and suggesting that tuberculosis was sent by God to remove people who would "weaken the race."[14]

To most doctors at the turn of the century, institutional segregation was the best way to balance their duties of care, training, and prevention. As early as 1895, one doctor advocated asylum care for feebleminded young women who might have disabled children. A separate institution dedicated to training the feebleminded, doctors argued, made economic sense because it would prevent feebleminded people from becoming prostitutes, spreading disease, producing defective children, and becoming "charges upon the communities for life." But financial considerations alone should not determine the state's response, one doctor remarked, since "we cannot estimate human souls in dollars and cents. Nothing marks a Christian Commonwealth more than her provision for afflicted ones."[15] In many cases, these institutions were able to provide better material care than families could, although at the expense of inmates' freedom of movement and connections with family and friends. There was also an authoritarian side to these institutions: for many Progressives, defective or delinquent people should be secluded in institutions unless or until they could become useful members of society.

Although medical doctors were the first audience for eugenics, social welfare professionals were not far behind. Welfare officials Daisy and Claude Denson made similar calls for separate institutions for each type of mental defective. Enmeshed in national discussions about the newest approaches to social problems, the Densons focused on the potential of segregation to reduce crime and poverty, provide humane care, and stretch meager welfare resources. As early as 1898, Claude called for an institution for "that most unfortunate class, the feeble-minded." As he argued to the legislature, there was very real need for better care of people suffering from insanity, epilepsy, or mental disability. His long career as an educator drove his view of the purpose of institutions, which he thought could train feebleminded people to be somewhat self-supporting.[16] When Daisy assumed her father's duties, she continued his calls for an institution but with a more explicit eugenic focus. While Claude saw mental defect as a product of bad environment, Daisy was firmly convinced it was a hereditary problem that could best be attacked with principles of eugenics.

Like other social workers who followed her, Denson's interest in eugenics grew out of a mixture of genuine concern for the feebleminded, religious duties, financial pressures, and assumptions about Anglo-Saxon superiority. She worried about feebleminded people who sat "in utter neglect" on the doorsteps of county poorhouses, their world "empty nothingness," "their rush-light intellects gradually going out." At the same time, she believed that care alone was futile and that only "the newest science, eugenics" could reduce "the burden the stronger half of the race is staggering under at the present time." Because "there is no hope of normal progeny from imbecile parents," preventing their reproduction was a key to reducing disease, crime, and poverty. Like her father, she believed segregation would ultimately save money by "preventing the transmission of hereditary taint," particularly since counties were already paying to care for many feebleminded people.[17]

In keeping with her thirst for professional knowledge, Daisy Denson learned about eugenics from professionals in other states, and she studied and advocated eugenic solutions during her decade and a half as secretary of the Board of Public Charities. For example, a few months after she took office, she went to Atlanta for the annual meeting of the National Conference of Charities and Corrections. There she heard the superintendent of Indiana's school for the feebleminded argue that states should segregate all "degenerates" to prevent them from passing on their "burden" to future generations. Denson's report to the legislature a few months later echoed similar conclusions. She soon conducted a "census of the insane and defectives," hoping to underscore the need for more institutional space for both populations. Every year she called for a school for the feebleminded, although she initially placed higher priority on providing for adequate hospital space for "the insane," another group that she believed might pass their condition on to their offspring. In 1908 she endorsed another common eugenic strategy: "stricter marriage laws" to prevent "imbeciles and epileptics" and "the congenital deaf" from reproducing. Denson was certainly aware of eugenic sterilization from discussions at the NCCC, but she never publicly advocated it, perhaps seeing custodial care and segregation as sufficient.[18]

Denson, medical doctors, and Progressive reformers saw an institution for the feebleminded as part of a chain of caring institutions that would provide specialized care for distinct populations. National discussions among Progressive social reformers emphasized that the best treatment required separating these populations to deal with their distinct needs.[19] Institutional staff trained in addressing specific populations' needs, they hoped, could reform delinquents, heal mental patients, and help the blind become self-supporting. Reformers developed an optimistic but authoritarian vision of society in which feebleminded, insane, or criminal people could be secluded in institutions until they could become useful members of society, allowing the rest of the populace to achieve new levels of prosperity and happiness. At the turn of the century, North Carolina already had a mix of public and private institutions to care for people who were deaf, blind, orphaned, insane, or very poor. The state's reformers hoped to follow a national pattern of expanding these institutions to house other populations. Reformers won a notable victory in 1907 when they created Stonewall Jackson Training School, a reformatory for delinquent white boys. The King's Daughters and other white clubwomen, who led the campaign, rejoiced that the state could now send white boys arrested for petty crimes to a training school, rather than jailing them with hardened adult criminals or even sending them to the chain gang. The legislature and governor recognized the importance of women's contributions by appointing nine women to Jackson's fifteen-member Board of Trustees—the first time women were appointed to such a state institution board.[20] Other reformatories took years to establish: eventually the state created Samarcand for white girls (1917), Morrison for Black boys (1921), and Efland for Black girls (created by clubwomen in 1925, although not supported by the state until 1940).[21]

The legislature did make some attempts to provide for people with mental defects in response to persistent calls for separate institutions for the insane, epileptic, and feebleminded. The heads of the state's schools for the deaf and blind often noted in their reports to legislators that they were not equipped to handle feebleminded children and had turned them away. They estimated that there were hundreds of such children in the state. One bill in 1905 to care for "idiots and epileptics" got a favorable committee report but was not passed. During the 1907 session the legislature created a Hospital Commission, with broad powers to provide for all mental defectives. Its intent was to enlarge mental hospitals and create new institutions to care for all mental defectives, including epileptics and feebleminded people. Denson and other observers were hopeful that it would help the state to "soon meet ... our needs." The funding provided, however, was not sufficient to fulfill the bill's intent, and all the funds went toward expanding care for the insane. Two years later, new legislation established buildings for epileptics at the Raleigh mental hospital, rather than at a separate institution.[22]

Ira Hardy's "Humanitarian Cause"

One doctor pushing for an institution for the feebleminded was Ira M. Hardy. Born in 1874 near Kinston, he attended both North Carolina A&M (later North Carolina State University) and the University of North Carolina. In 1901, he graduated from the Medical College of Virginia, then completed brief postgraduate work in New York City. He married his wife Mamie that year and began practicing medicine in her hometown of Washington, not far from Kinston.[23]

Although Hardy's rationales for an institution for the feebleminded were similar to other doctors' reasons, Hardy had a personal connection to the campaign that both drove him and made his case more compelling. Hardy's eldest daughter Hattie, born around 1903, was mentally disabled. Hardy's experience with her persuaded him to investigate the possibilities for care for the feebleminded. Around 1906 Hardy visited New Jersey's Vineland Training School, which was emerging as the nation's foremost center of research on feeblemindedness. There he likely heard about Vineland's eugenic research program and met Henry H. Goddard, who directed psychological research for the school and would soon bring the Binet-Simon method of intelligence testing to the United States.[24]

Four years later, inspired by this visit, Hardy started a campaign to create a similar institution in North Carolina.[25] He began by presenting his idea to the Seaboard Medical Society, a regional group that included doctors from North Carolina and Virginia.[26] On December 8, 1910, Hardy took the podium in Kinston before the assembled one hundred doctors and gave a paper entitled "What It Costs." Hardy's paper echoed many of the arguments aired among doctors for the past decade, including earlier that year at gathering of the North Carolina Medical Society, of which Hardy was an active member.[27] In his address in Kinston, Hardy proposed the creation of a training school "for the care of our Feeble-Minded children." Hardy argued that North Carolina's lack of such institutions had significant social, individual, and financial costs. He spoke of the feebleminded in compassionate terms, but he also forecast peril. No matter how much the institution improved the lives of children, its main purpose was to protect society from the "vast army" of feebleminded people. Although feebleminded children were often looked on "as harmless and inoffensive creatures," he warned that they were in fact quite dangerous—and even more so because the threat was "often unnoticed." Outside of institutions, he stated, feeblemindedness could lead to pauperism, crime, and even murder. He warned that their "sexual instinct[,] uncontrolled by will and reason," would surface as feebleminded children aged, almost inevitably leading them to become parents, in or out of wedlock. Their children, he said, "are almost certain to be mentally defective," because, as he reminded his audience, "Feeble minds cannot beget strong minds."[28]

The response to Hardy's paper was overwhelmingly positive. The *Kinston Free Press* reported that Hardy's paper "produced a sort of mild sensation" among the members of the Seaboard Medical Society. The society printed hundreds of copies of the paper to distribute in both Virginia and North Carolina and voted to work with the incoming legislature to establish an institution in North Carolina. The public reaction to Hardy's paper was also swift and positive. An editorial in the Kinston paper picked up on Hardy's assertion that feeblemindedness could strike anywhere, offering this as a reason that every citizen had an interest in creating an institution to care for "imperfect children," who were a "source of constant care and anxiety to their families." The institution, they argued, would "lift great burdens off numerous households." Hardy's address also received attention from newspapers around the state, all of which discussed his idea approvingly, mostly for humanitarian reasons. Even Governor William Kitchin spoke in support of a school in his message to the legislature when it convened in January, and the state Teachers' Assembly added their support.[29]

Hardy, whose daughter Hattie had died of pneumonia barely a week after his speech in Kinston, took advantage of this surge of favorable public opinion. He asked Raleigh insiders to draft legislation creating a school for the feebleminded, which supporters introduced in both the House and Senate. Hardy also spent a month in Raleigh lobbying for the bill and testifying about the need for a school.[30]

At the same time, unbeknownst to Hardy, Daisy Denson was leading a parallel effort. She had long been interested in creating a school, and she intensified her efforts after she began to correspond with an influential like-minded ally, Charles Coon. Coon was an educator and reformer who at the time was superintendent of schools in Wilson County. In December 1910, Coon set out to gather information about the number of feebleminded children in the state, hoping to build a case before the legislature. He sent a circular letter titled "Will You Help Find Out the Facts?" to school superintendents and other educators around the state, asking them to report on the number of "feebleminded and otherwise mentally defective children" in their schools. In dozens of replies, they told him that their schools or counties had anywhere from one to hundreds of feebleminded children. Based on the replies, Coon estimated that there were around seven hundred feebleminded children in the state. Coon also requested information from heads of institutions in other states, including Michigan, Wisconsin, Massachusetts, and New Jersey. He wrote to Denson with his findings, and they began to work together with friendly legislators. Their bill took a slow approach, first creating a commission to study the need for a school, with plans to bring their findings to the 1913 legislature for action.[31]

Daisy Denson was surprised by Hardy's bill, despite her constant proximity to legislators in her office in the Senate gallery. Nevertheless, Denson and Hardy met and decided to unite behind Hardy's bill but keep Denson and Coon's as a substitute in case Hardy's met with resistance.[32] Over the next month Denson and Hardy met frequently to strategize, and Denson began to collect information to support Hardy's case, including reports of schools in other states and notes about specific cases of children who could benefit from the school. After the Senate passed the bill and the decision came to the House, Denson lobbied on its behalf, including visiting members of the House and persuading the editor of the *News and Observer* to print an article underscoring the Senate bill's broad support.[33]

The bill passed in the House on March 3, 1911, with supporters crowding the chambers for an evening session. For nearly two hours, numerous representatives spoke in favor of the bill, with only the speaker of the house questioning them, likely out of concern for the cost.[34] Finally, at 10:30 p.m., the bill passed overwhelmingly by a roll-call vote. Even before officials announced the tally, there was "loud and prolonged applause from the crowded lobbies and galleries" from "an immense number of . . . sympathetic men and women" who had lobbied for the bill. With the school assured, Denson's version of the bill was quietly tabled two days later. She later called the school legislation the "most notable act" of that legislative session and rejoiced that the school completed "the chain of institutions caring for our defectives."[35] With the creation of what soon was called Caswell Training School, North Carolina became the first state in the South to charter a public institution for the feebleminded.[36]

One of the first actions of the new school's trustees was to look north for models, hoping to align their institution with national standards. This kind of tour was a common strategy in institutional planning; Georgia officials made a similar trip in 1919, as did leaders of North Carolina's reformatory for white boys a few years earlier. In April 1911, Hardy—now appointed superintendent of the institution—and three trustees spent several days inspecting public and private institutions in the Northeast to learn about their facilities and management.[37] Their stops included schools for the feebleminded in Maryland, New Jersey, Pennsylvania, and Massachusetts. At each institution, they met with the superintendent, toured the grounds, and made notes about the physical labor done by the inmates. They spent the most time at Vineland and left impressed with the staff and particularly enamored of Goddard's research laboratory, which they deemed "of inestimable value to society."[38] They also invited experts to North Carolina. Hastings Hart of the Russell Sage Foundation gave the school's executive committee a two-hour lecture about running an institution, and a doctor from New Jersey's institution visited the future site of the school in the fall of 1911.[39]

In one respect the existing institutions could offer no guidance: how to accommodate racial segregation. The school's charter made no explicit mention of race. In fact, it mandated that the school was for *all* feebleminded people "capable of being benefitted by school instruction."[40] But white officials never seriously considered providing space for Black children in their early plans. For one thing, as historian Steven Noll argues, Northern institutions had a more homogenous population, and in looking north for models, Southern institutions "simply did not account for race."[41] Some white advocates of the institution, steeped in myths of Black inferiority, may have assumed that Black children were not, in fact, "capable of being benefitted" by the training the school offered. There was also the consideration of cost: Jim Crow law and practice dictated that housing Black children would require separate buildings. Even that arrangement—having Black and white children at the same institution—might have horrified some white people, since schools and hospitals were usually rigidly divided along racial lines. Instead, plans were set to build dormitories for different "grades" of feebleminded white people (see figure 2.1). School officials and other reformers later called for a

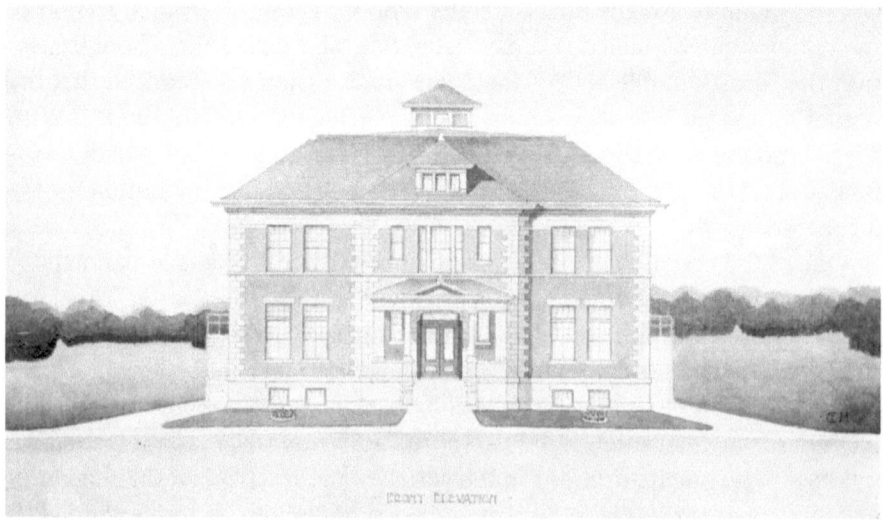

Figure 2.1 Artist's sketch of Caswell dormitory, 1911. *First Biennial Report of the North Carolina School for the Feeble-Minded, 1911–12*, 6, North Carolina Collection, Louis Round Wilson Special Collections Library, University of North Carolina at Chapel Hill.

school for feebleminded Black children, but it was not until after World War II that the state built dorms for them. In the meantime, feebleminded Black people wound up in segregated mental hospitals or were left in the care of their families, the usual arrangement in the South.[42]

Now informed about institutional best practices, the trustees' next task was to choose a site for the school. At least four towns vied to host the school, including Hardy's town, Washington.[43] The winner was Kinston, whose rural location aligned with the pattern nationally to choose pastoral settings.[44] Kinston's victory, however, was just as much the result of local people's concerted campaign to bring the school. Kinston citizens—mostly doctors, businessmen, and their wives—organized local residents to make their case to the state, including escorting the trustees to visit the proposed site in June.[45] Kinston's interest in hosting the school was primarily economic. Although Kinston's taxpayers had to service the bond that paid for their donation of agricultural land for the institution, Kinston's businessmen hoped to benefit from the proximity of the school, and some residents found employment at the school as housekeepers, laundry workers, or farmworkers.[46] It seems that Kinston residents were proud of the institution; they turned out in force for the dedication, and local women helped beautify the new campus with forsythia bushes and crepe myrtle trees.[47]

These responses of Kinston citizens were typical of North Carolina's middle class: their primary interest in the school was *not* based on eugenics; rather, the custodial goals of the institution meshed nicely with their economic motives and their social assumptions. When the state teachers' assembly endorsed the school, its members were likely thinking about removing difficult students from their classrooms. Similarly, families who sought to place a child at the school were driven by their own concerns about the inadequacy or expense of in-home care or by fears about their child's sexual urges. For many supporters, the most important justification for the school's establishment was simply that the state had a duty to provide for its less fortunate white citizens. Acknowledging this public sentiment, when Hardy and others testified about the need for the school, they often talked about "caring," "training," or "providing for" feebleminded children.[48]

But Hardy, Denson, and the school's trustees—many of whom were doctors—were also explicit about the school's eugenic purpose. The lack of opposition to the institution's publicly stated eugenic goals demonstrates that the general public, while not necessarily enamored of eugenics, did not find these goals unreasonable or repugnant. Now that the school was chartered, its creators hoped to take it one step further toward being a model eugenic institution. One of the school's trustees told the state medical society in 1912 that the school's custodial role should be secondary to its role in prevention, arguing that "it is a greater work to have prevented the birth of one of these unfortunates, than to have provided shelter for ten of them." In order to stop the "endless chain of reproduction" of the feebleminded, he argued that the school must conduct research on the causes of mental defects and the best ways of preventing their "propagation."[49] Hardy took a similar stance in a long paper for the medical society, calling for "more persistent laboratory research into the causes of feeble-minded[ness]" and for closer study of the "science of eugenics."[50]

Hardy took an important step toward giving the school credibility as a research institution by making connections with the Eugenics Record Office (ERO). Founded in 1903 and led by biologist Charles Davenport in Cold Spring Harbor, the ERO researched eugenic principles and attempted to coordinate state-level efforts to pass eugenics laws. Beginning in 1910, they also trained eugenics fieldworkers in order to advance eugenics research and spread the gospel of eugenics. Davenport hoped that the availability of trained eugenics fieldworkers would legitimize and spark interest in eugenics research, which would in turn fuel the desire for more fieldworkers.[51] Although it is not clear how Hardy first became acquainted with Davenport, he used their mutual interest to secure a fieldworker for six months' work in North Carolina. When Hardy contacted him, Davenport was particularly interested in the "opportunity to open the work in the South," where the ERO had not yet made inroads but where Davenport was convinced feeblemindedness was endemic.[52] From

Hardy's perspective, hosting a eugenics fieldworker could enhance the scientific reputation of the school among its peer institutions in other states.[53] As he wrote to Charles Davenport in 1913, "My heart is with you in the work and will do anything assigned me.... Inestimable good is sure to be the result of this humanitarian cause."[54]

Sybil Hyatt and the Importance of Pedigree

Sybil Hyatt, a white woman from Kinston, became Caswell's eugenics fieldworker and one of the first ERO-trained fieldworkers in the South.[55] Born in 1877, Hyatt was smart, energetic, and well educated. She came from a family whose wealth had been made from enslaving people. After the Civil War, Hyatt's family remained comfortably middle-class, thanks to her father's well-established medical practice. After attending a private school in Kinston and a Catholic women's collegiate institute in Baltimore, Hyatt kept house for her family, worked as a bookkeeper, and finally became a teacher and school principal in 1908.[56]

At some point during her teaching career Hyatt developed an interest in psychology and decided to pursue a master's degree in the field. Perhaps her interest grew from her observations of her own pupils, or perhaps she was intrigued by stories that her younger brother Anderson told her on holidays at home while he trained as a physician. In 1911, Hyatt spent the summer in New York taking courses at Columbia University, including experimental psychology and comparative and genetic psychology.[57] When she returned home, she resumed work as a teacher but must have been fascinated by the new institution slowly taking shape in her hometown. By the fall of 1911, when Ira Hardy started in earnest to figure out how many feebleminded children were in the state, Hyatt wanted to help.

Eugenics training likely appealed to Hyatt for a number of reasons in addition to her interest in children and psychology. Surrounded in her family by medical men, Hyatt may have seen training in eugenics as a way to achieve her own professional distinction. Learning about the inheritance of traits probably appealed to her because of her long-running interest in genealogy. Like many other North Carolinians of means, Hyatt and her family placed great stock in their lineage. In 1901, Hyatt joined the Daughters of the American Revolution, which required her to submit evidence of her ancestry. She apparently enjoyed this exercise enough that she continued to research the history of the Hyatt family.[58]

In the summer of 1912, when she was thirty-five years old, Hyatt once again went north, where she took more psychology courses at Columbia but also attended the ERO's fieldworker training on Long Island. During each summer throughout the 1910s, ERO founder Davenport and his deputy Harry Laughlin trained students in heredity, psychology, physical anthropology, and statistics. The vast majority of the fieldworkers were women, mostly unmarried, recent college graduates with some training in biology or other sciences. In 1912, Hyatt and thirty-five other ERO students practiced collecting information on heredity by interviewing each other and filling out "pedigree" cards that described personal and family history as well as physical, mental, and temperamental traits. To understand their future role as researchers embedded with institutions, they took field trips to nearby institutions for the feebleminded.[59]

Hyatt returned to North Carolina to apply her training. From October 1912 to June 1913, she traveled throughout the state, completing at least twenty-seven family pedigrees and over two hundred pages of accompanying description, which she dutifully copied and forwarded to Davenport and ERO officials.[60] In her fieldwork, Hyatt played a peculiar role. Hardy intended for her to spread the word about the school and convince families to send their feebleminded children. Some families seemed to welcome the relief the school provided. One mother told Hyatt that she was unable to care for her other children properly because of the burden of taking care of her twelve-year-old, whom Hyatt described as a "slobbering idiot." With parents who were reluctant to send their children to Caswell, Hyatt took a hard line. She believed that mothers became too attached to their feebleminded children and that they should be "separated early and forcibly, if necessary."[61]

At the same time, Hyatt's responsibility to the ERO was to trace "cacogenic and feeble-minded" families. Doing so required her to invade the privacy of every family, as well as some of their neighbors and relatives. One of Hyatt's fellow ERO trainees reported that she had an easier time getting information when she prevaricated and said that she was "studying questions of health" rather than "mention[ing] directly the mental side." Perhaps Hyatt adopted this tactic, too. Judging by her notes, her process seemed to be getting families to spill gossip about all their troubles—infidelity, a fight about a dog, stealing food or washtubs, burning a house to collect insurance money and then leaving town to escape the insurance agent's prosecution. Hyatt also made notes about each potential patient's siblings, parents, and other relatives, noting whether people were illiterate, "had funny ways," were "all smart," or "like[d] music." Although many details Hyatt recorded seem totally irrelevant to her mission, they were in accordance with Davenport's instructions to fieldworkers, which included encouraging them to use rumor.[62] And they ultimately served the purposes of the ERO: Hyatt transformed all of these details about odd or unsocial behavior into evidence that families were feebleminded, entering it in the appropriate places on pedigree charts.

Hyatt's work—the first systematic study of feeblemindedness from a hereditarian perspective in the state and likely in the South—helped educate North Carolinians about eugenics. Shortly after she began her research, Hyatt made a presentation to the school trustees about her study of North Carolina's feebleminded families, which was later picked up by newspapers. Her report echoed eugenicists' standard refrains about the "alarming increase in the number of defective children." She implicitly emphasized her training and credentials, citing academics from New York University and Columbia University on the significance of the problem. For readers unfamiliar with eugenics, she explained the hereditary nature of feeblemindedness, which appeared when "two affected strains have crossed each other." And she reminded readers of the eugenic nature of the school's "ultimate aim": eliminating feeblemindedness through segregation and through her own efforts to educate "every family that has produced a case."[63]

Hyatt's training in eugenics affected her other political views. In January 1913, she and Hardy went to Columbia, South Carolina, for the American Breeders' Association meeting. There Hyatt heard a paper by Dr. Ward about the eugenic threats of immigration, which she liked so much she said it justified the expenses of the entire trip. Her response to this paper is the first signal of what became her rabid anti-immigrant feelings. Back home, Hyatt reprinted Ward's paper in the state publication of the United Daughters of the Confederacy and followed it up with other articles warning of a looming immigrant menace in the South. Despite lower rates of immigration in the South, Hyatt was alarmed by developments such as a new plant in Kinston that planned to bring over a hundred Polish workers.[64]

Like many other ERO graduates, Sybil Hyatt stayed in touch with the organization for several years after her summer training course. In June 1913, on her way to Columbia for her final summer of psychology courses, she attended a fieldworkers' reunion at Cold Spring Harbor. At this session, fieldworkers presented papers on their findings, discussed research techniques, and compared their experiences as fieldworkers and as women.[65] Hyatt also maintained ties through the ERO's monthly *Eugenical News*, where fieldworkers submitted updates about their research, their careers, and their personal lives. Hyatt's subsequent career until her death in 1951 was conducting genealogical research, which she saw as linked to eugenics, but she did no more eugenics fieldwork.[66]

Hyatt's brief foray into eugenics research left a mark on the state. Hyatt shared her opinions about the shortcomings of the state's feebleminded families with legislators and Caswell's trustees, perhaps reshaping the ideological framework with which they confronted the problem of the state's feebleminded youth. The state medical society appreciated her work, and in

1913 its members passed a resolution assuring the ERO of their "hearty cooperation in their efforts for racial betterment." Hyatt's research also exposed dozens of North Carolina families to principles of eugenics. One of the school's staff later described her as crucial in increasing the number of applications the school received. By late 1913, even before it opened, the school had received 138 applications and reported that another 250 were pending, already exceeding the planned capacity of 130 beds.[67] The demand for the school was clear. Less clear was whether it would actually be built.

Caswell Training School

While Sybil Hyatt was interviewing families and filling out pedigree charts, Ira Hardy was trying to ready the school for students. Costs were higher than expected, and even though the school was established, debate continued about its mission. The constant struggles for money and the need to justify the school's existence to legislators remained a pattern for decades.[68]

Hardy had the nearly impossible task of opening a school with an inadequate appropriation, and the difficulties compounded until he was forced to resign. Despite the small initial appropriation, Hardy managed to start the construction process, but progress was slow. Several months after the ceremonial cornerstone laying, the legislature questioned whether anything was being done. They appointed a committee to investigate and barred Hardy from hiring staff or admitting patients in the meantime. The committee found that Hardy's bookkeeping was inadequate, and, perhaps most egregiously, that he spent money the institution did not have, putting it in debt. Still, the committee recommended that the school be expanded, and in the fall of 1913 they provided additional funds to finish construction. The school's trustees were bitterly divided over what to do about Hardy. In February 1914, embroiled in accusations of mismanagement that led to a libel suit, Hardy was forced to resign.[69]

The school's new superintendent, Dr. C. Banks McNairy, rushed to finish buildings and hire staff for the school. McNairy was the son of a farmer from Guilford County and had founded the first hospital in Caldwell County, in the foothills of the Blue Ridge Mountains.[70] Now in his late forties, McNairy firmly believed in the school's potential as a site for eugenic segregation and research. He took his new staff on a train trip to New Jersey and Maryland, where they visited similar institutions. As with the trustees' visit three years earlier, Vineland was the highlight of the trip. Each department head visited the branch of the school relevant to her job, and the staff spent time with Goddard and watched him give a Binet-Simon test to a young boy.[71]

Armed with this experience, the staff opened Caswell in June 1914, making North Carolina the first state in the South to operate an institution exclusively for the feebleminded. The first inmates were sixteen "higher grade girls," reflecting the widespread concern about the threat of seduction posed by charming, feebleminded girls on the loose as well as the greater difficulties of caring for more severely disabled children.[72] In its first year the staff of fifteen supervised 122 children. At least a hundred more were on waiting lists, and Denson and school officials made regular pleas for funding to expand the school's capacity.[73] Even at the current capacity, the staff found itself overwhelmed by the "herculean task" of providing food and clothing and meeting the population's basic needs. McNairy had hoped to administer mental tests to each new inmate, but the more pressing demands of basic care superseded his research agenda.[74]

With demand far outstripping capacity, Caswell's admission policy became a point of contention, reflecting larger debates about the school's ultimate aims—a common problem for institutions for the feebleminded, particularly in the South.[75] Stakeholders disagreed about the ages and types of mental disabilities the institution should prioritize. Legislators wanted to house young children and adolescents, both boys and girls. Reflecting the views of the public at large, they saw the institution's primary purpose as "caring" for and "training" idiots and imbeciles, the lower grades of feebleminded. To the extent they were interested in supporting the school, it was because they wanted to show "kindness to little children."[76]

School officials and state welfare officials, on the other hand, wanted to admit older children and even adult women. Although they believed that the school's inmates needed protection and training, they also believed that the goal of the school was "the ultimate decrease" of the feebleminded through permanent segregation. As Denson wrote, their plan was to admit women up to age forty-five and "keep them all their lives if we can." Legislators acceded to these arguments in 1915, capping the age of residents at twenty-one for men and thirty for women.[77] But the struggle over whom to admit would continue in later years. Voicing their constituents' concerns, the legislature pushed to prioritize lower-grade children, while Denson and McNairy made the case that women of reproductive age were the biggest danger to society and should be housed for more of their reproductive lives.[78] McNairy and his staff also continued with limited success to push for funding for psychological research at Caswell, with the goal of understanding hereditary feeblemindedness.[79]

Many parents of disabled children were not interested in these debates; for them, sending their child to Caswell was simply a relief. A disabled child was an economic burden for a family, who had few other options for care. The school promised some basic education and vocational training, in addition to constant supervision. With long waiting lists, some families petitioned the governor in hopes that he could help them. Other parents were reluctant to part with their children or concerned about whether they would be cared for lovingly at the school.[80]

Once children arrived at the institution, their care was far from ideal. Despite some observers' criticisms of "extravagant management," the reality of institutional life was harsh. Limited funding was at the root of most of the institution's problems, as was the case for other Southern institutions. Low salaries made it hard to keep trained staff. In 1924, McNairy noted that on his staff of fifty, he averaged two new staff members each week. Although the "teachers" for higher-grade students had college degrees, the ward attendants likely had little training and might resort to physical punishment. One child died from a head injury after falling from a high bed, where a negligent nurse left the child.[81] As at other institutions, inmates were expected to work to keep the institution running, substituting for paid laborers. Boys grew crops or cared for livestock, while higher-grade girls were trained to sew their own clothes or helped ward attendants in the kitchen or dorms. Staff framed this work as educational: "each child had a job, and he was expected to keep trying until he could perform it."[82]

The institution's biggest need was more space. With 190 inmates by late 1916, the "dignified" but simple buildings were at capacity. Beds were crowded into dorms with less than twelve inches between them. The twenty-two lowest-grade girls spent their whole lives in one room that measured twenty by forty feet. For higher-grade girls, the classroom space was bare except for desks and blackboards, and they had no comfortable "home space" with chairs or books to help fill evenings or rainy days.[83]

McNairy and his staff conducted a constant public relations campaign, hoping to paint a rosier picture of the institution, combat parental anxieties, and address the ongoing scrutiny from state lawmakers. A staff member at the time remembered that their efforts to educate the public about the school's work included "giving dinners, inviting many interested and potentially interested key people." Sundays, when the children were neatly dressed for church services, were open to visitors. The staff hosted mayors, county medical societies, and clubwomen. In at least one case, Caswell served as a model institution, when officials from South Carolina included it on their tour of Vineland and other institutions.[84] Superintendent McNairy gave talks across the state and beyond state lines to audiences of teachers, clubwomen, fairgoers, medical societies, and Progressive reformers, focusing on "the cause and consequence of mental deficiency." Although attempts at public relations never secured funding adequate to run the institution properly, Caswell officials did succeed in educating the public about mental deficiency and "the appalling fact of its menace to society."[85]

The Appeal of Eugenics

As Progressive reformers were drawn into the continuing battle to build and open the school, a growing number of people were exposed to the precepts of eugenics. The state's existing experts on eugenics—medical and social welfare professionals like Ira Hardy, C. Banks McNairy, and Daisy Denson—became crucial portals of information for lay reformers in several influential white organizations in the 1910s. Members of these organizations spread the word about eugenics through conversations, publicity efforts, and newspaper coverage. All these organizations passed resolutions in support of eugenic policies, from greater funding for Caswell, to teaching eugenics at colleges, to stricter marriage laws. Experts' explanations built on their own understanding of the science of eugenics and its potential as a social tool, but lay reformers tended to understand eugenics in terms of agricultural metaphors, the social gospel, white supremacy, and racialized maternal duties.

Experts and laypeople mixed within several influential Progressive-leaning organizations. Most notable was the Conference for Social Service, which claimed to be the "social pulse" of the state. Its members included many doctors, six of the initial Caswell trustees, and Denson, who continued to study eugenics throughout the 1910s. The "problem of feeblemindedness and eugenics" was one of the Conference's early concerns.[86] The group frequently heard from experts and became an incubator for eugenic ideas, which spread outward as Conference members went home to their offices, churches, and neighborhoods.[87] The state Mental Hygiene Association, founded in 1913 after a weeklong exhibit in Raleigh, was another forum for discussions about eugenics. Its primary concern was insanity, a topic that drew attendees who might not have otherwise been exposed to eugenics.[88] Middle-class white women were also a sympathetic audience, both among Conference members and in the Federation of Women's Clubs, where they hosted debates or speakers on eugenics as part of their investigations into health and social welfare.[89]

These organizations shared many members, but three people in particular—Daisy Denson, Louis Burgin McBrayer, and William Louis Poteat—linked them closely together. All three were founding members of the Conference for Social Service, and all three were officers of the Mental Hygiene Association.

Louis Burgin McBrayer was one of the state's most respected physicians. After receiving an MD from Louisville Medical College in 1889, he practiced in his hometown of Asheville until 1914, when he became head of the state tuberculosis sanatorium. McBrayer held a number of roles among the state's doctors, including as president of the state medical society in 1915. He was a devoted Caswell trustee, joining the 1911 trip north to look at model institutions, and he led the Conference's committee on eugenics until Caswell superintendent McNairy took over in 1915.[90]

William Louis Poteat was a self-trained biologist, born to slaveholding parents and raised in a strict Southern Baptist household. Poteat was president of Wake Forest College, and he was an important public intellectual and frequent lecturer. He served as president of both the Baptist State Convention and the North Carolina Academy of Science. His interest in eugenics grew from his fascination with social regeneration, a topic about which he often spoke and wrote from the 1880s through the 1930s. He was also interested in Mendelian genetics and was one of the South's earliest defenders of evolution, often explaining basic principles of inheritance to his audiences.[91]

Within the state's reform-minded organizations, perhaps the most common explanations of the "science" of eugenics used agricultural metaphors. Such metaphors worked well in a state with so many farmers, particularly when Progressive reformers were also interested in developing better farming techniques based on science. McBrayer argued that the farmers of North Carolina knew how to breed "thoroughbred and pedigreed" animals but were failing to apply this understanding to a more important animal: their children. One psychologist explained that as the quality of corn depends on its seed, so the quality of individuals depended on the quality of their "stock." Just as a farmer would throw away *all* "bad ears of corn" rather than using them as seed for the next season, society must use eugenics to stop the reproduction of all feebleminded people.[92]

Christian rhetoric, a common language for most Progressive reformers, also permeated many discussions of eugenics. Social Christianity provided a framework of shared goals across denominations, and within that framework eugenics became a possible means for creating an ideal society, one step on the path toward the kingdom of God.[93] Denson, for example, believed "there is no higher earthly aim" than shaping and strengthening the human race for God's kingdom on earth. Some experts combined religious rhetoric with agricultural explanations. McBrayer explained the process of heredity through an agricultural analogy in which humans were God's farmers, breeding the human race on His behalf. In the past, McBrayer wrote, God had created mankind "out of the dust of the earth. But . . . he is not doing that stunt any more. He has turned that job over to us."[94] These statements must have struck a chord among Conference members steeped in the social gospel's optimism.

Another important way that reformers understood eugenics was in terms of their beliefs about racial difference and white supremacy. At the time, many white Americans and Europeans thought there were multiple races, even within the category of "white."⁹⁵ Some even described the feebleminded as a race of their own. White Americans across the country were afraid of "race suicide," or "race deterioration," particularly as immigration surged and the birth rate of native-born white people fell.⁹⁶ Although North Carolina had low rates of immigration, some white elites watched with fear as immigrants from Asia and southern and eastern Europe arrived in other parts of the country. Unless something was done soon, one doctor warned in 1915, the human race would become insane and then extinct.⁹⁷ Other reformers urged proactive recruitment of "thrifty white settlers" to supply the state's labor needs so that other kinds of immigrants would never become a reality.⁹⁸

Fears about race suicide took on special resonance for white elites in the Jim Crow South, linked to both their pride in their Anglo-Saxon heritage and their fears of losing economic and political power that they felt was their birthright. Some reformers believed there was a distinct "North Carolina type," the product of both their "ancestral character"—a mix of white immigrant groups—and their environment. Poteat, for example, believed North Carolinians were "sterling, self-reliant, frank, [and] conservatively progressive."⁹⁹ Although some Northern eugenicists disparaged poor white Southerners and particularly disdained residents of Appalachia, local white reformers' faith in the vitality of the North Carolina type spanned the state and crossed class lines. Denson saw even "submerged whites" as redeemable through economic opportunity because they had inherited the superiority "of the best Anglo-Saxon stock." For reformers like Hyatt, Denson, and McBrayer, an interest in the state's Anglo-Saxon heritage was also personal. They were raised to revere their white slaveholding ancestors, they belonged to organizations like the Daughters of the American Revolution and the United Daughters of the Confederacy, and they were fascinated by their own genealogy.¹⁰⁰

While white reformers were proud of the state's supposedly ideal Anglo-Saxon heritage, they firmly believed that African Americans were a separate and inferior race, and they vehemently opposed racial mixing. They often expressed their concerns about both immigrants and African Americans in terms of fears about young white women, whose sexual purity was the ultimate bastion of white supremacy. White women who crossed racial lines, particularly those who bore children, threatened the racial order. Reformers worried particularly about white feebleminded women, who might be susceptible to rape or who simply ignored racial boundaries.¹⁰¹ To Denson, one instance of a "weak-minded" white woman having a second "negro child" was an example of the need for Caswell, to her a story "so horrible I would not like to be quoted as repeating it." She hoped the institution would do a better job of "protecting" white women while also protecting the community from "idiots who are dangerous."¹⁰² While reformers hoped Caswell would provide special care for the white feebleminded, they also hoped it would shore up racial barriers.

To preserve the white North Carolina type and create a "Race of Godlike Americans, perfect in face and form and intellect," as McBrayer proposed, reformers believed they needed to embrace both negative and positive eugenics. Poteat warned that if problems such as feeblemindedness, insanity, alcoholism, and epilepsy were not countered with negative eugenic policies such as segregation, the danger was "the ultimate decay of the race." He also celebrated the state's high white birth rate, praising the state's children as North Carolina's "best crop." Reformers believed native-born white children—"of a vigorous strain, now pure-bred and native"—were vastly superior to immigrants, and they wanted to protect their "infant industry" with positive eugenic policies. The combined results of various eugenics efforts, reformers hoped, would lead to the "upbuilding of the race," which they equated with having the "best citizens, physically, mentally, and morally."¹⁰³

Many white women's interest in eugenics grew from their sense of duty as mothers of the Anglo-Saxon race. In the same way that women entered the political realm under the mantle of extending their maternal duties to the realm of public housekeeping, women espoused eugenics as part of their roles as caregivers, as mothers of white babies, and as guardians of young white girls' sexual purity.¹⁰⁴ Women showed active interest in eugenics principles in the Conference for Social Service, making up almost half of the Conference's committee on feeblemindedness and eugenics, and women's clubs frequently hosted speakers who discussed eugenics. Many women were genuinely concerned about the well-being of feebleminded children as part of their desire to protect all children. They were particularly interested in young white women. One speaker urged Federation of Women's Clubs members to go out in their communities to find feebleminded girls and work to get them admitted to Caswell. She also asked them to lobby legislators to expand Caswell until "every feeble-minded girl" in the state could be "cared for so that she may not become a mother."¹⁰⁵

One of the most visible ways white women engaged with eugenics was in organizing "better babies" contests. These contests were the brainchild of a journalist from the *Women's Home Companion*. For the clubwomen and health department officials who organized the contests, they served the dual purposes of educating mothers about proper infant care and hygiene and setting physical and mental standards for white babies. The first contests in North Carolina, held in 1913, attracted hundreds of mothers from across the state who competed for a total of $300 in cash prizes. Newspaper coverage emphasized that the contests were "a scientific movement and not a beauty

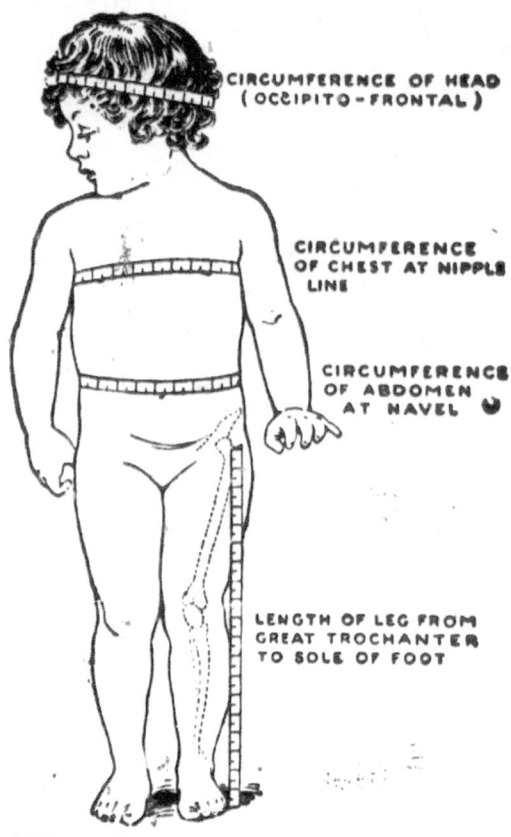

Figure 2.2
Image from a newspaper article showing parents how doctors and nurses would measure their child at a Better Babies contest. "Better Babies Health Contest," *Greensboro Patriot*, October 16, 1913, North Carolina Collection, Louis Round Wilson Special Collections Library, University of North Carolina at Chapel Hill.

show" because they featured expert assessments by "the foremost doctors and children's specialists of the State." During the competition, doctors and nurses—including Louis Burgin McBrayer—examined children's naked bodies, weighed them, and measured them (see figure 2.2). They also administered a "delicate mental test," such as asking a two-year-old to point to their eyes and ears. The medical staff assigned each child points on a scorecard for various categories. For parents who entered their children, the chance to get free health care was at least as great an incentive as a chance at prize money, a professional photograph, and public recognition. At the contest, doctors instructed mothers of "deficient" children about what treatment they needed, and every parent received a scorecard in the mail afterward.

The organizers were open about the eugenic goals of the contests, which one newspaper called "a big idea for race betterment." Often taking place at state or county fairs, where North Carolinians were used to having their livestock judged, the contests were billed as a chance to improve the "greatest crop, the finest blooded live-stock the Old North State produces, her babies." Because these fairs were segregated, white organizers were hoping to target white babies for race betterment. Better physical health, organizers hoped, would allow children to be better pupils, who in turn would become "normal, self-respecting, and desirable citizen[s] in the factory, store, or office." Newspaper coverage for the contest at the 1915 state fair emphasized that the ultimate goal of the contest was a "higher type of men and women" and "a more robust race physically and a stronger race mentally." As one scholar has remarked about similar work in Indiana, for participants "the line between public health and eugenics was nebulous or nonexistent." For the decade while they were popular in North Carolina, better baby contests educated hundreds of white parents about both proper medical care and the importance of physical and mental fitness, in service of creating "better babies and a better race."[106]

More broadly, the remaining evidence of the public reaction to eugenic principles in the 1910s shows that there was skepticism but little overt opposition. To be sure, eugenics was never a grassroots movement with wide popular support. The main problem, to some observers, was that many North Carolinians were reluctant to speak openly about sex, viewing such matters as "foul vulgarity."[107] Even among the middle-class or elite audiences who were spared from being targeted by coercive negative eugenic policies, there were skeptics. Some people derided eugenics as "faddish" and scoffed at its application to realms beyond reproduction.[108] In a small piece published in 1914, one newspaper seemed to joke that upwardly mobile middle-class people were laughably ignorant about eugenics: "'Have you any taste for eugenics, Mrs. Comeup?' 'I've never tried 'em. Do they taste best fried or boiled?'" Another critique ridiculed eugenics as just the latest manifestation of social "hysteria" and questioned humans' ability "to breed by law a race to order," in the face of nature's overwhelming power. Usually, to the extent that people offered substantive critiques, they simply called for the discussion to be more specific and practical, or they debated whether one eugenic strategy was more effective than another.[109]

But for proponents, the capacious reach and malleable logic of eugenics ideology was part of its appeal.[110] It was easy for reformers to see a number of other social problems as somehow connected to eugenics, particularly because eugenic principles addressed marriage and reproduction, institutions fundamental to society. For some, for example, teaching eugenics principles in schools was a way to address the otherwise taboo subject of "sex hygiene." Most laypeople and even many doctors did not care that the "science" of eugenics was fuzzy at best—that experts could not agree on whether mental defects were due to heredity or environment, whether cousins could safely marry, or how many feebleminded people lived in the state.¹¹¹ McBrayer enthused that people across the state were interested: they "are studying it, are asking questions, are reading everything that is printed about it." He optimistically argued that they would, "if given the proper information, form proper conclusions."¹¹²

When Caswell had been open for almost three years, Mattie Parrott, a young white mother of three from Kinston, visited the institution. As she described her visit to women assembled at the Conference for Social Service, the institution had come a long way but still needed more support from the legislature. Parrott's description of the institution showed the mix of attitudes that characterized North Carolinians' reactions to Caswell. Describing the "lowest type of girls," Parrott assured her listeners that "there is nothing repulsive here." Instead, "there are twenty-two little white beds, each immaculate." These girls cannot speak and they "hold out their arms to be caressed just as our babies do." Parrott drew lines of common cause between herself and mothers of the children at Caswell, who despaired for their "hopeless offspring."¹¹³

Yet Parrott ended her presentation with dire warnings about the dangers of "allowing the high-grade defectives to mingle, unrestricted, in society." She declared, "Your children, mothers, and mine, sit beside them in the schoolroom, and converse with them daily. . . . Are you willing that a mind capable only of distorted views shall influence your child in his tender years? No!" To Parrott, the "lowest grade" of feebleminded children deserved sympathy, care, and protection. All women could pity the mothers of such children. But when supposedly feebleminded children, souls already "blackened by sin," strayed into the sanctified territory of normal childhood, their feeblemindedness became a "crime." Although she framed her emotional reactions to feebleminded children in terms of her role as a mother, she proposed solutions that drew on the authority of scientific experts. She called for "McNairy and his assistants" to undertake "further study of the prevalence and effects of these conditions from a scientific standpoint, in order that correct facts may be widely disseminated." Through research, she hoped that the public might gain a greater understanding of the dangers of feeblemindedness and "a knowledge of its prevention."¹¹⁴

Parrott's description of Caswell demonstrates some of the ways reformers viewed the problem of feeblemindedness and eugenic solutions in the 1910s, a critical decade in building public support for a variety of eugenics measures. Progressive reform networks mobilized around a shared understanding of eugenics as a noble calling for all who cared about Progressive efficiency, Christian care, and the purity of the white race. In their efforts to create Caswell, the first eugenically driven institution in the state, North Carolina's reformers refashioned and interpreted eugenics for a broader audience. Over the course of the 1910s, policymakers—and middle-class white North Carolinians in general—accepted and even embraced eugenic principles that resonated with traditions of Christian charity, racial segregation, and celebration of the state's mythical Anglo-Saxon heritage. Like Governor Bickett, many reformers came to believe that eugenics was part of a suite of Progressive reforms that could help the state "assume her rightful place in the march of civilization." They envisioned that "from the blue of the mountains to the blue of the sea there will spring up a hardier, holier race."[115] Yet by the time Governor Bickett spoke these words in 1917, the limits of eugenic segregation were becoming apparent. Soon reformers would turn to other eugenic measures.

Chapter 3

Save the Feeble-Minded Girl

The Limits of Institutions and the Logic of Sterilization

In 1918, Lydia Spruill was "the most talked-about young woman in North Carolina."[1] Four years before, when she was about eleven, Lydia had been legally removed from her parents' custody. Since then she had been through a dizzying number of foster homes and institutions for white children. Officials finally declared her a "moron" and sent her to Caswell Training School. There, she escaped repeatedly and was accused of setting fires that caused extensive damage. These fires, combined with other inmates' unruliness, led to an investigation of Caswell. They also led to intense scrutiny and public fascination with Lydia herself, centering around the question of which institution should have control of Lydia. Ultimately, the actions of Lydia and other inmates also led reformers to rethink even the fundamental role of institutions.

This chapter focuses on the late 1910s, a pivotal moment in social policy for "defective" and "delinquent" people. The state shifted from relying on institutions alone for physical segregation to assembling several eugenic-inspired policies, including marriage restrictions and eugenic sterilization. These policy changes happened because reformers took advantage of a sense of acute social crisis that reopened the question of whether institutions alone could contain people who threatened the social order. The changes were also possible because the state and nation were at the height of a wave of reform, signaled by Woodrow Wilson's election in 1912. By the end of the decade, the state's reform coalitions, including the Conference for Social Service, had organizational strength, political experience, and connection with national organizations. The state's citizens, moreover, had become familiar with the language of Progressive reform from campaigns for prohibition, public schools, woman suffrage, child labor protections, public welfare, and public health. The advent of World War I boosted many of these reforms, opening opportunities for reformers both nationally and locally. Their efforts expanded North Carolinians' ideas of what a modern state could and should do.[2]

In the context of rapid social change, "problem girls" like Lydia Spruill were a primary cause of distress for reformers. They grew increasingly concerned with adolescent female sexuality during the 1910s as urbanization and industrialization allowed young women more autonomy. Many people fascinated by Lydia seemed to be grappling simply with the changing norms of adolescent girlhood: newspapers commented that Lydia "chews gum like a movie actor, dotes on pretty clothes and talks at an alarming rate."[3] For white reformers, white girls whose behavior diverged from the strictures of Southern white ladyhood presented a problem, a potential chink in the armor of white supremacy. Above all, they feared white girls' unsanctioned sexual activity, a direct challenge to claims of white female purity. Lydia Spruill's story captivated the state at the same time reformers were building a new institution to contain and hopefully reform delinquent white girls. The institution that became known as Samarcand Manor, chartered in 1917, was part of a nationwide movement for girls' reformatories. Like Spruill, though, many of Samarcand's new residents refused to be contained or reformed.

Officials' inability to control residents' behavior at Caswell and Samarcand led many reformers and legislators to reconsider the purpose and efficacy of state institutions. Reformers were already aware that Caswell's physical space was not sufficient to house all the white children they thought were feebleminded, much less Black children. Lydia Spruill's case reopened a question that had shadowed Caswell from the beginning: What kinds and ages of people should the school house and train? The evidence suggested that some people could not be contained in institutions, and the institution had no space for others. As successive waves of challenges battered institutions in the late 1910s and highlighted the limits of institutional solutions for complex social and mental problems, some white reformers turned to other solutions.

Within this context, North Carolina's reformers began to discuss a wide range of eugenic policies during the 1910s, including marriage restrictions, immigration restrictions, and educating youth about heredity. With Caswell filled to capacity, by the second half of the decade they began to consider more drastic eugenic measures, including sterilization and even euthanasia. Support for eugenics grew during these years, as reformers gradually became accustomed to new ideas. More extreme discussions paved the way for what had once seemed radical, and reformers turned to more drastic measures because existing policies had failed to meaningfully stem "the menace of the feeble-minded." Reformers envisioned a set of eugenic policies, both positive and negative, interlocking like pieces of a puzzle to address different types of people or defects.

By the end of the decade, reformers took advantage of a sense of social crisis to enshrine more eugenic principles in state policy. A series of fires at Caswell—with Lydia Spruill the alleged arsonist in at least one—intensified all of these concerns at a moment when Progressive sentiment was at its peak in the state, leading to the passage of a sterilization law in 1919. In 1921 the state passed a more restrictive marriage law. Throughout the debates about these policies, reformers used ideas of "fitness" to express their broader concerns about maintaining the social order.[4] This language was particularly striking in wartime discussions about soldiers' readiness, but it extended to their concerns about the average American's ability to participate in democracy. In the crucible of war, many kinds of people apparently failed to measure up, including delinquent girls, camp followers, and children with mental defects. This rhetoric of fitness seemed to resonate with many people in power, even those who were not interested in eugenics per se. The result was that even as the state was asserting a greater degree of responsibility in supporting its citizens—through broader public education, public health measures, extensive road-building campaigns, and other Progressive reforms—legislators also sought new ways to identify and control people who they saw as unfit for citizenship. Ultimately, decisions made in response to crisis had lasting effects in transforming beliefs about the social order—particularly fitness for parenthood—into a policy designed to reinforce the status quo.

"The Most Modern Scientific Methods": Marriage Laws, Sterilization, and Euthanasia

By 1919, when the fires at Caswell sparked interest in how the state was dealing with people who disrupted society, white Progressive reformers had spent the better part of a decade considering a range of solutions. Progressive laypeople had already learned basic principles of eugenics from social work and medical professionals in venues such as the Conference for Social Service, with one result being the creation of Caswell Training School. In the late 1910s, North Carolina's reformers continued to explore other eugenic measures in service of their social vision. They discussed the full range of eugenic policy options then circulating around the nation, including marriage education and restrictions, sterilization, and even euthanasia. They increasingly saw these policies as puzzle pieces that would interlock with institutions such as Caswell, which could house a limited number of people, sometimes for a limited period of time. Reformers believed they needed other policies to address mental defects, particularly to address people there might not be sufficient grounds to institutionalize. They worked to pass these policies singly as a matter of political expediency, but they almost always discussed multiple strategies in a single breath. Ultimately, reformers aimed to use several entwined policies to promote marriage among the "fit" and discourage reproduction among the "the state's delinquents, defectives, and dependents," as the 1917 Conference for Social Service program theme put it.[5]

Eugenicists endorsed marriage laws as one way to prevent procreation between people who were feebleminded, insane, or diseased. Some states began changing marriage laws on explicitly eugenic grounds in the late 1890s, and by the 1910s the effort was widespread. These eugenic marriage laws were part of a broader, coordinated effort during the 1910s to standardize marriage statutes and make it harder for people to cross state lines in search of more permissive laws. By 1914, around thirty states had added restrictions to their marriage laws. Most states' new laws declared that marriages between idiots or the insane were invalid. Others required health certificates in some cases or voided out-of-state elopements. By the 1920s, many states also enacted laws that required a waiting period before the marriage ceremony. These laws, however, were not only about eugenics. They were part of a broad push to regulate racial categories, control sexuality, and surveil social problems through the creation of new bureaucracies, which in turn gave the state new tools to define citizenship.[6]

North Carolina's white reformers showed consistent concern with preventing the marriage of white people deemed "unfit," whether for reasons of mental fitness or because they were infected with venereal disease. The state's medical doctors and Progressive reform organizations often discussed marriage restrictions in the 1910s as one piece of the puzzle to ultimately restrict procreation and protect the health of the nation. In 1915, for example, the Mental Hygiene Association recommended restricting marriage for "defective" people, aiming to have "a people well born." The state's medical association heard proposals to ban marriage between two blind people, marriage between cousins (because such unions supposedly produced children who were feebleminded, blind, or deaf), and marriages of idiots, criminals, syphilitics, and alcoholics. As one doctor in support of these changes argued, "you cannot raise thoroughbred people without a careful, practical study and application of blood strains and mating."[7]

The Conference for Social Service headed a more coordinated campaign for marriage laws. In 1916 its members charged a committee with studying legislation that would prevent "feeblemindedness, insanity, and crime." The next year they invited other social service groups to join them in their study, hoping to present the 1919 legislature with "a sane, scientifically based eugenic marriage law" that could "prevent many of the social ills" the Conference battled—in particular, through preventing the reproduction of "defectives."[8] The state orphanage association backed these calls, and the state welfare board also pushed for a law to prevent marriage between inmates of county homes. The state's director of child welfare told Conference attendees in 1918 that "one sensible marriage law of prevention" would be "worth more than all the humanitarian institutions of care and cure the State is supporting today." Such a law could prevent hereditary disease and produce children who were "well born"—not in terms of their wealth or social position, but a "newer, holier meaning": that their parents "stood the test, that their blood is pure." After hearing this address, the Conference once more urged a "eugenic marriage law to prevent increase of feeble-mindedness."[9]

At Clara Lingle's urging, white clubwomen followed the lead of the Conference for Social Service on marriage laws. After attending the 1916 Conference gathering, Lingle, the president of the Federation of Women's Clubs, declared that the "child's right to be well born" was an integral part of child welfare. On behalf of clubwomen, she wrote in the Conference's journal that "there would be fewer child problems if there were fewer human wrecks among parents.... Almost we are ready to say fewer children if need be, but better children for North Carolina. Children that will start life with better health, better moral instincts, better mentality will give us the class of citizens the State needs."[10] Following the 1917 Conference meeting, the executive council of the Federation of Women's Clubs approved Clara Lingle's motion that their legislative committee "cooperate with other organizations in framing a safe, sane eugenics law."[11] At least one individual club also joined the call to "prevent marriage of 'undesirables'" after hearing from Caswell superintendent C. Banks McNairy about "Race Betterment." Reformers' efforts partially paid off in 1917 with a law that centralized marriage records and prevented double first cousins from marrying, although they would have to wait several more years before passing a more restrictive marriage law.[12]

North Carolina also followed the national pattern in considering stronger miscegenation statutes, which were propelled in part by eugenics arguments. In the West, miscegenation statutes focused on preventing unions between white and Asian or Mexican people. In the South, white leaders tried to police the boundaries between Black and white, with eugenic ideology positing the need for racial purity and condemning racial mixing. North Carolina already had a miscegenation law passed in 1903, but a 1917 proposal would have strengthened it by nullifying existing interracial marriages and disallowing children of the unions from inheriting property.[13]

In the absence of comprehensive marriage laws, many reformers saw better education about eugenics—which quickly blended into education about sex—as critical. William Louis Poteat, the Wake Forest College biologist, condemned the South's reluctance to discuss reproductive matters because "under this cover of silence, the rot in the roots of humanity spreads." He exhorted his listeners to form a "conscience on marriage" and called for a more candid discussion of reproduction. The state's director of child welfare urged parents to tell their children about "the marriage relation," asking whether parents had "the moral courage" to tell their children that their "life-partner" was also "a parent for the children who were to come," and that "the continuance of the race is the divine reason for the marriage relation."[14]

In the late 1910s North Carolina reformers discussed sexual sterilization, which was on its way to becoming normalized in many states. Indiana passed the country's first law allowing sterilization in 1907. By 1916, fifteen states had passed a eugenic sterilization law. Most of the statutes were in states in the Northeast, Midwest, or West, but in 1916 Virginia passed a law that allowed the superintendent of one of its institutions to sterilize inmates.[15] At national social work conferences, too, sterilization gained traction. North Carolina's leading social welfare reformers witnessed in-depth discussions about eugenic sterilization at the National Conference of Charities and Correction and the Southern Sociological Conference.[16] As early as 1903 Daisy Denson attended an NCCC gathering where several people discussed sterilization, including Alexander Johnson, then head of the Indiana school for the feebleminded.[17]

Doctors, social workers, and institutional officials who brought the topic of sterilization to North Carolina audiences framed it as part of a suite of eugenic reforms: it was a logical extension of segregation or marriage restrictions, to be used when other measures failed. By 1912, one doctor at the state medical society meeting argued that North Carolina should adopt "vasectomy after careful scrutiny" modeled after Indiana's law, as part of a slate of recommendations that also included institutional segregation, census questions that would trace "defects," and laws requiring notification about venereal disease. His paper prompted effusive discussion, including a visiting doctor from Alabama who said the discussion of this "splendid" paper alone made "the trip worth while" and argued that every state should adopt a sterilization law. Reformers spoke about sterilization in similar terms to eugenic segregation: as a way to care for low-grade feebleminded people who could not protect themselves from sexual abuse, and as a policy supported by religious, economic, and racial imperatives. Like the doctor in 1912, they were usually careful to point out the differences between vasectomy, which they painted as humane and even potentially beneficial, and castration, which many people believed was brutal and could "unsex" a man. For a woman, they argued that salpingectomy (tubal ligation) was a protection from pregnancy. One clubwoman (later the principal of Caswell Training School) argued in 1920 that women had a duty to protect helpless girls whose virtue might be in danger. "Care of the feeble-minded girl" was not enough, she argued. Efforts needed to go beyond care to prevention, with sterilization as one option that could "stop the Feeble-minded from increasing."[18]

One of the foremost proponents of sterilization was Caswell's C. Banks McNairy, who seemed to chafe daily at his inability to sterilize people for whom he lacked space at his institution. He saw sterilization not as a sole panacea but as part of a group of necessary policies, arguing that a combination of segregation, education, and sterilization was the "only way to wipe out this menace to the population." McNairy believed that the feebleminded affected society "socially, politically, financially and religiously," and he marshaled arguments for each of these categories. In 1916, his official report to the state focused on economic imperatives, calling for sterilization of lower-grade inmates as a partial solution to the "alarming" lack of space, saving room to institutionalize higher-grade girls. At other times he told medical colleagues that mental diseases were the result of sin. While souls could be redeemed through Jesus, he said, no religion could "prevent the children from suffering mentally and physically as a consequence of the sins of the fathers." His solution was to "segregate the girls, higher grades especially; sterilize the lower grades (the hopeless and helpless)." He used these arguments frequently in attempts to build support for sterilization among members of the Conference for Social Service.[19]

McNairy and some other doctors expanded the conversation by exploring an even more radical solution: euthanasia. As with other discussions about eugenic policies, they painted euthanasia as a continuation of the logic of sterilization, appropriate for the most extreme cases. Doctors first discussed euthanasia in 1913, when ERO fieldworker Sybil Hyatt's father, Dr. Henry Otis Hyatt, presented a paper whose title "Physiological Psychology" echoed the title of one of Sybil's courses at Columbia. The ostensible focus of his paper was the need to study inherited physical traits that contributed to feeblemindedness, but he framed the stakes in sweeping terms. "The glory of a country is dependent on the average quality of its citizenship," he said, and America's "subnormal citizenship" threatened to overwhelm "normal people." In part of his paper, he argued that "our Anglo-Saxon ancestors" periodically rounded up the feebleminded and "destroy[ed] them," as well as applying capital punishment to 223 types of offense. He saw these methods as effective ways to eliminate "scrub stock," but admitted that they were "brutish" and impossible to implement in an age of "higher ethics." In this framing, eugenics education and laws were the essence of enlightened science. The audience did not take issue with the principles he described. Instead, the discussant called it "brilliant," "sane," and "mature." He called for more eugenics education to prevent "neurotic mothers" from giving birth.[20]

McNairy, too, proposed euthanasia of feebleminded people before a medical audience. In a paper submitted to the 1915 meeting of the Tri-State Medical Association, he expressed immense frustration with society's inability to teach people to marry with eugenics in mind, which resulted in racial mixing and "mongrels" who were allowed to "run at large and disseminate their kind, as numberless as the stars, without any regard for future generations."

"Would to God we were permitted" to chloroform feebleminded people, he lamented, as in many cases it seemed to be "the most humanitarian act." But, he acknowledged, both society and religion opposed euthanasia. Instead, he saw segregation, education, and sterilization as more politically viable alternatives.[21]

In 1917, McNairy presented a similar proposal to kill "abnormal human animals" at the Conference for Social Service, opening a window into laypeople's views of the range of acceptable eugenics policies. At a Conference session in Raleigh in January 1917, with war looming on the horizon, McNairy participated in a panel on "the care of the dependent child." He argued that in the case of "unfortunate" or "afflicted" humans, society should "apply the most modern scientific methods for that specific case—medicine, surgery, environment, segregation, [a]sexualization, and castration." Judging from the lack of debate these principles generated, most of the audience agreed. McNairy's next proposal went further: He "told how wild geese, migrating from North to South, bear above them the injured members of the flock, and how, when this is impossible, they administer a deadly narcotic." Rats, he said, exhibited similar behaviors. McNairy suggested that humans should be at least as "wise" as animals in nature. He asked, "May I be permitted to suggest that in extreme cases of abnormal human animals in body, and mind, where there is no ray of hope or escape, that society should be as broad, as tender and as merciful as the fowls or the rat to their own, to permit his taking the narcotic that would produce the sleep of eternal peace?"[22]

McNairy's tentative phrasing indicates that euthanasia was not quite acceptable, but the response to his proposition demonstrates that neither was it out of the realm of possibility. His proposal drew applause from the audience until another speaker took the podium and chastised them.[23] While sterilization was necessary, this speaker argued, he did not support killing people with physical and mental defects. During the "stiff debate" that followed, some Conference members condemned the proposal as shocking and criminal. McNairy defended himself by saying he sometimes got requests from parents to make such actions legal. When one respected Conference member proposed a resolution "against putting defectives out of the way," McNairy finally backtracked, claiming he had been misunderstood and that he merely meant to raise the "question of its preference."[24]

Conference attendees thus stopped short of condoning euthanasia, but did so only after prompting from several leaders. Their negative reaction to McNairy's extreme idea forced him to claim that he had been misunderstood and possibly curbed his desire to explore the possibilities of euthanasia. The Conference was nevertheless in favor of eugenic measures short of euthanasia, including McNairy's suggestion of sterilization, which drew no objections.

Two days later, panelists in the closing session on "race betterment" issued a "slashing denunciation" of "the mating of defectives." They discussed the problem of "bad stock," the breeding of humans, and restrictions on marriage. One former state senator and Caswell board member, John R. Baggett, advocated giving heads of penal or charitable institutions the authority to sterilize inmates when in their "wisdom" it was "necessary to protect society from an increase of defectives."[25]

Despite the lack of any recorded objections to the principle of sterilization, Conference members chose for the moment to focus their lobbying efforts on "a sane, scientifically based eugenic marriage law," probably following the advice of the committee that had studied the issue.[26] Their choice of language—emphasizing sanity and science—indicates their awareness of potential opposition to such a measure or their own worries about the slippery slope leading from sterilization toward more sweeping measures. In 1917, even reformers convinced of the merits of sterilization thought it worth trying a marriage law first. Moreover, most still hoped that institutions could contain enough defective people to reduce the burden on society.

The "Girl Problem": Female Delinquency, Feeblemindedness, and the Limits of Segregation

In the first years after Caswell was built, many reformers remained optimistic that institutional segregation would make a meaningful difference in the number of feebleminded, insane, and epileptic people who were able to reproduce. To accomplish this goal, however, they thought institutions needed far more space, since they estimated that the state had several thousand feebleminded people.[27] Other institutions, including mental hospitals and schools for deaf and blind children, faced similar space constraints. Intertwined with the debate over how many state dollars to spend on new institutional facilities were debates over the missions of each institution. Was the primary purpose to treat patients, care for them permanently, or contain them in sex-segregated facilities to prevent their reproduction? More fundamentally, to what degree were taxpayers willing to fund these institutions?[28]

As the newest institution, Caswell was a focal point of debates, with nearly every legislative session adjusting details of its charter. While many reformers saw the school's dual eugenic and caring purposes as complementary under ideal circumstances, the limited number of beds at Caswell meant that officials were constantly caught between their desire to implement eugenic principles of permanent segregation and the real need for adequate care for severely disabled children. Institutional officials were more concerned about containing women of reproductive age, but the legislature and the broader public wanted Caswell to provide care and training for children, whose families were often unable or unwilling to care for them.

In 1917 Caswell's trustees requested a quarter of a million dollars to build another dorm and improve the current infrastructure, looking to increase its present capacity of 190 inmates by fifty or more in the next two years. Even adding fifty more beds would fall far short of meeting the needs of the state's feebleminded population, according to McNairy's projections. That spring Caswell's staff hosted two dozen members of a special legislative committee who visited to investigate the school's needs. Caswell did not receive what McNairy wanted in 1917, instead getting funds that allowed only a small addition to the girls' building and the construction of dining and storage rooms.[29]

That same year, the state created a new institution for delinquent white girls, which was soon embroiled in similar questions about the possibilities of institutions to solve larger social problems. Progressive reformers had long pushed for a reformatory for "wayward" white girls as part of a chain of institutions that would care for, contain, and control the state's "dependent, defective, and delinquent" population, ideally in separate institutions. They often focused on children and adolescents, since they believed that by providing moral instruction, health care, and education to youth, they could make the next generation stronger, more productive, and less deviant.[30] At Caswell, although officials and legislators battled over the age limit and specific mental types, children were always a priority. Children elicited pity from the public, while also showing some potential of benefiting from the school's training. A similar logic lay behind the establishment of the state's first reformatory, the Stonewall Jackson Training School for white boys, created in 1907. Clubwomen hoped to provide a place where boys arrested for delinquency could be retrained, both protected from the hardened criminals they would encounter if sent to jail and removed from the corrosive influence of whatever friends or family had led them astray.

With white boys provided for, North Carolina's white reformers turned to an institution for white girls. The "girl problem" was not new; the growth of industry and urbanization created new opportunities for working-class girls to work and socialize. Factories, dance halls, or movie theaters lacked family supervision, allowing young women new possibilities for flirtation and sexual activity. Late nineteenth-century reformers had worried about young white girls' morality but painted them as victims of male seduction. After the turn of the century, Progressive reformers and social workers increasingly blamed young women for their sexual activity, reframing them as delinquent and immoral.

"Wayward" white girls emerged as a particular concern for reformers in the first two decades of the twentieth century because they challenged the logic of white supremacy. In straying from middle-class behavioral norms of sexuality, these girls undermined the myth of the white Southern lady, which posited that pure white women deserved and needed white men to protect them from the base sexual desires of Black men. Feebleminded women and girls were seen as particularly dangerous not only because they could pass on their mental defects to their children, but also because middle-class reformers understood them to be more sexually excitable. By containing deviant young white girls in a clean, orderly, Christian environment where they learned homemaking skills for their future as mothers, proponents of a reformatory hoped to redeem young white girls before they disgraced the race.[31] In establishing a reformatory for white girls only, the state doubled down on notions that it was both possible and necessary to save white girls from moral decay. On the other hand, white reformers believed that Black girls were inherently promiscuous and did not deserve saving. Black female reformers pushed back against these assumptions, seeing Black girls' respectability as vital to their reform efforts. They created and privately funded Efland, a reformatory for Black girls, for two decades before the state supported it.[32]

Samarcand Manor for white girls was the product of a long, cooperative crusade, as the campaign for Jackson had been a decade earlier. Early lobbyists included the Woman's Club of Raleigh, the King's Daughters of Durham, and various benevolent societies. The Federation of Women's Clubs joined the campaign by 1915, but women's organizations were making little impression on lawmakers. Beginning in 1915, Presbyterian preacher A. A. McGeachy began calling for a home for "bad girls," and at his urging the Conference for Social Service threw its weight behind the idea. In 1917, Alfred M. Scales, a Conference member and experienced state senator, drafted a bill for an institution to house and reform young white prostitutes, drunkards, vagrants, or other petty criminals. Scales helped shepherd the bill through "the most liberal-minded" legislature in recent memory, where it passed despite some opposition.[33]

The critical context for the passage of the bill was the Great War, which shadowed the horizon across the Atlantic. While the legislature met during the spring of 1917, newspaper headlines were dominated by the threat of conflict, leading up to the official declaration of war on April 6. As Americans prepared to join the Allied forces in Europe, they also confronted their fears about the nation's fitness, mental health, and the strength of American civilization. The US Army's program of administering psychological tests to recruits gave psychologists a chance to prove the worth of intelligence tests to the public at large, but the test results raised an alarming specter of national decline. Biased toward men with formal education, the tests produced distressingly low scores among native-born white men, particularly in the South.

According to tests, the average mental age of the white draftees was 13.08 years, barely higher than the benchmark for feeblemindedness. Rather than question their testing protocols and definitions of feeblemindedness, some psychologists concluded that feeblemindedness was far more pervasive than they had believed. Cynics took the results of the army's extensive testing program and ran with them, expounding on the "masses" of "morons" who imperiled American democracy. The *Charlotte Observer* ran a special feature proclaiming that "too many" men had been rejected from the armed forces in South Carolina for being feebleminded—and that North Carolina's rejection rate was higher than South Carolina's, at 16.5 men per thousand.[34]

The war also intensified concerns about female sexuality, focusing attention on young white women who flaunted their sexuality and, in flouting the norms of white ladyhood, presented the possibility of feeblemindedness. Venereal disease was a substantial threat to public health during the war, and military officials took it seriously. As federal and state officials clamored to contain the threat, they focused their attention mainly on women as vectors of disease. They cracked down on prostitutes, camp followers, and even alluring working-class girls, whom they saw as an enormous threat to soldiers' moral and physical health. They also associated prostitution with feeblemindedness, particularly for white women; genteel constructions of white womanhood left no room for "normal" white women to be sexually active outside of marriage, much less to engage in prostitution. Increased extramarital sexual activity around army camps brought reformers' attention to the presumed underlying problem of female feeblemindedness.[35] When Governor Thomas W. Bickett addressed the Conference for Social Service and the Federation of Women's Clubs in the spring of 1918, for example, he began his address by talking about venereal disease but almost seamlessly wound up advocating sterilization of mental defectives, whether that defect was the product of venereal disease or other causes.[36]

Beginning in April 1917, the federal government coordinated a campaign to root out "camp followers." The War Department's Commission on Training Camp Activities published pamphlets about the need for America's male fighting forces to remain pure, and they targeted red-light districts and prostitutes, fully embracing a sexual double standard. The Chamberlain-Kahn Act of 1918 strengthened this work, creating the Interdepartmental Social Hygiene Board, which sent funds to the states to combat prostitution near military camps. This campaign (and these federal funds) spurred the national reformatory movement: Samarcand was part of a wave of twenty-nine reformatories for delinquent girls created between 1910 and 1924.[37]

These social and policy changes intensified the demands on space at Caswell and other institutions, where wartime needs took precedence over institutions' chartered missions. In mid-1918, the US Justice Department, apparently unwilling to wait while the state prepared Samarcand to open, asked Caswell to accept feebleminded young women who were arrested for prostitution near military bases. The state welfare board seemed to share the federal government's fears, publishing articles during the summer of 1918 highlighting the dangers of leaving feebleminded girls loose in communities where they might become prostitutes near army camps.[38]

Thus when Samarcand opened in September 1918, its mission—rescuing and redeeming young girls *before* they could go down a path of immorality—was already compromised. The head of the institution, Agnes MacNaughton, who had worked at Pennsylvania's reformatory, tried to emphasize the girls' peaceful gentility and their healthy, bucolic surroundings. The institution sat on 235 acres of farmland in the Sandhills region, and the girls were taught "garden and domestic work," plus basketry, weaving, and "scientific poultry" management. They had access to a library of 1,200 volumes, plus hikes, swimming, picnics, and music. In contrast to this uplifting image, federal and state officials pressured the institution to make space for girls or women, including prostitutes, whose diseased bodies might threaten the health of the troops. Financial problems further compromised Samarcand's mission, similar to Caswell's experience. Samarcand had received an initial annual appropriation of $10,000, which MacNaughton later claimed was intended for only thirty girls.[39] These challenges amplified reformers' sense that institutions were not a sufficient answer to defect and delinquency.

"Matches and a Craving for Excitement": Lydia Spruill and Unruly Inmates

By 1918, North Carolina faced challenges on many fronts. The war continued. Influenza tore through the nation. And even as Samarcand Manor opened, many reformers began to reckon with the shortcomings of custodial institutions they had longed for, recognizing that they were incapable of preventing social rupture. Limited space made clear that institutions were not enough to prevent the spread of venereal disease, feeblemindedness, or bad behavior. The blurring of lines between institutions undermined reformers' goals to separate different populations. On top of this crisis landed a growing problem: the reality that many of the "delinquent" and "defective" people placed in institutions did not want to be there and went to great lengths to get away.[40] Lydia Spruill, the young white woman who attracted so much public attention in 1918, was one of these "unruly inmates."

Lydia was born around 1903 in New Bern, where her father, the son of an Irish immigrant, worked in a sawmill. When Lydia was about eleven, a judge committed her to the care of the North Carolina Children's Home Society, believing that her parents Hilbert and Laura were not taking care of Lydia and her younger sister Blygh. Lydia was placed in a series of foster homes in Greensboro, but she repeatedly ran away. While officials saw her as "incorrigible," she claimed that she had been mistreated in every home. In one episode around 1916, she showed up on a cold evening at the large home of typewriter salesman Henry Wharton and his wife, asking for a place to stay. Mrs. Wharton was sympathetic to her plight, and the couple found her to be "very bright" and "a good conversationalist." But the Whartons soon discovered that Lydia was telling neighbors that the Whartons were keeping her against her will. After two weeks, she "became unmanageable." With Lydia repeatedly returned to the Children's Home Society because no family would or could keep her, the society sent her to a reformatory in Baltimore, Maryland. After a few weeks, officials there also rejected her, finding her "influence and example in the institution" to be unacceptable. Finally, around 1916 or 1917, the Children's Home Society applied for her to be sent to Caswell, supplying a certificate from a physician who had examined her and found her of a low enough IQ to be classified a "moron." As the president of the Caswell board later argued, institutionalization was necessary for Lydia's "own protection and the protection of society."[41]

Naturally, Lydia did not agree. In the summer of 1918, she ran away from Caswell and sought refuge with a member of the Salvation Army in Kinston, the closest town. Lydia accused Caswell officials of neglect and abuse, including whippings. The Salvation Army took her claims seriously, publishing her charges and publicly questioning why she had been sent to Caswell in the first place. She was not feebleminded, they argued, merely a juvenile delinquent whose behavior was the product of the foster-care system. Thwarting Caswell's authority, they secretly moved her to Durham and kept her there for several weeks while refusing to tell Caswell superintendent C. Banks McNairy where she was. They may have even attempted to send her to Georgia to prevent her return to Caswell.[42]

Lydia's "sensational charges" of abuses at Caswell sparked a minor scandal. McNairy and other officials insisted that she had not been mistreated, although they admitted that they sometimes used "the rod" to "coax unruly inmates" into "modest behavior." They insinuated that anyone who believed Lydia's charges was merely being taken in by her "fanciful stories." Aware of the need for public support, McNairy asked the governor to open an investigation to prove the institution free of misconduct. The governor agreed, but the investigation never materialized because Lydia's supporters in Durham failed to bring forward an official charge. Meanwhile, Lydia's mother Laura asked to have her returned to Caswell until the family was able to take care of her, but for the summer she remained out of the institution.[43]

The public's fixation with Lydia Spruill was part of widespread public confusion about how to categorize various so-called antisocial behaviors. Of course, experts themselves defined terms such as "feeblemindedness" or "delinquency" in many different ways, and often an individual diagnosis reflected the whims of the person assessing them. Many laypeople were even more perplexed about the lines between feeblemindedness and delinquency, two conditions often linked to concerns about female sexuality. Her supporters lamented that in the summer of 1918 the state had not yet opened an institution to reform white girls who, like Lydia, were the product of a "depraved and impoverished" environment. They argued that the lack of a girls' reformatory did not "under any circumstance" justify sending a delinquent to Caswell instead. Others, including Caswell officials, argued stridently that behavior such as Lydia's was the product of her mental deficiency. The debate about what to do with "problem girls" such as Lydia was far from academic, since officials' decision about whether someone was normal, insane, a moron, or delinquent could determine whether the person spent months, years, or the rest of their life at an institution.[44]

In Lydia's case, Caswell officials managed to have her quietly recommitted after several months—but the school's troubles were far from over. Although McNairy grudgingly admitted that Lydia had been well-behaved since her return, he was "not exactly" glad to have her back. On December 8, 1918, a fire broke out just before lunch, destroying the old girls' dormitory. Authorities immediately assumed Lydia was responsible: she had boasted about starting the fire, although other girls said she was not responsible. Veracity of the claims aside, Lydia was locked in a room until she could be examined to determine whether she was insane or feebleminded, which would determine which institution might become her permanent home. On Christmas Eve of 1918, three days before the scheduled examination, she made another sensational escape from her locked, second-story room. Newspapers reported on her "human fly stunt," in which she broke the window pane and jumped from her window ledge to the ledge outside her friend Clara's room. Together, they sneaked off the Caswell grounds, perhaps to seek refuge with Lydia's stepfather, who lived near Kinston.[45]

One night less than two weeks later, while Lydia and Clara were still missing, four other girls "with matches and a craving for excitement" sneaked quietly out of their rooms. They stuffed rags into an elevator chute and lit them with stolen matches. As the flames surged through the building and lit the night sky, the school's staff evacuated the dorm's 124 residents and dragged furniture out onto the lawn. Fire trucks raced toward the school, but the school's water supply was too low to stop the fire, and even with the firefighters' help, the building was destroyed. Officials estimated the damage at $25,000, equivalent to over $750,000 today. Luckily, no lives were lost in this fire on January 7, 1919. Although Lydia had not been at Caswell when the second fire started, the state's deputy insurance commissioner nevertheless wanted to speak to her, viewing her as a prime suspect in the first fire and probably also a bad influence on the other girls. With the aid of McNairy and the local sheriff, he managed to track her down almost twenty miles away and capture her "after a lively chase."[46]

After the second Caswell fire, the plight of the children sleeping on floors in classrooms and in "spare corners" drew the attention of the state legislature. Superintendent McNairy found room for some displaced Caswell residents, including Lydia and the other "firebirds," at the mental hospital and other state-run institutions in Raleigh, but this solution was at best temporary. Governor Bickett urged the legislature to make an emergency appropriation of $75,000 to replace the buildings destroyed in the fires at Caswell. Groups from around the state joined the appeal, including Rotary Clubs.[47]

At the same time, the war's horrors also put indirect but significant pressure on the capacities of mental hospitals, adding to a sense of looming crisis. In January 1919, as troops demobilized, federal officials in the Bureau of War Risk Insurance asked state officials to prepare to house veterans whose sanity had been shaken by wartime trauma. Even with the governor pressuring institutional heads directly, solutions were piecemeal at best. The head of the Raleigh hospital for the white insane agreed to take twenty-five returning veterans, while the head of the Goldsboro hospital for the Black insane had room for only ten. The superintendent of the Morganton asylum voiced the crux of the problem: admissions of "mental cases discharged from the Army" would "be at the expense of the civil [civilian] population, since at present we are unable to accommodate all applicants for admission."[48]

The legislators declined to make an emergency appropriation for Caswell, but they did appoint a special joint committee to consider its needs, using this moment to resolve long-standing debates over the institution's capacity and mission. Fast-talking, gum-chewing Lydia soon became part of the legislative committee's evidence. To them, Spruill was the emblem of the problem girl—definitely delinquent, likely feebleminded, and possibly insane. In late January 1919, state officials asked an outside expert to examine Spruill and confirm a diagnosis of feeblemindedness. Dr. Martin W. Barr, an eminent psychologist and superintendent of a Pennsylvania institution for the feebleminded, spent a week in North Carolina as an adviser to the legislative committee. The day after his testimony in the capitol building, Barr completed a "painstaking examination" of Spruill in front of several institutional officials. He also examined Sally Bryson, a seventeen-year-old girl accused of killing her mother. He found both to be feebleminded.[49]

Barr's examination process merits as much attention as his verdict. His scrutiny of the girls, which was covered by the local paper, exposed their minds and bodies to public inspection. Barr reported finding physical "marks which he considers unmistakable evidence of imbecility," including the shape of their ears, faces, and even the inside of their mouths. Although the newspaper mentioned that Barr conducted "various mental tests," it focused on his physical findings, suggesting that feebleminded people were abnormal enough to be identifiable by sight alone. Barr also commented on the girls' lack of a "sense of moral responsibility," and noted that "in such cases the sex impulse frequently appears to be irresistible."[50]

Barr's diagnosis undercut Spruill's legitimacy and countered attacks made against Caswell: How could a feebleminded young girl with no moral compass be an accurate and trustworthy judge of institutional conditions? For a decade, reformers had been spreading awareness about the social problem of feeblemindedness and building public support for taking more drastic action than institutional segregation. Barr's focus on links between feeblemindedness and delinquency echoed welfare experts' claims that antisocial behavior was often rooted in mental deficiency.[51]

Sterilization and the Limits of Institutions

The fires at Caswell and the work of the special investigative committee forced the problem of feeblemindedness into the public view once again in the 1919 legislative session. The committee's primary response to their investigation of the situation at Caswell in the aftermath of the fires was to call for more beds, but the fires also led to changes McNairy and some other reformers had long desired. In a letter to the editor in the *Charlotte Observer*, a member of the Caswell board encouraged readers to write their representatives in favor of an emergency appropriation to Caswell; he also asked his readers to consider McNairy's idea for a statute prohibiting feebleminded people from marrying. The joint committee on Caswell, too, favored establishing an outreach bureau and studying feeblemindedness.[52]

Following some of the committee's recommendations, the 1919 legislature used the fires and subsequent investigation as an opportunity to revise Caswell's charter once again. The new charter "more correctly" and explicitly defined Caswell's goal as preventing the reproduction of feebleminded people, labeling eugenic segregation as its primary function. The charter also gave Caswell officials the responsibility of educating the public about mental deficiency, as well as "initiat[ing] methods for its control, reduction, and ultimate eradication from our people." Although the new charter created an outreach bureau, the legislature failed to fund it. They did appropriate money to rebuild Caswell at a larger size, although not as much as the trustees had hoped. At the same time, lawmakers sought to create more oversight of the institution by consolidating its management under the state hospitals for the insane.[53]

The flurry of events surrounding the fires at Caswell fueled legislators' sense of urgency and pointed toward sterilization as an alternative to the shortcomings of existing institutions. Within a month of the second blaze, the Caswell investigative committee's work led to the introduction of a eugenic sterilization bill. When Barr came at the committee's invitation to scrutinize Spruill, he also visited Caswell. He left convinced that sterilization would be appropriate for some inmates there and at other state-run institutions. When the committee reconvened in Raleigh, Barr met with them for an informal conversation focused mostly on "methods employed in dealing with imbeciles, idiots and moral imbeciles," and he recommended sterilization. At least one newspaper linked his study of Spruill to the committee's recommendations with the headline "Examination Shows Need of Legislation to Protect Feeble-Minded and Society." McNairy's report on the fires also went straight from describing the fire to demanding the power to sterilize inmates, along with increased space to segregate inmates.[54]

The following week, Speaker of the House Dennis G. Brummitt introduced a bill that would put into effect Barr and McNairy's suggestions for sterilization of inmates. Brummitt, a native of Granville County and graduate of Wake Forest, was a lawyer and leader of the state Democratic Party who would become state attorney general in 1925. Local media declared him "progressive without being radical" and noted that he supported measures "calculated to set the State forward morally and educationally." Brummitt would have welcomed those descriptors, as he saw the sterilization bill as falling into that category. The bill he introduced on February 1, 1919—after several boys at Caswell started a *third* dormitory fire—was entitled, "An Act to Benefit the Moral, Mental, and Physical Condition of Inmates of Penal and Charitable Institutions."[55]

The title of the bill did not indicate its purpose, and the text itself merely instructed institutional officials to perform "any surgical operation" that would "be for the improvement of the mental, moral or physical condition of such inmate." Newspaper headlines, however, left little doubt of the bill's real goal, which was to "permit sterilization."[56] Supporters of the bill framed sterilization as merely an improvement on segregation, not as a radical divergence in strategy or consequence.

Meanwhile, physicians, including the head of the state's health board, continued to educate legislators about eugenics. Several doctors supported the sterilization bill's passage, including the chair of the House health committee and a legislator who was also a physician. A psychiatrist stationed at Camp Greene wrote that the sterilization law was "far in advance of almost any of the eastern or southern states." Although welfare officials did not speak out in favor of the sterilization bill, the Conference for Social Service, which met in Raleigh in the middle of February, passed a resolution broadly endorsing measures that would advance "principles of child welfare and social progress."[57]

Progressive reformers' political connections paid off during the 1919 sterilization debate. The support of Governor Thomas Bickett, who had been an active member of the Conference for Social Service since 1913, was crucial to the bill's introduction and passage. Bickett saw the sterilization bill as the "most important" of the session's public health or medical measures, using his opening message to the General Assembly to frame it as "the essence of humanity and common sense." He likely asked Brummitt to introduce the sterilization bill, and he pushed the bill along at key moments, such as when it was stalled in the Committee on Health. Aware that some lawmakers were "aghast at the thought of any such legislation," Bickett worked behind the scenes to persuade them of its merit, drawing explicit connections between existing eugenic-tinged restrictions on marriage licenses and this new measure of sterilization. As he later told the state's doctors, "I called those members down into my office, and put the question squarely to them, man to man and face to face, as to whether or not the State of North Carolina could justify its position in refusing to issue a marriage license to an incurable mental defective and, at the same time, permit the unlimited and lawful perpetuation of these infirmities." His arguments behind closed doors apparently won over some of these reluctant legislators, while others might have owed the governor their vote as a political favor.[58]

Bickett also made public appeals to the legislature, seeking to focus public opinion and use it as additional leverage. On March 7, after the Committee on Health unanimously approved the bill for a second time, Bickett interrupted the session with a special message. Addressing both houses, Bickett begged lawmakers to pass Brummitt's sterilization bill. Interestingly, he claimed that the Conference for Social Service and the Federation of Women's Clubs supported the principle he described, although both groups had resolved only to support a "eugenics law" or "eugenic marriage law." Bickett, at least, seemed to assume that consonance of goals was more important than the means used to achieve them. And reformers did agree that, as Bickett said, "It is not punishment. It is mercy to make provisions of this kind."[59]

After the governor's urging, the bill was approved, although not without resistance. In the House, the vote was sixty-seven to twenty-five, with

Democrats more favorably disposed than the chamber's few Republicans.[60] The only vocal opposition came from Representative Julius Brown of Greenville, whose characterization of the bill as "barbarous and cruel, and made in Germany" was apparently based on an objection to its procedure, not its content, as he thought a jury rather than a board of specialists should judge individual cases.[61] In the Senate, the bill passed easily despite attempts to table it on the grounds that "it was not the sort of document that should be read in the senate," presumably because it referred to matters of sex and reproduction. Supporters, including a senator who was also a medical doctor and state health officer Watson S. Rankin, argued in its favor for both medical and economic reasons. In order to "remove objections" to the bill, a member of the legislative committee on Caswell offered an amendment to require approval of the governor and head of state Board of Health before institutional authorities could sterilize inmates. The amended bill then passed "without a dissenting vote" on the penultimate day of the session.[62] Supporters rejoiced. At a joint meeting of several professional associations that drew hundreds of physicians and their wives, the president of the state Health Officers' Association praised the new law as "a step in the right direction" and even called for "further legislation." A combined program of segregation and sterilization, he argued, would decrease feeblemindedness and crime within "a few decades."[63]

The same spirit of mingled crisis and opportunity led to a raft of other reform-minded legislation in 1919 and soon after. The 1919 legislature passed several laws addressing venereal disease and prostitution. The state created a juvenile court system, which allowed courts to treat young offenders outside of the adult court system and send them to reformatories rather than jails. The law also allowed the court to order a mental exam, and if the child was found to be feebleminded, they could be committed to Caswell. There were also some near misses, including a bill to castrate prisoners convicted of rape, which failed in committee.[64]

Significantly, a failed attempt to pass a marriage law in 1919 also led to success in the next legislative session. In 1919, a pair of failed bills would have required health certificates for men before marriage and prohibited marriage of people with venereal disease. But a comprehensive marriage bill finally passed in 1921. It required both men and women to get health certificates addressing tuberculosis and mental fitness, as well as certifying men were free from venereal disease. One newspaper called it "the new eugenics law," commending its general purpose but questioning whether it was possible to enforce it.[65]

Institutional officials also soon gained some support to address the pressing lack of space. McNairy began rebuilding Caswell at a larger size, then was much aided by a 1921 bond issue of $6 million, about $240,000 of which went to Caswell. In 1922, new dorms and a new dining hall went up at the school. Samarcand also grew. In early 1920, North Carolina's welfare officials turned to the federal government for help supporting Samarcand. Bolstered by Superintendent McNaughton's evidence about overcrowding, unexpected medical expenses, and a lack of equipment, the state secured a total of almost $60,000 from the Interdepartmental Social Hygiene Board. The funds, however, were specifically to care for girls with venereal disease who were a "direct and certain menace" to troops. Inmates of these two institutions were still subject to the whims of officials' diagnosis, and officials continued to see significant overlap in the conditions of mental defect and delinquency. In 1920, the state brought an expert from the National Committee for Mental Hygiene, who found that two-thirds of the inmates at Samarcand were feebleminded.[66]

While McNairy tried to rebuild Caswell, Lydia Spruill remained at Dix Hill, the Raleigh mental hospital where the "firebirds" and other Caswell inmates had been transferred. In January 1920, she once again escaped from state custody and sought refuge with her stepfather's family near Kinston. Her infamy continued at least until 1922, when the state welfare board recycled the story of her supposed arson.[67] After that, her story disappears from the historical record, like those of many inmates of these state institutions.

Scholars have dismissed the 1919 sterilization law as unimportant since there is scant evidence that it led to any sterilizations.[68] It was, however, the first statewide eugenic sterilization law in the South.[69] Its very existence signals that North Carolina's reformers had built sufficient public support to pass a law far earlier than the standard narrative of eugenics in the South suggests. Of equal note, the 1919 sterilization law was part of a broader campaign for eugenic policies, the results of the growing appeal of the ideology for influential North Carolinians. Led by doctors and social workers, these white, educated, upper-middle-class North Carolinians brought their own experiences to their understanding of eugenics and set the stage for sterilization by educating the public about the presumed necessity of eugenic interventions.

As reformers recognized the limits of institutions to reform or contain defective and delinquent people, Progressive leaders transformed support for abstract eugenic principles into concrete laws that allowed the state to restrict people's choices about marriage or surgically sterilize them. The turn toward the latter of those, sterilization, followed the same pattern as the spread of eugenics ideas more generally. Although sterilization provoked more opposition than eugenic segregation, its advocates prevailed because they linked the goals of sterilization to ideas that already had broad support—humanitarian and religious concerns, racial purity, scientific efficiency, and a focus on children as the future of the race—while downplaying the expansion of state power their new programs entailed.

Supporters of sterilization were responding to what they saw as real social threats. Caswell had been their first attempt to solve those problems with a eugenic approach, but the Lydia Spruill case and constant overcrowding at Caswell indicated the limits of a strategy based on institutional segregation. In this moment of policy innovation and wartime fervor, events converged to produce a sense of crisis, focusing attention on an ideology that had already gained ardent supporters because it promised simple policy solutions to seemingly intractable social problems. In this sense, the move toward sterilization was merely an extension of earlier efforts to control the entwined problems of crime, poverty, and mental defects. The evidence, clear in hindsight, that reformers' tools were poorly fitted to this work highlights the poignancy of their failure to find politically feasible policy solutions for complicated social problems.

Chapter 4

The Root of Social Problems

Eugenics and the Training of Social Workers

Kate Burr Johnson, the state welfare commissioner, had an unexpected flair for comedy. In the midsummer heat of 1922, she led her staff into an improvised courtroom at the University of North Carolina. There they performed a mock trial for an audience of white social workers, who would later dissect it for proper procedure as part of a two-week welfare training institute. A heavyset, middle-aged county welfare superintendent played "Willie," an "undernourished" boy accused of stealing a pistol.[1] Other social workers played the roles of a judge, a welfare superintendent, witnesses, and Willie's parents. Johnson, however, stole the show. She became "the clown of the piece" as she improvised the lines of Willie's chatterbox neighbor, dishing on the family's domestic relations.[2]

Jokes aside, Johnson hoped the social work trainees would pay close attention to the next "witness," state psychopathologist Dr. Harry W. Crane. Dark-haired, blue-eyed Crane began questioning Willie in his "clear, strong, pleasant voice." Although Crane loved satire, he must have felt a professional obligation to conduct this mock mental examination with an air of decorum. Giving mental exams and testifying in juvenile court proceedings fell under his regular duties as head of the state welfare board's new Bureau of Mental Health and Hygiene. Crane and the state welfare board believed that examinations of juvenile delinquents such as "Willie" were of paramount importance, since, as they claimed, "mental deficiency" was one of the biggest contributing causes of delinquency. They had recently published estimates that less than a quarter of delinquent boys had average or above-average intelligence. The rest were "morons" or "borderline." When Crane wrapped up his mock questioning, he declared Willie to be a "high-grade imbecile." In this dramatic rendition, the judge wanted to send Willie to Caswell Training School but could not because it was full. Instead, he rebuked Willie's father for his son's thievery and entrusted the boy to a six-month parole under his parents' tutelage. The sham court adjourned, the institute's students and teachers dropped their assumed personas, and everyone chattered and laughed about the good fun had during the performance.[3]

These were not mere moments of amateur theater. Instead, they reveal one of the many ways social workers were trained to see mental defect as "the root of all social problems," part of their broader training in preventive social work methods for rural areas as part of North Carolina's growing welfare apparatus. Beginning in 1917, North Carolina established a welfare infrastructure that fulfilled the goals of many Progressive reformers and functioned as another puzzle piece in maintaining the "fitness" of the white population. An alliance of academics and professionals fashioned principles of social work that suited their analysis of the rural Southern situation. The growing welfare infrastructure provided stronger guarantees of support for the deserving white poor, including children, widowed mothers, and the elderly. At the same time, it promised more state supervision of others, including poor African Americans, delinquent youth, and "mental defectives." Officials in a centralized state office ensured that welfare programs were widespread and that county-level staff administering these efforts had some amount of professional training. The new welfare board embodied reformers' aim to provide government protection for certain groups through centralized oversight, as well as a commitment to using trained professionals, which later enabled them to implement eugenics policies. Their work on rural social welfare became a model for rural areas beyond the South. Although growth was slow, the Board of Charities and Public Welfare eventually became a clearinghouse for experiments in reform on multiple fronts and significantly expanded welfare services before the New Deal.

At this turning point in the growth of a statewide welfare system, old assumptions about poverty continued to hold sway despite new standards for professionalization of social workers. A family's fate at the hands of county boards of welfare—whether they received cash assistance, were sent to the poor home, or got nothing—had long depended on county officials' appraisal of whether they were "deserving." Although eligibility for welfare benefits was not yet formally defined at a state level, state officials encouraged local social workers to systematize their decisions by using casework methods and relying on the state's mental testing services. These new tools to assess poor people's "fitness" for using relief, however, produced similar decisions about who was deserving. As one scholar argues, eugenics "tossed the mantle of science over the ancient distinction between the worthy and unworthy poor," but it did so within a new bureaucratic context that allowed increased surveillance and supervision of its targets.[4]

As state welfare officials attempted to standardize poor relief across the state, they were forced to grapple with ideas of citizenship, including the role of social welfare in cultivating their ideal citizen as an economically productive member of society. In 1926, the future state welfare commissioner wrote about this ideal citizen for members of the League of Women Voters. At the apex of her ideal was a family unit that provided for itself by "work[ing] industriously" and "liv[ing] thriftly." Citizens in such a family should also read and "think straight," "use leisure fruitfully," and act honestly, responsibly, and "with self-control." Such traits were even possible for children, whose obedience to authority was a sign of good future citizenship.[5] If such a model family fell on hard times, temporary assistance might return them to self-sufficiency. Similarly, reformers saw merit in providing cash assistance to worthy widowed mothers who followed sexual mores and had impeccable character. This select group of women, almost all white, received mothers' aid so they could afford to stay home, rather than seeking gainful employment elsewhere—and thus be present to rear their children as good citizens. Even delinquent white youth showed some promise; rehabilitation at an institution was the key to preventing further slumps into crime and moral degradation. These groups of dependent and delinquent white people received some state support, albeit with supervision, in hopes that they and their children could be redeemed as good citizens.

The state also supported social work among African Americans, but only as second-class citizens. To justify this expansion, welfare officials highlighted that the services would be segregated and reminded critics of Black aid that the fates of the two races were intertwined. This argument appealed to white leaders, who recognized that the state's economy rested on Black labor but believed that Black people were inherently lethargic and ignorant and would remain so unless white people led them toward social salvation and economic productivity. Even so, white conservatives remained reticent to spend money on any welfare services. In response, welfare officials demonstrated the potential of social work in Black communities by using private funds, hoping that eventually the state would finance the work. They succeeded in persuading legislators that investing in trained, efficient social workers would save money in the long run by helping both Black and white people become self-supporting, law-abiding members of society.

But there was another group whom welfare officials considered unable to meet the obligations of citizenship in a competitive world: "mental defectives." Those people, welfare officials believed, simply lacked the ability to *be* citizens—to support themselves, avoid crime, and obey sexual and racial codes. Because welfare officials saw many mental problems as hereditary, they often labeled entire families as defective and therefore unfit for citizenship. In this light, proponents of eugenic segregation were convinced that eliminating "propagation among the feeble-minded" would result in the "betterment of citizenship in the state."[6] State officials castigated county welfare workers for wasting relief funds on such families, encouraging them instead to remove feebleminded people from county homes and admit them to state-run institutions, or to remove children from homes where the environment might allow bad character traits to develop unchecked.

In the end, the state welfare board's success in alleviating poverty and other social problems was constrained by two main factors. Externally, constant pushback from conservative corners checked the Board's reach. Although the growing welfare board expanded citizens' expectations of the government's role in their lives, traditions of individualism and localism persisted. County-based social workers struggled to translate state policy into local practice while they traveled long hours over miles of rutted lanes, fettered by their lack of resources, often entangled in small-town political skirmishes.

An internal, and ultimately more problematic, factor was that reformers' plans for social transformation were premised on maintaining race and class hierarchies. As the state's agricultural industry faced strain in the 1920s, North Carolina's leaders faced a burgeoning economic crisis—indeed, a crisis of the capitalist system. Rather than addressing the underlying problems of massive inequity and limited economic opportunity for the majority of the state's population, reformers turned to publicly funded professional social work to dull the sting of social problems. In other words, instead of reshaping society, they set out to smooth the ragged edges.[7]

Kate Burr Johnson and Public Welfare for North Carolina

Kate Burr Johnson was the epitome of the homegrown white social workers who staffed the state welfare agency during the 1920s. She was born in 1881 in Morganton, North Carolina, to parents with deep political and economic ties to the state. Her father, who worked for the railroad, died when she was young. Kate and her two sisters were raised by their mother, whose antebellum ancestors included wealthy slaveholders in the Morganton area. After education at a private school in Morganton and at Georgetown High School, she spent two years at Presbyterian Female College in Charlotte (later Queens University). In 1903 she married Clarence A. Johnson, a North Carolina native four years her senior. They moved to Raleigh, where Clarence owned a successful ice and coal company. With their two sons, born in 1905 and 1907, they enjoyed a middle-class standard of living in downtown Raleigh. By the early 1920s, they moved to the exclusive new suburban neighborhood of Hayes Barton, claiming a home on one of the grandest streets. But in September 1922, Clarence died. Kate soon returned downtown, probably to a more affordable house.[8]

Before and after her husband's death, Johnson exercised her considerable energies in improving her city and state. She began her "public career" as president of the Raleigh Woman's Club and was soon drawn into statewide

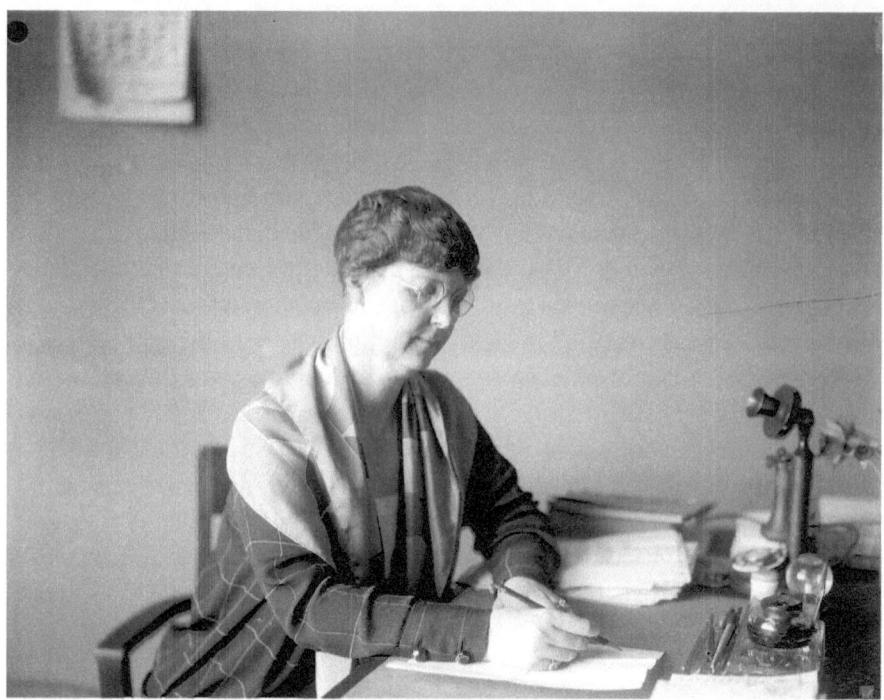

Figure 4.1 Photograph of Kate Burr Johnson, ca. 1930. Photo by Albert Barden. From the Albert Barden Photograph Collection, N.53.15.4757. Courtesy of the State Archives of North Carolina.

leadership roles. In 1917, as the president of the white Federation of Women's Clubs, Johnson guided the clubs' work through the upheaval of the war and the ensuing influenza epidemic. At her urging, the FWC endorsed woman suffrage at its 1918 convention, and as she finished her presidential term at the June 1919 convention, news arrived that Congress had passed the Nineteenth Amendment, granting suffrage rights to women. Her high-profile wartime leadership in the FWC brought her an appointment on the state's Central Liberty Loan Committee.[9]

Johnson also became a leader in the state's Progressive push for social welfare. She joined the Conference for Social Service soon after it formed, serving as a member of the committee on dependent and delinquent children and by 1918 as vice president. In a parallel effort, during the war she encouraged clubwomen to continue their work in public health, education, and child welfare, arguing that this work built morale and contributed to the war effort.[10] In June 1919, as Johnson finished her term as FWC president, she moved fully from being a social reformer to becoming a social worker, joining the staff of the state's newly reorganized welfare board.

The new Board of Charities and Public Welfare was intended to tackle social problems such as poverty, crime, and mental illness by equipping a modern bureaucracy with trained staff. Progressive reformers had long recognized the inadequacy of the Board of Public Charities, where Daisy Denson had soldiered on alone for years. Many lamented what they saw as needless spending on *results* of crime, insanity, and poverty, when they believed these were preventable "social sores." The peak of Progressive sentiment around World War I gave them an opportunity for more sweeping changes aimed at preventive social work. The crucial push came from a Greensboro-based businessman and Conference member, Alexander W. McAlister, whose father had been a member of the Board of Public Charities for a decade.[11]

McAlister and his allies believed that a modernized welfare board could maximize the efficiency of both social workers and, crucially, their clients—the laboring masses critical to the success of the New South's economy. The current system of charity, McAlister argued, was inefficient; a business would never be run with so much loss. An effective social welfare system run as a "public business," on the other hand, could be a pillar of "happiness and prosperity" in the New South.[12] Of particular interest to McAlister were children, who he argued were too often exposed to poverty, illiteracy, and immorality, leading them to become delinquent, depraved, and dependent adults. McAlister believed that children's plasticity offered reformers an opportunity to remake the world—to "reform, regenerate, reconstruct society."[13]

McAlister's plan relied on a stronger role for government. He used the term "public welfare," a term that had traditionally signified the commonweal but that, beginning in the 1910s, connoted a broader vision of welfare. As the field of social work set professional standards, "public welfare" signified a system that moved away from philanthropic aid to the poor toward preventive measures based on social scientific research.[14] McAlister drew inspiration from a board of public welfare in Kansas City, Missouri, founded in 1909 by Leroy A. Halbert to coordinate private and public welfare activities. Halbert saw particular promise in his model of public welfare boards for rural areas. McAlister drafted a public welfare bill for North Carolina based on Halbert's vision, with an interlocking system of state and county bureaucracies staffed by trained professionals.[15] He called this new iteration of the state welfare board the Board of Charities and Public Welfare. McAlister then built a formidable political coalition in support, including teachers, religious organizations, white clubwomen, and the Conference for Social Service. Even the new governor, Thomas W. Bickett, supported the bill in his inaugural address.[16]

In 1917 and 1919, McAlister's efforts came to fruition with laws that restructured the state's welfare system. Together, the laws committed the state to supporting the "public welfare," hiring professional staff who could research social problems, and supporting the county-unit model that extended social workers to every corner of the state.[17] In espousing this new board of public welfare, North Carolina's lawmakers and reformers signaled their optimism. They shared a belief that through research and centralized planning, they could extinguish many social problems at the root. In the words of McAlister, "the end will be the stamping out of such social diseases as poverty and crime, with the inspiring spectacle of deserted almshouses and empty jails."[18]

With this legislation, North Carolina became the first state in the nation to establish a state board of public welfare and a statewide county-unit plan, which supported the development of social welfare in a rural environment.[19] At this time, models of social work—as seen in welfare statutes, professional standards, and schools of social work—assumed urban environments were the context for the work. The county-unit system offered a new model: a limited number of trained workers could cover vast rural territories with efficiency, reaching even the most secluded parts of the rural countryside while also coordinating their plans statewide.[20] In adopting this model, North Carolina moved to the forefront of innovation in rural social work. The newly appointed welfare commissioner, newspaperman and former legislator Roland Beasley, believed that with "time and wisdom," the state's plan would be "the model" for the nation.[21] The "North Carolina Plan" had a "wide run of popularity" at national meetings of social workers, including high praise at the 1918 National Conference of Charities and Corrections.[22] Other Southern states were particularly drawn to the plan.[23] Even the federal government took note: in 1924, in response to demand from other states for information about the county-unit system, the US Children's Bureau studied the plan in North Carolina and Minnesota, the two states where it was most successful.[24]

The "North Carolina Plan" did not explicitly mention race but was nonetheless part of a raft of early twentieth-century legislation in Southern states that enshrined a racial hierarchy. Legislators wrote the new welfare laws in the context of a legal scaffold that already denied Black men voting rights, segregated Black and white people, and provided substandard (if any) services for Black people. So while prisons, county homes, and state custodial institutions were already segregated by race, the new welfare law required these institutions to report on the race of inmates and to submit building plans for new jails and almshouses, allowing the state to enforce physical segregation of inmates by race. If a white member of a county welfare board violated any norms of white supremacy, such as placing a white child with a Black foster family or providing county relief funds to a white woman who lived with a Black man, the state board now had the power to remove that member. In this context, welfare laws did not need to specify the race of welfare officials or their clients.

Everyone in power understood that welfare services would be administered by white people and that funds would go primarily to poor white people, particularly those who complied with the racial order.[25] Welfare programs became part of a broader pattern, similar to the segregated education system, in which the fruits of Black people's labor (sometimes in the form of extractive labor systems, sometimes in the form of tax dollars) were claimed by or redistributed to white people.

Kate Burr Johnson's work as the director of the new state division of child welfare reflected these racial hierarchies. The child welfare division was the first unit of the new state welfare board, as it was crucial to carrying out a vision of an agency dedicated to protecting children and thereby regenerating society. The children to be protected or rehabilitated were white. A large part of Johnson's work involved helping county officials deal with tough cases, most commonly children who were deemed defective or delinquent. Johnson helped admit delinquent white children to Jackson Training School or Samarcand Manor and white children with mental defects to Caswell Training School—but the state had no public institutions (apart from mental hospitals and jails) for Black children. In other cases, Johnson helped place children in orphanages or foster homes. Even as Johnson called for a training school for delinquent Black boys and facilities for Black children with mental defects, she also eschewed any government responsibility to support Black children who were orphaned or deserted, claiming that their relatives and friends usually took care of them.[26]

In July 1921, Johnson took over as head of the state welfare department. Although the welfare board appointed her unanimously, she was not their first choice, being neither a man nor "a trained investigator of social service problems," as the law required.[27] To be fair, the first welfare commissioner, Roland Beasley, had no training apart from a trip to Indiana to learn about their welfare programs.[28] Johnson had at least completed six weeks of "special studying" at the New York School of Social Work in 1919 when she began her work with the state board. She lodged with an old friend in New York City and spent her time reading books, observing social welfare machinery at work in a juvenile court and an orphanage, and meeting with notables such as Dr. Hastings Hart of the Russell Sage Foundation.[29] Despite Johnson's shortcomings, she became the best option because the Board had little luck finding a trained man willing to take the job.[30] Board member Clara Lingle teased Johnson that she was "the best prepared *man* in the state for the work," and the Federation of Women's Clubs endorsed her for the job, arguing that "Public Welfare is near to the hearts of all women."[31] Daisy Denson, on the other hand, was appalled that the Board had overlooked her and resigned the instant Johnson was appointed.[32]

From "Natural Talent" to Trained Professionals: White Welfare Officials in the 1920s

When Johnson took over as commissioner in July 1921, she confronted many of the challenges that had perplexed Beasley before her: scarce funding, a tiny state staff, and a shifting group of untrained county superintendents. Even so, Johnson was "a most influential and capable woman," and under her leadership the Board grew quickly.[33] Her first priority was establishing new divisions, each headed by an expert who could develop that aspect of the Board's work.[34] The divisions were bare-bones, each at first comprising only the director and some part-time clerical help. Johnson first solidified the work of the division of County Organization, whose goal was to meet with county superintendents in situ to educate them about their duties.[35] Johnson also expanded the Board's work in child welfare. In September 1921, she created a third division, on Mental Health and Hygiene, employing a psychologist from the University of North Carolina to work part-time with the Board.[36] Next she created a division of Promotion and Education and a division of Institutional Supervision. By the time of her first report to the legislature in June 1922, Johnson had assembled a full staff and moved to new office space, with five rooms.[37]

During the 1920s, Johnson oversaw a staff that included, on average, nine executive members and three clerical employees. There was near-constant turnover, with thirty-one people in those positions during the decade. Like the Board members who had hired her, Johnson confronted the challenge of finding and retaining qualified staff by hiring local people who were "capable and tactful and gradually train[ing] them to do their jobs rather than [experimenting] with outsiders."[38] Two of her first employees, Mary G. Shotwell and Wiley B. Sanders, illustrate the range of experiences that new employees brought, as well as the ways their career paths diverged.

Johnson hired Mary Shotwell to replace herself in leading the child welfare division. Born in Oxford, North Carolina, Shotwell was a college graduate with a background in teaching and an avocation for social service.[39] Despite her lack of specific social work training, Shotwell succeeded in her position. Her recommendations to orphanages in her 1922 report reflected best practices at the time, such as adopting the "cottage system" (housing children in numerous smaller units rather than a single massive building).[40] She used her connections with other white clubwomen in service of the Board, such as organizing lectures for Raleigh clubwomen on social hygiene and "the state's duty to her mental defectives."[41] After a few years of work with the Board, Shotwell moved to New York to study for a year at Columbia University, then officially resigned to take a job in New York. Her career in child welfare and education lasted another two decades, including serving as Southern regional director for the National Youth Administration.[42]

Shotwell's career illustrates several characteristics of the Board's dozen female executives during the 1920s. Most were unmarried and likely self-supporting. Although many had attended college, only one had an advanced degree before joining the Board.[43] Most had little prior training in social work, but rather relied on their local networks and their experience in education, social service, and war work. Some sought training after joining the state board staff, such as one staff member who took a course on child welfare at Columbia University before taking on Mothers' Aid work.[44] For many women, the exposure to professional social work on the Board redefined their lives and careers. Even their volunteer efforts transformed, as these women shared the latest social science research with their networks of clubwomen. Although most women stayed with the Board only a few years, when they left it was to take other positions in the field of social welfare.[45]

Wiley Benton Sanders was another of Johnson's early hires. Originally from Georgia, Sanders moved to Chapel Hill by 1920 to complete a master's degree in sociology at the University of North Carolina (UNC), studying "maladaptation to environment" and poor relief in North Carolina. Perhaps as an extension of his research, he was appointed part-time superintendent of public welfare for Orange County, surrounding Chapel Hill.[46] In the spring of 1921, he also began doing some work for the state board, including a study of children at Jackson Training School and an investigation of conditions in mountain counties.[47] Although Sanders was already deep into his graduate work in sociology, Johnson wanted him to have additional training in public welfare administration. The Board paid for Sanders to study for three quarters at the University of Chicago's Graduate School of Social Service Administration. Sanders enjoyed his time in Chicago, where his courses ranged from advanced casework to a course on "the child and the state" with Sophonisba Breckinridge, a founder of the school and a luminary of the settlement house movement. On one memorable night, he accompanied an officer from the city's Social Hygiene Board on a visit to two cabarets, where they "obtained first hand evidence" of "immoral dancing" and illegal liquor sales.[48] Sanders returned to North Carolina in July 1922 to head the state board's work in county organization, but he was already thinking of how his work there might count toward a PhD degree.[49] When he received his master's degree in sociology a year later, he quit the Board to join UNC's faculty, teaching in the new School of Public Welfare. Although Johnson hoped Sanders would eventually return to the Board, he remained at UNC until his retirement in 1963.[50]

Sanders's career was typical for a male member of the Board's staff. To begin with, the Board had trouble recruiting male social workers, and several worked only part-time or as advisers.[51] They tended to have more education upon entering the Board's employment than the women. In fact, many came from academic backgrounds, and when male staff members left the Board they moved into the academic world or other positions of greater authority.

The rapid departures of both Sanders and Shotwell were symptomatic of a larger problem for Johnson: she hired untrained workers, spent months or years educating them about rural social welfare practices, then lost the workers to other jobs. Part of the problem was that North Carolina would not provide competitive salaries. In September 1926, shortly after Shotwell resigned, Johnson pointed out that her staff was paid less than counterparts at other state agencies, even when they had graduate degrees. Some staff remained out of loyalty to the state despite the low pay, but Johnson fumed that more often, North Carolina "act[ed] as a training school" for people who were then lured by higher salaries elsewhere.[52] The state's refusal to increase welfare workers' salaries signaled continued resistance in some quarters to the new "public welfare" bureaucracy.

While Johnson struggled with staff problems in Raleigh, she also had to consider county welfare officials. County welfare superintendents were critical to the success of the new "county-unit" welfare plan, each one a node in the network of welfare officials who together would blanket the state. But county officials who appointed local superintendents were slow to help the state welfare agency with this grand plan, most often because the funds for their salary had to come from local tax revenues. By November 1920, fewer than a third of the counties had appointed a full-time superintendent. At least a dozen lacked a superintendent entirely, and others had only part-time superintendents.[53] On top of these problems, a 1921 law passed by skeptics of the new system required county superintendents to be reelected every two years, opening numerous possibilities for continued debate about the welfare system in every county.[54]

Given the political challenges she faced, Johnson decided early on that hiring and training local people with "natural talent and capacity" was preferable to bringing in trained workers from other states.[55] Accordingly, many of the first superintendents lacked training, experience, and education. In 1922, seven superintendents had only an elementary school education, and only two of the superintendents appointed in 1919 and 1920 had served on their county welfare boards before the reorganization in 1917.[56] The superintendent of Forsyth County was typical: a retired hardware dealer with a high school education, he was a "patient, kindly soul, who literally worked himself to death." His cases "never seemed to get anywhere" because he "had no conception of organization in the field of social work."[57]

Incorporating dozens of untrained locals into a statewide bureaucracy meant that the Board needed to *train* them. One of the new divisions of the Board was dedicated to standardizing that process. The first goal was simply to teach superintendents about basic casework methods, the core method of the emerging field of professional social work. The state's training manual focused on proper recordkeeping procedures and provided sample case files.[58] In addition, the Board used its quarterly *Bulletin* to educate superintendents about best practices in North Carolina and in other states.[59]

North Carolina's desire for trained social workers reflected a national trend but also highlighted shortcomings in existing social work models. In the 1920s and 1930s, government agencies began to require professional training in "social work." By 1919, seventeen accredited schools of social work served the swelling ranks of would-be white social workers who wanted credentials. For residents of North Carolina, however, few options were readily available. Most schools were in the Northeast and Midwest, and the South had only two schools for white students and none for Black students. Moreover, the field of professional social work was born in an urban environment, and most social work training was based on urban casework. Although North Carolina's cities had typical urban social problems, many of its citizens lived in rural poverty. North Carolina and the rest of the rural South needed social workers trained specifically for work in rural areas; as the Board remarked in 1920, "the city training is not what the county workers need." In addition to knowing the basics of casework, social workers in rural counties needed a distinct set of skills to navigate local customs and rural conditions. Kate Burr Johnson believed that a trained worker used to having "adequate facilities" would be "exceedingly discourag[ed]" when placed in a rural community where they had to not only "solve the problems, but be ingenious enough to make the facilities." Existing social work programs, like the one Wiley Sanders attended in Chicago, simply did not provide this sort of training.[60]

North Carolina began to fill this gap for white students in 1920 with a school of public welfare that emphasized rural environments, calling it "the first training school of social work designed especially for the rural social worker."[61] The school's creator was Eugene Cunningham Branson, a professor of rural social economics at the University of North Carolina. Branson wanted to create a school devoted to the study of Southern social problems, but gradually reframed it from a school of "social sciences" to a school of "public welfare," which he and his allies deemed less likely to be condemned as socialist.[62] In early 1920, UNC decided to offer courses in public welfare. The Red Cross funded instructor salaries, part of an effort to provide training for its own personnel and jump-start rural social work in the region.[63]

To lead UNC's school, Branson chose Howard W. Odum, then a professor at Emory. A native of Georgia, Odum had doctoral degrees in sociology and social psychology. He also had seemingly endless energy and a penchant for grand plans. In Chapel Hill, Odum fostered a community of likeminded social scientists who were dedicated to addressing regional conditions.[64] Odum and his colleagues saw themselves as providing desperately needed training for rural social workers. Jesse F. Steiner, a former Red Cross instructor who became a professor of social work at UNC, wrote that the fundamental problem in rural conditions was their lack of uniformity. Not only were rural communities unlike urban communities, he argued, they were unlike each other. Some rural communities were in fertile areas and prospered, while others were characterized by a "poor housed and inefficient tenant population," and still others were sparsely settled hilly regions with rocky soil and difficult transportation. Moreover, Odum and Steiner argued, social work administrators had little "scientific" knowledge of the conditions in rural areas. On top of these problems, rural workers faced geographic challenges of large areas with bad roads, cultural attitudes that were skeptical of social workers, and few existing private organizations with which social workers could cooperate.[65]

Under Odum's direction, the School of Public Welfare drew its faculty from the departments of sociology, psychology, and economics to create a curriculum in rural social work. The faculty fashioned training from their own theoretical expertise and the experiences of North Carolina's welfare officials, who, along with outside social welfare experts, gave guest lectures. By 1922, the school had six faculty in addition to Odum, who offered courses on topics including rural economics, rural social problems, statistical methods, community surveys, juvenile delinquency, social pathology, and family casework. The school offered several programs, including one- or two-year courses of "professional training" for college graduates, a four-year baccalaureate program in social sciences, and special quarter-long courses for county superintendents.[66]

UNC's most important contribution to the Board was its summer welfare institute for county superintendents. For the first summer institute in 1920, twenty-two county workers attended the full six weeks, and another ten attended some part of the course.[67] Many superintendents, already paying work-related expenses out of their salaries, could not afford to come, even though there was no tuition charge for the program. Some superintendents decided the program was worth paying their own way; one wrote that "If I have to go at my own personal expense, I am determined to become efficient in serving the people."[68] The students who converged on Chapel Hill heard lecturers from leading social work schools, including Columbia, Yale, and the University of Pennsylvania, as well as UNC faculty and regional Red Cross officials.

Classes ran each day from 8 a.m. to 4:30 p.m., with a taxing schedule of six 50-minute lectures on theories of rural sociology, family casework, rural economics, social problems, public health, and child welfare. Afternoon roundtable sessions focused on practical matters such as superintendents' duties, casework, and recordkeeping.[69] The institutes also offered chances for the welfare workers to mingle and socialize, as during a swimming party and picnic at the 1923 institute.[70]

Summer institutes became a mainstay of the state's training program for its white county workers, and the state issued certificates to superintendents who passed an exam at the end. In subsequent years, a shorter program allowed more county workers to attend. In 1922, the summer when state officials presented the mock juvenile court proceedings featuring "Willie," the institute lasted over two weeks. By 1927, the institute was only a week long, and 150 white social workers attended. In 1926, UNC further extended its reach by offering a correspondence course to continue the institute's in-person discussions. By the end of the decade, the state also changed the appointment deadline for county superintendents to spring so that all could have some practical work experience before they attended the summer institute.[71]

As Johnson and her staff offered more training, they gradually raised standards for superintendents. In 1921, Johnson merely listed general qualifications for superintendents, but she quickly realized that some of the best superintendents would not qualify for the highest grade of certification because they lacked education. Even worse, formal education seemed not to produce the best workers. One of the three PhD-holding superintendents in the state was incompetent and hostile to recordkeeping. In contrast, one superintendent who had "less than sixteen months of school during his whole life" did "a very good piece of work in his county" and wrote excellent reports.[72]

Johnson also had to consider emerging national standards for professional social workers. In 1922, the New York–based American Association of Social Workers had only eight members in North Carolina, with no local chapter. Johnson was simultaneously embarrassed and amused by the fact that she herself seemed not to qualify for membership, based on her limited experience and her brief education; in addition to her two years of college, she had taken only two summer courses, one in New York and one at UNC's School of Public Welfare. Association officials approved her membership application, however, probably anxious to have an organizer on the ground in North Carolina. They also seemed willing to bend the membership rules for other North Carolina social workers, recognizing that the circumstances in North Carolina differed greatly from those in the urban North.[73]

Trying to walk the line between the ideal and the practical, Johnson and her staff settled on a flexible list of minimum requirements, tweaking them as local officials became convinced of the value of trained social workers. In September 1923, they published a list of qualifications in their monthly newsletter. In addition to tact, sympathy, good moral character, and good physical condition, new superintendents thereafter had to have a high school education and preferably some college work. They also had to have shown a past interest in social work and be willing to come to summer training courses.[74] Within a month, Johnson had refused the appointments of four superintendents as unqualified: one for "immorality," one for having been a "habitual drunkard" in the past, and two whose appointments were solely political.[75]

The new requirements created opportunities for female social workers. In 1917, when superintendents were first appointed, there were questions about whether women were eligible. At the time, women were not allowed to vote or hold public office in North Carolina, except on local school boards. Nevertheless, officials in several counties named female superintendents, since many women's extensive experience in teaching, benevolent work, or wartime work outstripped men's relevant experience.[76] The Board decided to "endorse or reject the qualifications of a woman just as if she were a man," and see if anyone objected.[77] As professional standards increased, including a requirement of two years of college education, newly trained women replaced older, untrained men.[78] Twenty women served as superintendent in June 1926, and by 1932, fully half of the state's sixty county superintendents were women.[79] As counties in urban areas began to employ multiple workers—assistant superintendents, probation officers, and other caseworkers—about three-quarters were women.[80]

By 1924, the state board had made notable progress in creating a county-unit system, but welfare officials were constantly frustrated by their inability to force more significant change. Johnson had increased the size of the staff in the state office to twelve, but over forty counties still did not have a full-time welfare superintendent.[81] Most funding for relief came from counties, where local politics often stymied change. On both local and state levels, North Carolina's low-tax, low-expenditure philosophy shaped the possibilities. In the long run, Johnson believed that the only way local officials would understand the worth of a trained superintendent was to give them a living, breathing example of what a trained worker could do.

To provide these examples of trained workers, Johnson turned to Northern philanthropists for funding. In 1924, Johnson and UNC's Howard Odum secured funding from the New York–based Laura Spelman Rockefeller Memorial (LSRM) for a project that became known as the "Four-County Demonstration."[82] The plan provided the Board and the School of Public Welfare

$60,000 over three years, with specific support for trained workers who would follow professional standards of casework, including investigating families who received aid and keeping detailed records. Odum and Johnson hoped to show local officials that a trained worker could be more effective in helping poor families lift themselves out of poverty and thus would ultimately save money for counties.[83] They also promised LSRM officials that the demonstration would spur the state to increase its financial investment in their programs. They chose Orange and Chatham, two rural counties close to UNC; Wake County, home to Raleigh, "a large town representing varied social conditions"; and Cherokee County, a mountain county at the far western tip of the state, which had done little welfare work but clamored to be included.[84]

The project had mixed results. In Chatham and Orange counties, the demonstration faced "many serious handicaps," including "an almost total ignorance by the people of Orange of everything connected with public welfare." In addition, the workers were supposed to cover huge areas: Orange County was 390 square miles, and neighboring Chatham was 690 square miles—and there were no reliable maps of either. During the three-year demonstration, student trainees in Orange oversaw 330 cases, the demand far outstripping their ability to help. Ultimately, one observer called the project's goals "unduly optimistic." "Much has been learned," he said, "in regard to how not to proceed."[85]

In Wake and Cherokee, work went well enough that by the end of the demonstration, the counties assumed the costs of a trained worker. Cherokee was a particularly compelling example, as it was "absolutely virgin soil for social work" and provided a starkly contrasting example of the divergence in rural and urban social work.[86] The mountain county was little affected by the modernization of the New South, with only two small towns of about 1,500 people each. The remaining 12,000 people in the county, almost entirely white or Indigenous, lived in remote areas. Many roads were "impassable from November to May," when some areas were accessible "only on horseback or muleback. Even in summer it is often necessary to walk six or seven miles up a mountain trail to make a family visit." The social worker assigned there was Elizabeth Smith, who had completed an MA in social science at UNC. Smith managed to oversee eighty-five cases at once, although with no stenographic help, her case records were restricted to the basics. The bulk of her cases were family welfare, neglected children, and physical disability, with only a handful of cases of juvenile delinquency or adult probation. Transportation difficulties were a constant impediment to her work. In one case, she drove seventeen miles, walked ten, and found help to carry a crippled boy eight miles on a stretcher so he could see a doctor.[87] Smith's work proved the usefulness of public welfare work to county officials, who agreed unanimously to pay for a social worker after she left. Perhaps more important, neighboring counties and even the bordering states of Tennessee and Georgia expressed interest in Cherokee's new approach to welfare.[88]

The state board's efforts to provide training did pay some dividends, bringing the state closer to the vision of a network of local officials well versed in modern social work techniques. For many superintendents, training helped them gain confidence and efficiency, and they took to their duties with vigor. In one ten-month period, county workers from around the state reported doing a monumental amount of work. In total, they made 17,606 home visits, received 26,314 office visits, and traveled 263,660 miles.[89] Their training taught them how to keep records of all this work and helped them understand the resources the state or private agencies could offer for a difficult case. Their new background in casework might help them quickly glean the essentials of a family's situation before they had to jump back into their Ford to see the next client. And importantly, their training gave them a theoretical understanding of many social problems as intertwined but preventable.

Yet the limitations of the model of social work itself meant that the fundamental problem of widespread poverty remained. North Carolina's per capita income in the late 1920s was $394, far below the national average of $703 and below even the Southern average of $424.[90] Casework methods aimed to reduce the dependency of families, but often that meant cutting off support for a family rather than solving the underlying factors leading to their poverty. Broader change would have required increased funding for welfare programs or a challenge to long-standing fears of creating dependent paupers. In the absence of these changes, the most notable outcome of the state's approach of providing training in casework methods was that state officials now had better records about the families who did receive some meager aid. North Carolina's county-unit model and UNC's School of Public Welfare solved the problem of how to spread professional casework across a rural state, but it did not solve the larger problem of rural poverty.

The "Trained Leaders of the Race": Lawrence Oxley and Black Social Work

With many pieces of a welfare bureaucracy in place, Johnson began to consider how to extend the county-unit system to Black people, who constituted a third of the state's population. Johnson shared the views of many white people, including Progressives, who saw the white race as necessarily distinct from and superior to the Black race. Even those who were involved in efforts for "interracial cooperation" rarely questioned segregation. Many were deeply disturbed by any indication of miscegenation, seeing "any blending of race characteristics" as "a case of biological ungodliness."[91] At the same time, Johnson saw the need for social work in Black communities, at least in part to help the South achieve economic progress. Johnson saw an opportunity in the partnership with the Northern philanthropy Laura Spelman Rockefeller Memorial, which was willing to take a chance by creating a state bureau under Johnson's oversight that would coordinate social work among African Americans.

At the time, most of the state's welfare work was segregated along racial lines, and racial segregation had solidified as the state "modernized" its welfare system. County poorhouses, for example, had both Black and white residents, but state law required they be housed separately. Where the lines of Jim Crow split the poor, Black North Carolinians consistently received fewer or less-funded services, despite their greater need. For example, per-patient state spending at the two mental hospitals for white people in 1921 was roughly $198, while the equivalent figure at the mental hospital for Black people was $145.[92] In many cases an equivalent Black institution did not exist; the state founded Caswell for white feebleminded children in 1911 but made no provision for Black children.[93]

With little support from the state, Black communities had found ways to provide social services for themselves through clubs, churches, and mutual aid societies. For example, while the state built reformatories for white boys and girls in the 1910s, Black clubwomen built and privately funded a reformatory for Black girls for years before the state finally provided support. Despite the resilience of Black welfare efforts in the face of discrimination and overt hostility, white officials and reformers often found this self-support to be unremarkable. They failed to recognize that Black people were doubly burdened in paying taxes that mainly supported poor white people *and* contributing what they could to support poor Black people.[94]

Many white reformers in North Carolina saw basic improvements in the social and economic condition of Black people as necessary for the state's long-term success. As one white reformer told the state conference for social service in 1913, "we must lift up the negro or he will drag us down." He told his audience that they had considered Black people "a foreign body in our National organism eventually to be removed in some way or other," but "the negro race is with us to stay. . . . A study of the population statistics gives one no hope that the solution of the Negro Problem is the extinction of the negro race."[95] Commissioner Johnson had a similar attitude, writing in one report to the state legislature that "it is futile to make an effort to solve the social problems and raise the standard of living of one race and ignore the other when the two live side by side."[96]

Accordingly, Johnson and Odum included funding for a Division of Work Among Negroes in their plans for the Rockefeller four-county welfare demonstration almost from the beginning.[97] Such a bureau could build on existing Black self-help efforts and address shared Black and white concerns about social problems, while keeping firm the lines of racial segregation. While the demonstration placed a trained white worker in each of four counties, with a state-level supervisor of casework, it funded only one Black social worker to work in all four counties. Johnson's pick for this important post was Lawrence A. Oxley, a thirty-seven-year-old native of Boston who had served as a morale officer for Black soldiers during World War I. After the war he taught social science for several years at St. Augustine, a Black college in Raleigh.[98]

Oxley began his work in January 1925 with a charge to singlehandedly organize Black welfare services for the four demonstration counties, a charge that soon expanded to more counties because of high demand. His usual strategy was to first receive the blessing of the local white welfare board, then to recruit local Black leaders. These leaders served as an advisory committee that studied local needs as well as a group of fundraisers who could canvass their churches and neighborhoods, pooling the resulting funds to hire a trained Black social worker. Some counties also appointed a Black welfare board to serve in an advisory capacity to the white board.[99]

Oxley quickly produced impressive results, partly because he capitalized on existing self-help efforts, bringing them into alliance with government officials in a new way.[100] Before the demonstration, only three counties had Black welfare boards, and only five cities had a Black social worker. Eighteen months later, nineteen counties had either a Black worker or board. Black organizations and individuals around the state gave an astounding $35,190 in that time period, compared to $14,810 paid from public funds. Oxley's success spurred other investments, including a $15,000 donation from the Duke family for a Black children's ward at the state orthopedic hospital. In his nine years working with the Board, Oxley helped a total of thirty-eight counties organize.[101]

Oxley worked to provide opportunities for Black social workers to receive training. Black social workers in the South had few avenues for professional education, with only Fisk University in Nashville and the Atlanta School of Social Work admitting them. In 1925, St. Augustine's College in Raleigh established the Bishop Tuttle Memorial Training School of Social Work, which offered a two-year professional program in theory or fieldwork for Black women.[102] But, as Johnson had discovered in trying to train white social workers, many Black social workers lacked the education to complete college-level coursework, and shorter courses of study like summer institutes were more effective in quickly orienting social workers to a new bureaucracy. By unwritten rule, only white social workers could attend the state-sponsored summer institutes, since courses were held on the racially segregated campus of the University of North Carolina.[103] In 1926, under Oxley's leadership, the state began to hold separate, shorter public welfare institutes for Black social workers at Black colleges, with an average attendance of ninety Black workers.[104] Although these Black institutes covered similar materials, the white officials in charge particularly stressed the need for ingenuity and resourcefulness among Black social workers. The instructors were nearly the same as at the white institutes, including most of the Board staff, Odum, and other UNC faculty. The instructors also included guests such as white female representatives of the North Carolina Interracial Commission, an associate justice of the state supreme court, and a lecturer from the American Social Hygiene Association.[105]

Oxley quickly became a popular public figure among both white and Black North Carolinians. White leaders praised him as "a credit to his race," "the guiding genius," and "a Moses to the negroes of North Carolina." In 1927, the state's American Legion sent him to Paris as a delegate to the annual convention. Black newspapers praised his "fine work," which they projected would result in "increasing returns in family life, better race relations, justice in the courts, and larger opportunities." Oxley was invited to speak at Black and white colleges, national conferences, and on radio broadcasts in other states. In his first eighteen months of work, over one hundred articles about his work appeared in daily papers around the country.[106]

Part of Oxley's appeal to white people across the political spectrum was his willingness to leave unchallenged most of their racist assumptions. As one editorial put it, Oxley was not inclined to believe "the premise of those who come a-missionarying to our race problem—that the white man is deliberately unjust." Oxley was full of praise for North Carolina's "broadminded spirit toward the Negro," telling one audience of white college students that he "knew of no state in the union which was doing so much to bring about a better understanding between blacks and whites." He denied that "thinking negroes" even pondered "social equality; what they wanted was an opportunity to develop as God meant them to" through self-help and racial uplift.[107]

Oxley also seems to have held many negative views about working-class and poor African Americans. The masses, he said, were easily led wrong because of their "primitive beliefs, ignorances, superstitious fears and suffering because of an inferior social complex." He criticized lower-class Black people's housekeeping and living standards, blaming it on their "slothfulness, ignorance, and dreadful carelessness." Accordingly, he believed that the wrong kind of social work would simply be "submerged beneath a mass of social ills and problems of racial mal-adjustment."[108]

At the same time, Oxley believed that the responsibility to "rouse" Black people from their "lethargic state" fell to Black leaders. Echoing W. E. B. Du Bois's idea of the talented tenth and the philosophy of racial uplift, Oxley wrote that social welfare for Black people "must come about through education and the efforts of the trained leaders of the race for their poorer and less intelligent fellows." He criticized North Carolina's Quakers for having "helped the negroes too much, rather than taught them to help themselves." As for the Black leaders who were so crucial to his fundraising success, Oxley consistently praised their "hearty response and cooperation."[109] Like many white North Carolinians, Black North Carolinians were invested in racial improvement, and Black leaders felt a sense of responsibility for the fate of the race as a whole.[110]

To most white people, Oxley's dim views of African Americans made sense. Even the state's white racial moderates treated Black people with condescension and paternalism. One white member of the state's Commission on Interracial Cooperation patronizingly compared the intellectual development of Black people to that of "a growing child." "We have no Negro problem," she said, "we have a problem of human striving." If Black people deserved justice, it was only because God entrusted people with authority to "administer equal and exact justice" to the "weak."[111]

Welfare publications and news reports treated poor white and poor Black people in distinctly different ways. When welfare officials discussed the state's welfare work generally—meaning primarily work with white people—they were much more likely to focus on worthy families who benefited from constructive welfare work. When white families had problems, welfare officials were quick to point to hereditary mental problems, often arguing for eugenic segregation or sterilization as a solution. When Oxley or other welfare officials discussed the work of his division, they inevitably addressed crime, illegitimacy, rampant disease, moral failings, and other social "sickness."[112] In one telling story that received coverage across the state, Oxley rescued an old Black man from an almost literal state of savagery. The man, "as grizzled and brawny in his blackness as a savage," was found sleeping on a bed of "prickly boughs" in woods near a college campus in Raleigh. He "only occasionally at night crept from his wilderness home toward civilization for food." Oxley sent the man to a local hospital.[113] Welfare officials were also always careful to mention that the Division of Work Among Negroes was funded by *private* dollars, and they often noted that funds raised from Black organizations were turned over to white officials.

The overall logic—that social work among Black people, largely funded by Black people, was "an economical and sensible activity"—proved to be popular. By 1927 the state legislature appropriated funds for two assistants for Oxley.

Given this promising start, Johnson requested additional funds from the LSRM. Maintaining that North Carolina had done "pioneer work," she requested $27,000 to be spread out over five years. Johnson told the LSRM that "the negro work" was the Board's most pressing concern at the moment and was even the "most popular among citizens at large."[114] The LSRM continued to fund the Division of Work Among Negroes as a stand-alone project until 1931, when the state took over financial responsibility for it. Oxley continued working with the division until he left in 1934 to take a job with the US Department of Labor, working in various federal roles for over twenty years.[115]

Ultimately, the Division of Work Among Negroes was both a major change and a continuation of old ideas. With LSRM funding, Johnson and Oxley built an infrastructure for Black social work and increased Black access to some welfare services, allowing marginally more equitable funding. North Carolina became the first state to dedicate a state bureau to this work. A number of other states, including Georgia, Missouri, Michigan, Ohio, Pennsylvania, and Tennessee, created similar programs after consulting with Oxley. At the same time, the existence of the Division of Work Among Negroes was always a political compromise that left Black people in the position of second-class citizens. The arrangement, framed as allowing Black communities to lift themselves, funded by Northern philanthropists, did not force any North Carolinians to confront systems of discrimination. When the state took over the division in 1931, it was on the same premise of making Black people "useful and upright citizens," compliant laborers in an exploitive system.[116] This public–private partnership was an effective compromise between conservative legislators and more liberal reformers. But the partnership ultimately reified racist ideas, laying the groundwork for the continued discrimination against Black people and creating circumstances ripe for backlash.

Social Work Professionals and the Problem of Mental Defects

As they trained the state's new social workers, Commissioner Johnson and her staff faced several overlapping challenges: How could they justify spending taxpayer dollars? How could they train social workers to use the state's funds efficiently—in particular, to tell the difference between families who deserved their help and those who did not? And how could they continue to make claims that the white race was superior to the Black race when so many white people lived in poverty?

The answer they posited to all of these questions was that hereditary mental defects—feeblemindedness, insanity, and epilepsy—were "the root of most of the social problems" in the state.[117] In March 1924, Johnson's staff wrote in their newsletter that readers might "wonder why so many stories about the feeble-minded appear in this sheet when the subject is such a disagreeable one. The answer is that the State Board of Charities and Public Welfare believes that mental defectiveness in greater or less degree is to a very large extent responsible for delinquency, dependency and immorality... and that no social problem which North Carolina has to face is so grave as that which is presented by unrestricted increase of mental deficiency in the population." One study they conducted of the white residents of county homes found that only 4 percent were "mentally normal. State officials read in these numbers a clear link between white poverty and mental defects. The corollary was that to prevent social problems, to cut them off at the root, "mental defectiveness" had to be a primary target.[118]

Moreover, Johnson and her state staff believed that trained social workers could be an effective part of an apparatus that identified people with supposed mental defects and separated them from the rest of the population in the interest of preserving a genetically superior white race and protecting white supremacy. They framed their training programs for the state's new corps of county-level social workers, white and Black, in these terms. At summer institutes, in publications for county workers, and in correspondence with individual social workers, state officials tended to focus on hereditarian explanations for social problems. They underscored the vital need for social workers to recognize mental defects, conduct mental exams, and separate the "unfit" from the rest of the population—particularly for poor white people, who many reformers and social workers saw as critical to shoring up the so-called superiority of the Anglo-Saxon race. Eugenics permeated the very core of the state's policies and training programs for welfare workers.

In her first report as commissioner, Johnson explained why social workers needed to focus on inherited tendencies as keys to solving social problems. "The problem of the delinquent, the defective, and the dependent elements of population," she wrote, "affects the very mainspring of a commonwealth, the quality of its human material." Allowing "these inferior and unfortunate elements . . . to increase without restriction" would weaken the very foundation of society. It was the responsibility of the welfare department, she said, "to prevent their future promiscuous spread." She drew parallels between the goals of welfare and public health, maintaining that social workers prevented "social sickness such as crime, immorality, and poverty" in future generations.[119] Social work, in short, addressed the health of the body politic.

Similar explanations frequently appeared in the Board's publications, sent to every social worker in the state.[120] In one article about delinquent children, Johnson's staff argued that "bad heredity" was of equal importance to "evil

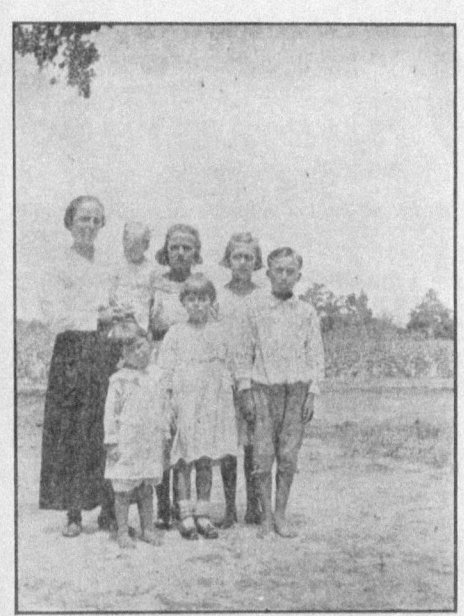
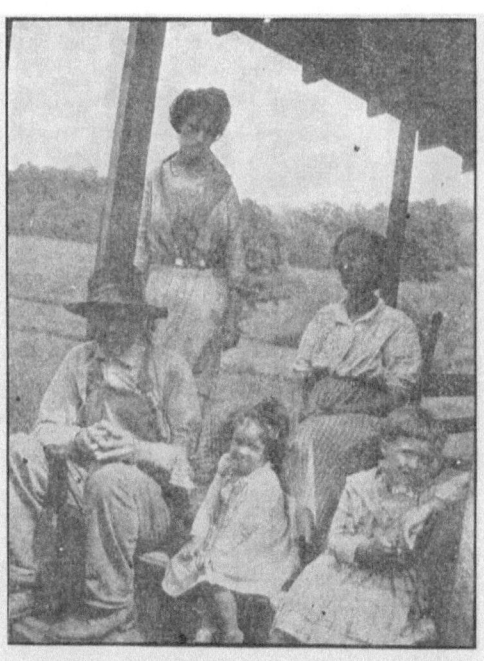

THIS MOTHER IS BEING ASSISTED IN KEEPING HER CHILDREN BY A SUPERINTENDENT OF PUBLIC WELFARE WHO BELIEVES IN SEPARATION ONLY AS A LAST RESORT.

A FAMILY OF WHICH EVERY MEMBER IS MENTALLY DEFECTIVE. NOT ONLY IS SUCH A FAMILY AN INCREASING EXPENSE TO THE STATE EACH YEAR, BUT A SOURCE OF VICE AND CRIME IN THE COMMUNITY.

Figure 4.2 Photographs and captions from a welfare bulletin comparing two types of families. *BCPW Bulletin* 4, no. 4 (October–December 1921): 24, North Carolina Collection, Louis Round Wilson Special Collections Library, University of North Carolina at Chapel Hill.

companions" and "broken homes." Quoting the Eugenics Record Office, they claimed that both feeblemindedness and criminal tendencies were inherited. Similarly, they reported that when the state provided relief to a widowed mother who then failed to emerge from poverty, there was usually "a weak spot somewhere in the past history of the family." Because of the importance of heredity, they encouraged superintendents to investigate "the family" as a unit. When a child was delinquent or a father unemployed, they believed, "the chances are that something is wrong with the whole family."[121]

In one edition of the *Bulletin*, the Board used photographs to demonstrate how mental defect could doom a family to poverty.[122] Two family portraits, side by side, were intended to typify different sorts of families (see figure 4.2). On the left, a white mother stands with one white child in her arms. Five others line up in stairstep fashion around her, neatly dressed in white clothing and with their straight, light hair combed or tied back. Though the backdrop is merely empty fields and a distant tree line, the photograph conveys a sense of

The Root of Social Problems 113

order. The photograph on the right is a stark contrast. Five members of a family, including two small children, crowd under what seems to be a ramshackle shed or porch. The diagonal jut of the roofline lends the image a haphazard feel, as does the tilt of the photographer's lens, which sets both the horizon line and the shed's support beams at a discomfiting angle. Through the shadows, most of the family members have curly hair and darker skin, traits that would likely suggest to contemporary viewers some amount of Black ancestry.[123]

In the photographs' captions, social workers found a moral tale. The mother on the left, readers learned, was keeping her children together with the help of a county welfare superintendent. The state had no official Mothers' Aid program yet, so she probably received outdoor relief from the county's poor fund.[124] The family on the right, however, was "mentally defective" and "a source of vice and crime in the community."[125] State board staff made no mention of attempts to help the family, despite their obvious poverty, and there was no discussion of what caused their dire economic straits. Instead, welfare officials implied that their mental defects consigned them to the category of hopeless cases. The best outcome for society was to somehow control the amount of money spent on the family and to mitigate the effects of their "vice and crime." The juxtaposition of these two photographs suggested that there were two types of families in North Carolina: those who might be helped by welfare professionals' careful assistance, and those whose mental defects made them unfit for such help.

As these photographs indicate, white assumptions about racial potential and a legal system of racial segregation framed conversations about feeblemindedness.[126] Similar to the way white middle-class reformers of the 1910s had celebrated a distinct "North Carolina" type of white people while assuming that Black people were inferior, white welfare workers in the 1920s saw African Americans, as a race, as beyond hope. Feeblemindedness and immorality were, they believed, naturally more common in the Black germplasm.[127] In their view, since Black feeblemindedness was unremarkable, it was also not worth using scarce state resources to identify. On the other hand, if feeblemindedness led to crime and poverty among white people, it would do the same among Black people. These sentiments combined with fears of uncontrolled feebleminded Black men to produce Progressive entreaties for an institution for the Black feebleminded. The Board and the head of Caswell Training School repeatedly called for an institution in the 1920s but never made headway in the legislature.[128] Instead, Black people with a range of supposed mental defects were sent to the state mental hospital or wound up in jail. For many white officials, witnessing Black criminality or mental illness simply reinforced their racial prejudices, and they saw these problems as unsolvable.

Lawrence Oxley, the head of the state's Black social workers, largely agreed. To Oxley, part of racial improvement was addressing feeblemindedness, which he saw as "the most menacing of all social dangers."[129] Not only did feebleminded African Americans endanger "law-abiding citizens' life and property," he argued that the constant menace they presented also soured race relations and impeded "racial adjustments in rural communities."[130] Although it is unclear whether Oxley or other Board staff were responsible for determining the program at the Black summer welfare institutes, the institutes did include lectures from Harry Crane, the head of the state bureau of mental hygiene. These lectures were probably condensed versions of his courses for white social workers, including information about how to recognize mental defects. Black social workers also spent a good deal of time learning about casework and recordkeeping—standard for the emerging social work profession, but also important to supporting the state's mental hygiene efforts.[131]

Black social workers' attitudes toward this training in mental hygiene are difficult to discern. Most Black social workers probably came from middle-class backgrounds, likely shared at least some of Oxley's prejudices and concerns, and might have found Crane's training sessions to be a valuable part of their project of racial uplift. The idea that feeblemindedness was a pressing social problem perhaps had no less resonance for them than for their white peers. At least some of them likely referred patients for mental testing, since the state did report testing some Black people.[132] At the same time, the state's Black population in general was less exposed to the ideas promoted by the Board, simply by virtue of the smaller number of Black public welfare officials. Most Black social workers worked for private agencies rather than in county welfare departments. In addition, Black social workers may have been less likely to request Crane's services because of suspicions of white officials' motives or simply because they were used to operating social service programs independent of white support. Perhaps Crane and other white officials also discouraged them from using the scarce time and resources of mental health experts.

In contrast, crime or mental defects among white people threatened to undermine notions of white superiority, and Johnson's staff trained white social workers to see feeblemindedness in white people as an aberration. According to Johnson, "segregation and prevention of increase of the mentally defective is absolutely essential to the purification of our blood stream."[133] She and her staff argued that such mental defects must be identified and rooted out in order to maintain the superior position of the white race. In the Board's view, one almost foolproof indicator of feeblemindedness was racial mixing. Their focus on white people who ignored racial boundaries played to the anxieties of white conservatives and lent urgency to their attack on feeblemindedness. The Board's descriptions of feebleminded white people, particularly women,

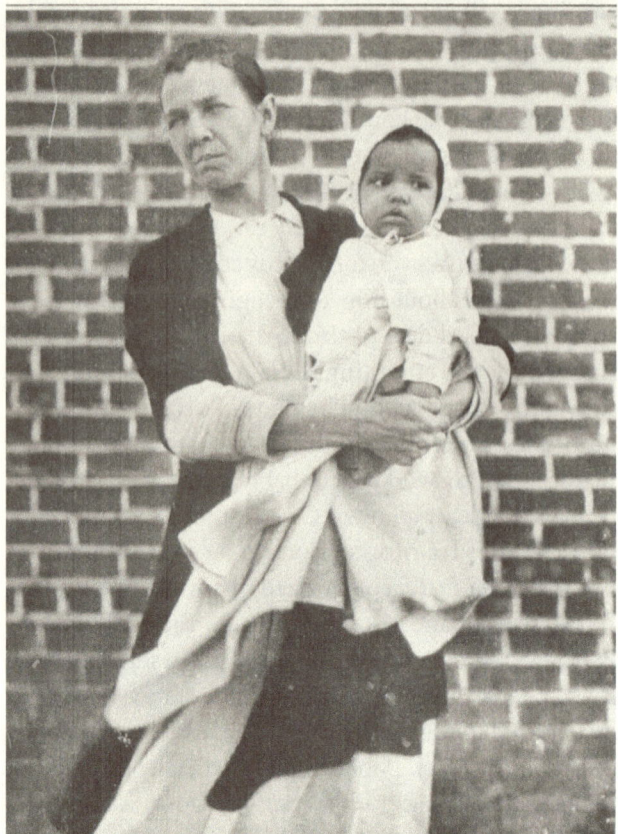

Figure 4.3 Photograph and caption from the welfare board's annual report, intended to show that county homes were inadequate to institutionalize feebleminded people. *BCPW Report, 1920–22,* 54a, North Carolina Collection, Louis Round Wilson Special Collections Library, University of North Carolina at Chapel Hill.

routinely noted their racially mixed children. One photograph in the 1922 report, the result of a survey of county homes, offered a visual representation of a feebleminded woman (see figure 4.3). The caption gave no further reason for the diagnosis of feeblemindedness except the woman's poverty and the description of her offspring: she lived in a county poorhouse, and "she gave birth to a child whose features suggest a negro father." Perhaps the unidentified woman in this picture had mental disabilities. We have no way of knowing. What matters is that the Board chose this image, of a white woman with a dark-skinned child, to make its argument that county homes were "breeding places for the feebleminded."[134]

State welfare officials told social workers that the imperatives of white supremacy demanded treating and controlling feebleminded white people, as well as "conserving" eugenically fit white people. The Anglo-Saxon race, in particular, was the hope of human civilization, and for the welfare of the state,

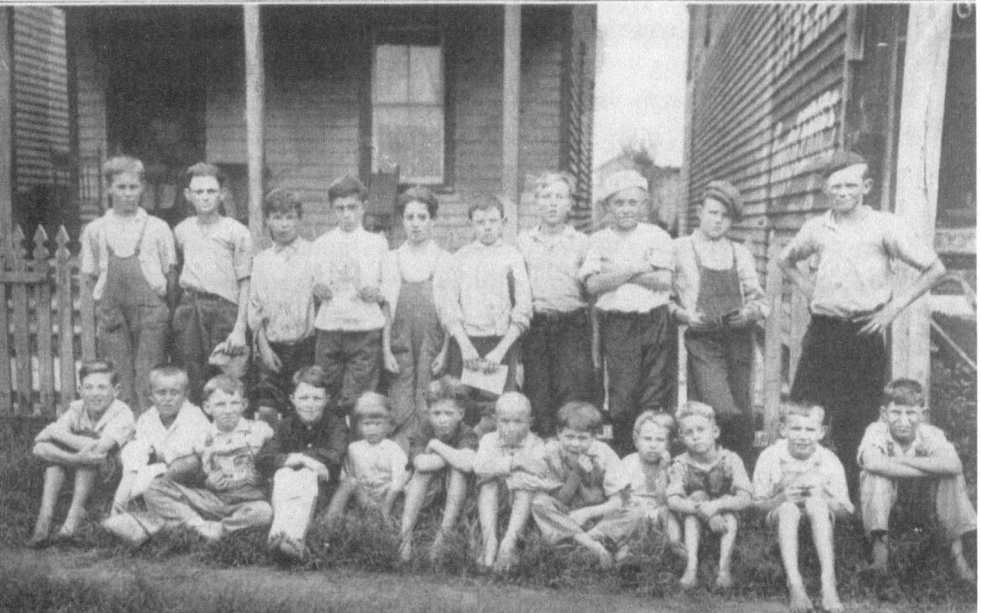

Figure 4.4 Photograph of white boys at one of the state's institutions, published in the welfare board's annual report. *BCPW Report, 1920–22,* 6a, North Carolina Collection, Louis Round Wilson Special Collections Library, University of North Carolina at Chapel Hill.

the nation, and the world, its racial fitness must be maximized. To do so required both negative and positive eugenics. Poor, "defective" white people were the targets of institutional segregation, mental testing, and other intrusive measures. At the same time, Johnson's staff claimed with pride that North Carolina's "native stock is the purest Anglo-Saxon of all the States in the Union," and noted that "the problem, therefore, is not one of assimilating foreign stocks, but of conserving native population—the sturdy, independent descendants of the hardy English, Scotch-Irish, and German settlers."[135] A photograph at the beginning of the 1922 report, entitled "North Carolina's best crop—her children," showed rows of white boys who came under the supervision of welfare officials and juvenile court judges (see figure 4.4). Although the text accompanying the photograph focused mostly on juvenile delinquency and environmental influences, the photograph's title left little doubt that the best kind of child was white and that children, like cotton or tobacco, should be grown from the finest seed and cultivated with care.[136]

A white Mothers' Aid recipient was the pinnacle of this category of deserving, "fit" white person. Mothers' Aid was created in 1923, funded jointly by the state and participating counties, to support women with children under age fourteen who had fallen on hard times. The program was optional, but by 1930, eighty-seven counties applied to participate, with a total of four hundred families receiving $50,000 in benefits. The program had strict moral standards. Its ideal recipient was a woman who was "mentally and morally qualified" to raise her children and held back only by her poverty, which might push her to work at the expense of neglecting her children's health and education. As welfare leaders acknowledged, the public saw this program, and the investment in citizenship it entailed, as an "economic one—the mother is a citizen employed to rear her own children as good citizens."[137]

The Board saw work with Mothers' Aid families as entirely different from their work with "defective" people. Officials routinely divided their reporting on Mothers' Aid cases from other sections of their annual reports. They believed that because these families were fundamentally fit in a physical and hereditary sense, they needed only "friendly supervision." Changing their environment with a small amount of aid could preserve the family's economic and moral integrity (see figure 4.5). The Board's reports rarely bothered to specify the race of Mothers' Aid families, knowing their readers would assume they were white—as, in fact, the vast majority were. In 1926, only four Black women received help from the program, compared to 260 white women.[138]

The state board hoped that white social workers would use their training about feeblemindedness to take advantage of the state's mental testing and institutions, with the ultimate goal of segregating the white "unfit" from the rest of the population. State psychopathologist Crane routinely addressed welfare superintendents and other social workers at the state's summer institutes, hoping to make mental testing a standard part of social workers' casework procedures. In 1926, for example, one of the four days of the summer institute was dedicated to "mental and social hygiene," with Crane a prominent speaker. County workers could thereafter read reminders in the *Bulletin* about Crane's services, which included examining and giving "advice concerning any special cases of defective or problematic individuals" who appeared in juvenile courts or came to welfare superintendents' attention.[139]

This eugenics-based mindset produced a welfare system in which social workers were taught to differentiate between different types of people. As Commissioner Johnson wrote, "unless the State's public welfare program is such as to segregate this defective and thus prevent his promiscuous breeding, society will be increasingly weakened by the perpetuation of the mentally defective." State officials' desire to segregate mental defectives extended even beyond eugenic rationales. In orphanages, for example, welfare officials believed that the very presence of feebleminded children in cottages or on

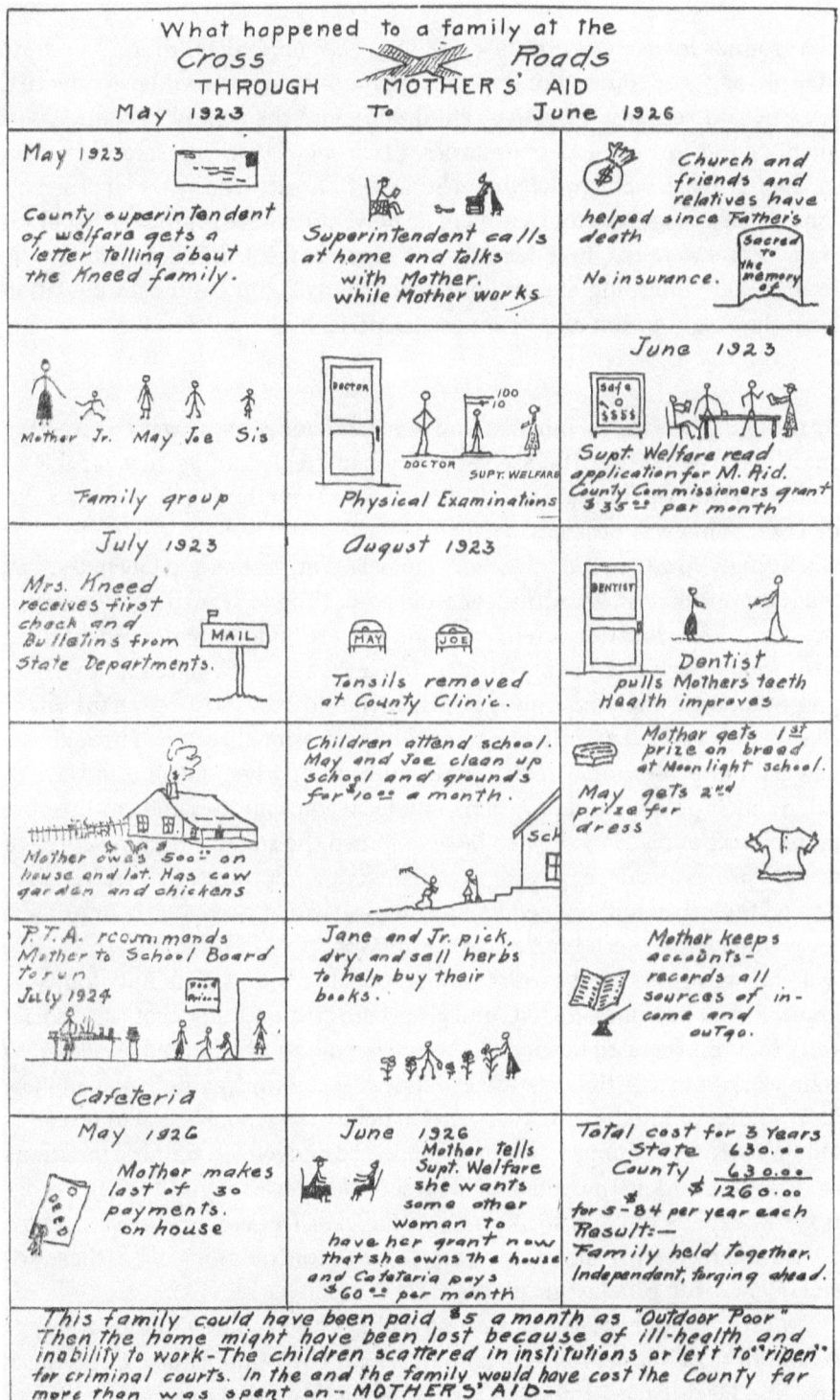

Figure 4.5 One attempt by the welfare board to illustrate the difference that Mothers' Aid could make for a deserving family—with ultimate savings for the state and county. *BCPW Report, 1924–26*, 53, North Carolina Collection, Louis Round Wilson Special Collections Library, University of North Carolina at Chapel Hill.

playgrounds interfered with the development of normal children.[140] Outside of orphanages or county homes, county superintendents could help identify, classify, and remove "defective" children before they could become delinquent or transgress racial boundaries. Black social workers were instructed to identify Black feeblemindedness because it threatened the racial order, although their resources for treatment or prevention were minimal. White social workers were taught to identify and separate feebleminded white people from society, marking them simultaneously as "unfit" and as a deviation from the Anglo-Saxon race's supposed superiority.

By the end of the 1920s, Johnson and her staff had, in many ways, solved the challenge they had set themselves. They had created an agency capable of administering welfare cases in a uniform way, from the state's mountains to its coast. This was no small victory, given North Carolina's size, its overwhelmingly rural population, many officials' commitment to low taxes, and that commitment's cascading consequences: limited transportation infrastructure, low education levels, and tight welfare budgets. Powerful political coalitions as well as affluent outsiders often sheltered the state's new welfare programs from the worst ravages, while the Board's most powerful offensive weapons were emerging standards of professionalization. Through the new field of professional social work, Johnson and her staff found ways to extend their policies and programs into local communities and cut through pernicious politics. For the people who joined the state's emerging corps of welfare professionals, exposure to social work and professional training reshaped their lives and opened new avenues—a trend particularly important for young women with limited career options.

In bringing McAlister's county-unit model to fruition, Kate Burr Johnson, her staff, and her allies at UNC and elsewhere created a model of rural social work that reverberated beyond the bounds of the South. Odum had set out to train workers in a distinctly Southern style of social work at his School of Public Welfare. Although many years passed before the school began to resemble Odum's dreams, Odum and Johnson pioneered and refined training programs in rural casework with the benefit of practical experience and became recognized as experts in rural social welfare. Officials from other states asked for advice about creating similar systems. Odum's contributions to Southern social science won him lasting eminence.[141]

Johnson, though relatively unknown today, also achieved national recognition. In 1929, she served on a committee for the White House Conference on Child Health and Protection.[142] According to a proud report in the *North Carolina Clubwoman*, "She was one of three women in the United States, and the only woman from the South, who was asked to head an important section in the White House Conference."[143] Johnson even had a chance to describe the "North Carolina Plan" to the nation's chief executive when she sat next to President Hoover during lunch at the White House in early November 1929. Although Hoover must have been preoccupied with the October 29 stock market crash and the looming financial crisis, he asked her many questions and knew a great deal about the state's public welfare system. In addition, Johnson helped to prepare guidelines for the White House commission about the proper division and relationship between the fields of public health, public welfare, and public education—an issue with which she had firsthand experience in North Carolina. A Rockefeller Foundation official passed on to President Hoover her recommendations for distinct but cooperating federal government departments.[144]

While news of North Carolina's welfare programs traveled far beyond the state, the programs' greatest impact was doubtless at home in the Old North State. With advice from experts in Raleigh, local officials helped provide education, financial support, and institutional homes to the state's neediest whites. Although welfare programs for African Americans were by no means equivalent to those for whites, North Carolina became the first state in the South to extend some modicum of official support to Black-run social welfare efforts. By the end of the 1920s, welfare officials and social reformers had taken notable strides in professionalizing and modernizing the provision of social support.

Yet the way reformers had defined social ills limited their success. They saw poverty, crime, mental illness, neglect, and other social problems as rooted in individual or family defects rather than as consequences of a political economy that offered security and stability only to a privileged few. Even the most effective social worker, striving diligently to maintain records and use public funds effectively, could provide only stopgap support for one family at a time. In many cases, the solutions social workers offered were likely not the solutions the families desired. In the best cases, families had to accept public funds with strings attached, such as a social worker monitoring their spending choices or criticizing their housekeeping. In worse cases, they might be institutionalized or they might lose their children if a social worker saw evidence of neglect, for example, and placed a child with a foster family.

Eugenics campaigns of the 1920s thus shaped the policies of a maturing social welfare bureaucracy. Dozens of new Black and white social workers learned that whenever they saw social problems—alcoholism, truancy, criminality, desertion—they should suspect mental problems and seek the expert help of state officials. They learned that feeblemindedness led to crime, poverty, and immorality and sapped state finances. They learned that the best way to deal with feebleminded people was to shut them in institutions or to deny them a marriage license. For white social workers in homes of white families, the imperative was nothing less than maintaining the fitness of the white race. Black social workers, who worked within a system that denied the basic potential and even humanity of poor Black families, may still have hoped that discovering hereditary mental problems could help uplift the race and prevent the worst allegations of criminality and insanity. Above all, social workers learned that some people were born to be a "burden on the rest."[145]

Chapter 5

The Burden of the Socially Useless

*Eugenics Research and the Campaign for
Sterilization Laws in the 1920s*

Each day during the state fair of 1922, crowds tramped through the dusty grounds, scrutinizing prize-winning cattle, reliving the excitement of the day's races, and waiting for the grand display of fireworks that careened crazily upward each evening. The fairgoers who wandered toward the clump of booths for various state agencies would have seen staff from the state welfare board—perhaps the Board's publicist Nell Battle Lewis, young and energetic Wiley Sanders, or even psychopathologist Dr. Harry Crane—ready to explain a series of large posters. On one poster was a photograph of the "Wake family," the villains of the Board's recent eugenic family study, conducted along the lines of famous models like *The Jukes* and *The Kallikaks*. The Board had spent six months studying Joe and Mary Wake and their descendants, a white family who "gave no end of trouble" to authorities and were reportedly deviant, alcoholic, feebleminded, or addicted to drugs. Officials claimed that the Wake family had cost the state $20,000, the equivalent of the Board's annual appropriation. For the exhibit, the Board had prepared brightly colored illustrated posters to show the "costly, criminal and disorderly history" of the family. The artist drew figures peering through black jail bars and blue-uniformed policemen to represent arrests, houses to represent institutions where they had been committed, and "wigged, black-gowned judges with startled expressions" to represent court appearances. The staff had brought placards about other elements of the Board's work, including Mothers' Aid and prison reforms, but the Wake family posters were the "most prominent feature" of the exhibit. Before the fair even opened, one reporter predicted that the welfare department booth would be "of special interest," and their display did attract "wide attention."[1]

The publicity surrounding the Wake family study was part of a broader campaign during the 1920s to educate North Carolinians about eugenics, beyond the circles of reformers and professional social workers who were conversant with language of mental defects and cacogenic families. The interest in eugenics reached its peak across the nation during the 1920s, and North Carolina was no exception. In the early 1920s an interinstitutional network developed among academics, social workers, and medical professionals who focused on the problems of feeblemindedness and mental defects. At the center of this network was the state welfare board's new Division of Mental Health and Hygiene, headed by Harry Crane. The division coordinated mental testing, conducted research like the Wake family study that reinforced arguments about the pervasive problem of mental defects, and carried out extensive publicity efforts. Their work gradually fed public fears about mental defects and helped define the problem in the minds of many powerful North Carolinians as one that deserved more attention.

At the same time, pro-eugenics reformers and their legislative allies repeatedly pushed for eugenic measures. Their primary goal was to pass a more powerful sterilization law. The existing sterilization law of 1919 included significant administrative hurdles, and no definitive record remains of anyone being sterilized under the law. Almost immediately after its passage, reformers and welfare officials began to lobby for a more "workable" sterilization law. Twice, in 1923 and 1925, sterilization bills ended in close defeats. These failures were due not to intense opposition to eugenics principles, but rather to a lack—yet—of enough outspoken champions who could make the bill a priority among the hundreds proposed. The repeated public discussions of these bills, along with a 1926 report on conditions at Caswell that called for greater use of sterilization, kept eugenic sterilization on policymakers' agenda and gave reformers and their allies a chance to refine their arguments.

In 1929, reformers succeeded in passing a sterilization law giving officials more power to sterilize people deemed unfit, in the name of the "public good." By that time, legislators who might have been concerned about the legal implications of the bill could look around the nation. The pace of sterilization legislation picked up in 1923, and by the end of 1925, seventeen states had sterilization laws. The US Supreme Court's 1927 decision in *Buck v. Bell* increased this activity. The now infamous Supreme Court opinion reassured leaders in North Carolina and other states that state-sponsored eugenic sterilization programs were constitutional.[2] In addition to these national trends, North Carolina's new law built on a decade of intentional educational work by reformers and welfare officials, who taught the public to see eugenic sterilization as a necessary preventive measure for multiple social problems. In the end, many white leaders were drawn to the idea that targeting "racial defectives" could maintain white supremacy *and* minimize public expenditures.[3]

The Division of Mental Health and Hygiene

At the center of reformers' legislative success in 1929 was a widespread belief among policymakers that inherited mental defects created many social problems. One agency was responsible for much of the work leading to that belief:

the Division of Mental Health and Hygiene, housed in the State Board of Charities and Public Welfare. With Harry Crane at the helm, the division quickly became central to the Board's work. Crane led a network of researchers who tested thousands of white North Carolinians for mental defects. The evidence they collected and the ways that they framed the problems of mental defects shaped the ways legislators framed the need for eugenic sterilization.

The creation of the division in September 1921 capped a sustained effort by welfare officials and medical doctors to expand the state's ability to study mental defects. It was not a foregone conclusion that such a research bureau would find its institutional home with the state welfare board. Caswell superintendent C. Banks McNairy had for years called for the establishment of a psychological clinic at his institution, including a pointed comment in 1918 that such a clinic would fulfill the "spirit and intention" of the welfare board's charter. Indeed, many other states consolidated psychological testing at their state's institution for the feebleminded.[4] The post-fire revision of Caswell's charter in 1919 (see chapter 3) included studying feeblemindedness and running a psychological clinic and outreach bureau, but the legislature was slow to provide funds for a psychological expert.[5] The Board of Charities and Public Welfare, on the other hand, had the law in its favor. The Board's first commissioner, Roland Beasley, had made a clear case that insanity, feeblemindedness, and mental hygiene in general were the bailiwick of the welfare board. The Board had a constitutional mandate to "investigate and report causes of insanity and feeblemindedness and kindred subjects," and Beasley pointed out that they could not properly study these subjects without a trained expert.[6]

The Board of Charities and Public Welfare also had momentum on its side, thanks to a damning study of mental defects. In 1920, Beasley arranged for an expert from the National Committee for Mental Hygiene, Dr. William McDonald, to conduct a study in North Carolina. Funded by the Rockefeller Foundation, the group had conducted surveys of mental conditions in five other Southern states between 1916 and 1920, sometimes leading to the creation of institutions. In North Carolina, McDonald's primary goal was to survey the insane, but in its annual report to the legislature, the welfare board focused on his findings about the feebleminded and epileptic. After observing institutions in fifty counties and all of the state-run institutions, McDonald claimed there were at least 1,426 feebleminded or epileptic people already in institutions and many more beyond, wreaking financial and social havoc. "No single class of persons," he argued, "draws so largely and increasingly upon the public purse as do the feeble-minded," particularly because they tended to be criminals. Moreover, he saw no room for redemption. "Not one" child of parents with mental defects could "by any chance possess mental potentiality higher than either of its parents, whereas many are below both mother and father in intelligence." To deal with the "grave concern" of the feebleminded, McDonald called for much more space at Caswell, use of eugenic sterilization, and a psychological clinic.[7]

Welfare officials used these findings to their advantage. Beasley cited them in requesting funding for a state psychiatric bureau with a "competent specialist" who could handle individual cases and conduct a statewide educational campaign. The legislature increased the Board's appropriation that year, but not by enough to hire an expert. When Kate Burr Johnson became commissioner in the summer of 1921, she was more creative: she recruited a psychologist from UNC to work part-time for the Board, thus establishing the division at minimal expense. The Division of Mental Health and Hygiene became the third division in the expanding state welfare bureaucracy.[8]

To head the new division, Johnson hired Harry Wolven Crane, who oversaw its influential research and educational work until 1933. Crane, who appeared in the mock juvenile court hearing in chapter 4, was both well-connected and well-qualified. Born in Michigan in 1885 to a middle-class family, Crane took degrees in psychology at the University of Michigan, including his PhD in 1913. After graduating he found a job as the chief investigator with the Michigan Eugenics Commission, for which he cataloged the extent of insanity, epilepsy, feeblemindedness, and other mental defects in the state.[9] In 1915, Crane went to New York to formalize his training as a eugenics fieldworker, becoming one of the few men at the Eugenics Record Office's summer training program.[10]

Crane began a professorial job at Ohio State University in the fall of 1915, but his doctorate in psychology made him one of the ERO's most valuable eugenics fieldworkers, and the organization soon called him back into service. In January 1916 he took a leave of absence from Ohio State and moved to Little Rock, Arkansas, where he worked under ERO auspices for the Arkansas Commission for the Feebleminded. From his work there he submitted voluminous records to the ERO archive, including information about over one thousand Arkansans. As a result of his efforts, the state established a school for the feebleminded the following year. Crane also took on two other postings for the ERO in 1916, in the Psychopathic Laboratory of the New York City Police Department and as the fieldwork director of a eugenic survey of Nassau County, New York. Following his leave of absence, he returned to Ohio State and taught psychology, reporting to other ERO fieldwork alums that his course in criminal psychology made "considerable use" of "eugenical material."[11]

While at Ohio State, Crane met his future wife, Mabel Ensworth Goudge. The same age as Crane, Goudge was born in Canada to a Canadian father and a mother from Massachusetts. She received her PhD in psychology in 1914 under the mentorship of Edward Bradford Titchener, a prominent psychologist at Cornell University. Her research focused on patterns and visual perception. In 1915 or 1916, she took up a position teaching psychology at Ohio State. She and Crane married in 1918, presumably having met while teaching in the same department. Around the same time, Goudge began working toward a medical degree at Ohio State, which she completed in 1922. When Crane moved to North Carolina in 1921, Goudge found a position at Watts Hospital in Durham and later opened a private practice as a clinical psychologist. She published at least one article, on abnormal psychology in general medical practice, and she attended the annual American Psychological Association meeting at least once, as did Crane.[12]

In North Carolina, Crane joined UNC's new department of psychology and became the director of the Board's new Division of Mental Health and Hygiene, which was housed in Chapel Hill. Kate Burr Johnson arranged for Crane to be jointly employed, with one-third of his time belonging to the Board.[13] Crane's work as head of the division reflected the expansive definition of "mental hygiene." Clifford Beers, the founder of the mental hygiene movement, had a personal interest in mental illness, but the term also encompassed prevention of feeblemindedness, nervous disorders, even anxiety and depression.[14] Medical and welfare professionals saw all these mental disorders as interrelated in cause and cure. The work of the Division of Mental Health and Hygiene reflected that breadth; its work included testing, research, and education and covered a range of mental disorders.

Testing was the core of the division's day-to-day activities, with requests coming from institutions, the court system, social workers, and sometimes families. Although many social workers believed they could identify feebleminded people by sight or common sense, their training from the Board emphasized the importance of expert psychological exams, which lent the imprimatur of science to their convictions. Exams also helped smooth the admission of a child to Caswell and offered judges an expert evaluation of the mental capacity of defendants.[15] Because testing had multiple uses, the Board tested an extraordinary number of people, usually individually but also in group settings. In the first eight months, Crane and his assistants carried out 575 mental examinations and reported that they did not have time to test even all of the "urgent cases." In the following two-year period, they examined 847 people and still felt that they had not been able to follow through on all the requests for tests.[16] The number of people they tested was dwarfed by the number of feebleminded people they believed lived in North Carolina, which Crane estimated at fifty thousand.[17]

State officials seemed to believe that mental problems in white people were abnormal and thus worth addressing, but mental problems were simply to be expected in Black people. The bureau's work aligned with these assumptions, focusing almost solely on white families. In their first year, they conducted a study of eight county homes but examined only white inmates. From 1922 to 1926, they tested a total of 1,183 people, only twenty-two of whom (less than 2 percent) were Black. Of course, the division's tally of mental tests reflected the general pattern of providing few services to African Americans. In the first complete biennium after the state created the Division of Work Among Negroes, the number shot up to forty-four Black people tested, 14 percent of the total. But their testing tally also reflected the attitudes of Crane and his staff. They explained their attitudes explicitly in one Board report, citing psychological research that purported to show that the intelligence of Black people "as a whole is definitely lower than that of the white." They also assumed that there was a higher proportion of feebleminded Black people. In later years, Crane continued to insist that the average mental ability of white people was higher than that of Black people, even as some professional organizations began to make public statements that research showed "no inherent psychological differences among 'so-called races.'"[18]

In the process of this extensive testing regimen, the Board created an enormous registry. Crane's staff aimed for completeness, trying to test every known feebleminded person and their relatives.[19] As Crane and his staff examined their subjects, they carefully entered information about each person on a white index card. They also produced pink cards with information about any known relatives who might be mentally defective, even though often their only information was hearsay. They even gathered information about suspected cases from newspaper articles, entering this secondhand information on buff-colored cards.[20] Crane believed that mental tests alone provided insufficient data to understand each person's case, so he likely trained his staff—as he had been trained at the Eugenics Record Office—to record other details of the person's social and family history. Their notes might include phrases such as "careless about personal appearance" or "evidences of neural instability in alcoholic and drug excesses of two maternal aunts."[21] Each case was cross-referenced with county and institutional indexes. The intent was to allow for systematized study of the transmission of mental defects, as the ERO and other eugenics researchers of the 1920s did. The volume of index cards mounted quickly, and each year Crane proudly reported new additions to the collection. Between 1922 and 1924, for example, they made 6,281 cards about individuals they had examined and 7,737 cards about their relatives. By the end of the decade, their files contained at least thirty thousand entries, each representing an individual suspected of being mentally defective.[22]

The Board's huge body of data was created in the name of research but ultimately enabled state surveillance. Crane and his staff not only collected information about thousands of people in North Carolina; as they recorded this information in a systematized way, they also made decisions about how to classify behaviors or test results. They assigned an IQ and a mental age to each person they tested to determine whether they were feebleminded. Their research, then, was part of the process of creating categories of mental defectiveness that enabled the state to monitor people of interest on a massive scale. Crane's staff willingly shared the information about individuals in their card file with other social welfare officials, both public and private. Welfare officials could then choose to act on this information about an individual and their relatives as they decided how to handle cases.[23]

Caswell continued to be a secondary hub of mental testing, and its staff conducted their own eugenics research. Superintendent C. Banks McNairy published a treatise on eugenics and incest, and he lectured around the state about mental deficiency. His successor W. H. Dixon kept up an active publicity campaign in North Carolina, frequently publishing articles about feeblemindedness in the welfare board's magazine.[24] Both were active members of the American Association for the Study of the Feeble-Minded (AASFM), including publishing articles in its journal, and McNairy become the first Southerner elected president of the organization.[25] Despite the public activities of its superintendents, Caswell's mental testing programs remained small compared to the work of Crane's bureau. One medical officer there, William Newbold, tested a few dozen people each year.[26] He also used the inmates for his own research purposes: he gathered blood samples from over three hundred Caswell patients and twenty-nine "normals," and for up to three years gave experimental treatments to the fifty-four Caswell children he believed were endocrine defective—all likely without their consent and perhaps without their knowledge. This work was the foundation for a paper on the relationship of endocrine levels to mental activity that he presented to the AASFM.[27] At least one of Newbold's successors was unfamiliar with mental tests, and Crane and a UNC graduate student thereafter helped conduct tests for Caswell.[28]

Crane's network produced evidence that helped establish the scientific credibility of the Board's policy proposals while simultaneously using the state's population as fodder for academic research efforts. For example, Crane used his study of mental defects in county homes to argue that at least five hundred to six hundred feebleminded people lived in county homes, then called for expanding Caswell's capacity to over a thousand inmates and allowing inmates of any age. While the Board's goal in this study was merely to quantify the extent of feeblemindedness, Crane was interested in learning more about group intelligence testing and the correlations between those tests and individual intelligence exams. Crane also presented papers to medical and psychology professionals on topics such as "heredity in relation to retardation" and the role of social adjustment in diagnosing mental deficiency.[29]

Many graduate students who studied under Crane's likeminded colleagues contributed their own research to the state. Margaret Brietz, a UNC master's student in sociology who worked with Wiley B. Sanders, is a case in point. Brietz arrived at UNC in 1926 after five years as a probation officer for delinquent girls in Winston-Salem and Forsyth County. She hoped to gain more formal training in social work, and with Kate Burr Johnson's help she secured a fellowship from the state Federation of Women's Clubs. In her 1927 master's thesis, she interpreted her previous work as a probation officer through the lens of her sociology education at UNC. She described the "complete life-setting" of eighteen "delinquent" white girls committed to Samarcand whose probation she had overseen from 1921 to 1925. Brietz organized their cases into four categories of her own invention that reflected her desire to disentangle environmental and hereditary causes of delinquency: adolescent delinquency; delinquency and bad surroundings; delinquency and homelessness; and delinquency and mental defectiveness, the largest category.[30]

Brietz tried to tackle her case studies scientifically as she invoked eugenic principles, but her comments are rife with contradictions and conjecture. One of her subjects was Carmine James, whom Brietz classified as "a defective delinquent with personality charm." Carmine had "keen insight" and appeared "bright, clever, and responsive." Brietz speculated that she "might easily have floated in a much higher strata of society, and might have married into stock much superior to her own." But because she worked in a mill, she was likely to marry a poor man whom Brietz assumed might be "as defective as Carmine herself," and their children would likely be "future liabilities to the State in defectiveness and crime." Brietz resolved the apparent tension between Carmine's charm and her diagnosis of "defective mental capacity" by noting that "the mental defective is not to be labeled at a casual glance." While Carmine appeared "bright, clever, and responsive," a mental exam at Samarcand gave her an IQ of 77, classifying her as a high-grade moron.[31]

In some cases, however, Brietz believed mental defect was obvious, with equally obvious eugenic solutions. Mandy Shivvers, deemed "a defective delinquent showing back-mountain degeneracy," seemed "distinctly feeble-minded" before a mental exam had been made. In such a case, Brietz believed that "even the wisest care of social workers cannot insure useful social adjustment" because mental defect could not be cured, merely "transmitted to future generations." To allow someone like Mandy to become a mother and add to the "toll of feeble-minded babies" was "anti-social." Brietz exclaimed, "What a price!" She argued that "the only reasonable thing in such cases" was to prevent procreation through segregation, sterilization, or marriage laws.[32] Brietz's thesis shows how tightly bound feeblemindedness and delinquency were for social workers. Eugenics ideology provided a unifying framework for her social work practice, her academic training in sociology, and her preconceptions about poor white women.

"Cacogenic Strains": Eugenic Family Studies

Among the most influential pieces of eugenics research emerging from Crane's network were eugenic family studies, which made explosive fodder for publicity efforts. In the 1920s the Board conducted "family studies" to show "the importance of control of cacogenic strains" and "the necessity for preventing propagation in such families."[33] Family studies were a common means by which eugenicists traced the transmission of undesirable traits from one generation to the next. The scandalous details in these studies garnered interest from readers, who also ingested a strong dose of eugenic logic.[34] Crane was familiar with the methods of constructing family studies from his training at the Eugenics Record Office, and through conducting these studies other staff became well versed in eugenics field research techniques. Board staff frequently used brief descriptions of families they saw as flawed to illustrate the importance of mental defect in creating social problems, but in at least three cases they went to great lengths to study entire families or communities.

The first study of note preceded the formation of the mental hygiene bureau and provides an interesting counterpoint. In the fall of 1921, the Board published a sketch of several white families living in isolation, followed by a special bulletin devoted to them, entitled "Swamp Island" (see figure 5.1). The story they laid out, they emphasized, was "not fiction," but rather a cautionary tale about the dangers of remaining outside the progress of modern civilization. The families they described were cut off from the outside world by a river and surrounding swamps, at least two miles from the nearest school or church. In the eyes of the county welfare superintendent who "helped" them, they were guilty of multiple transgressions: bootlegging, illegitimacy, rape, incest, polygamy, and clear child neglect. The people there also suffered from venereal disease (often linked to sexual abuse) and physical disability from work accidents. To the authors, the story showed "what isolation, ignorance, ill-health and idleness" could do in any community. The solution, they argued, lay in "science, common sense, and sympathy." Accordingly, their response was to jail adult perpetrators of incest and illegitimacy and send children to be retrained in foster homes or reformatories for a "normal moral life." In one family alone, seven children were sent away from the supposedly

> This bulletin is not fiction. The families studied and helped in these pages are living now in this State. A Superintendent of Public Welfare, a man trained in social work, knows these conditions and made this report. For obvious reasons all names of persons and places are changed. The facts are not pleasant, the story is not "pretty," but it is printed to show what isolation, ignorance, ill-health and idleness can do in a community probably not fifty miles from where you read this report. The second object in publishing the study is that of proving that real things can be accomplished even in so apparently "hopeless" cases when science, common sense, and sympathy combine in an effort to solve humanity's problems.

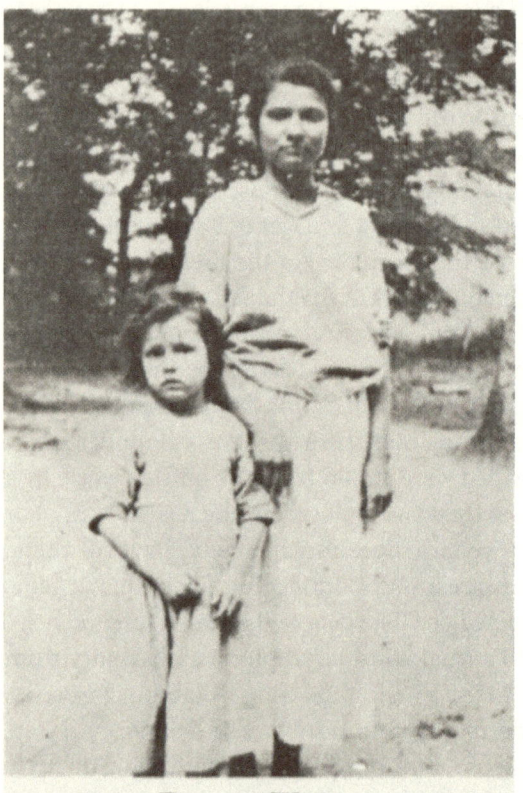

FANNIE WILKS
Delinquent girl, infected with gonorrhea—and her little sister.

Will the little sister follow in the big sister's tracks?

Figure 5.1a and b The text introducing the Board's report on a family in "Swamp Island" and a photo of two of the family members (with pseudonyms). BCPW, "Swamp Island," 3, 10, North Carolina Collection, Louis Round Wilson Special Collections Library, University of North Carolina at Chapel Hill.

corrupting influence of their family. The report did not use hereditarian language such as "degeneracy," focusing more on the effects of culture and environment, but the message was clear: there was a type of family who could not be allowed to raise their children if the children were to have a "chance to become good citizens."[35]

The next extensive study was of "Joe and Mary Wake" and their descendants, soon to find infamy in the colorful poster exhibited at the 1922 state fair. The Board published a lengthy description of the Wake family's "immorality, drunkenness, and filth" in its report that year. The Wake study focused on the costs of feeblemindedness to taxpayers. The Board wrote that Joe was "undoubtedly born feebleminded" and was suffering from general paresis, which the staff assumed was a result of his advanced syphilis. According to the Board's report, "absolutely no contribution has he made to civilization *except the repairing* of a few shoe soles." Joe's wife Mary was a "dope fiend" who allowed her children to play "in the green slime in the nearby ditch." The couple had eight children, two of whom had died. The children had been arrested for petty theft, sent to reformatories, or taken in by foster parents.[36]

The reality of the Wake family's lives was less sensational and perhaps more miserable than the Board described. Mary was born in Harnett County, part of a large family that moved to Raleigh in the 1890s. When she was around twenty, she married Joe, who was a shoemaker in Raleigh. Their first child was born soon after, but died in infancy. They moved frequently within East Raleigh, sometimes near Mary's mother, sometimes near one of Raleigh's red-light districts. Mary's encounters with the law began around 1909, when she was first charged with being drunk and disorderly, found lying on the ground with her child nearby. At her hearing, she said she drank to "drown her troubles." She pled with the judge not to "send me to jail with this child" and promised not to drink anymore. This child, like several of her other children in subsequent years, was soon placed in foster care; three of her daughters were sent to Caswell (and two were friends with Lydia Spruill, the center of the arson controversy in 1919). When Mary was committed to the state mental hospital in 1916 after serving a charge for public drunkenness, she protested to hospital officials that "I love them [my children] as good as I do myself." In the decade leading up to the Board's 1922 profile, Mary was sentenced to the county jail 242 times as she continued to struggle with alcoholism. She became a well-known figure in Raleigh newspapers, with one headline reporting "Terrible Mary Is in Jail Again." Only days before the exhibit disparaging her opened at the state fair, Mary may have tried to kill herself: she set fire to her mattress and lay "in a drunken stupor" while it burned, saved when police dragged her from the house. She died of unknown causes three years later, a month after her husband died in Dix Hill, a state-run mental institution in Raleigh, where he was being treated for his paresis.[37]

Welfare officials concluded that the couple should have been refused a marriage license "on the ground of feeblemindedness—as is done in a number of states," and sent to an institution, which would have saved the state "much expense and trouble." They also suggested Joe and Mary be sterilized: "had they been rendered incapable of having children they could not have been more diseased than they are, and still society would have been spared a second generation of their kind." Johnson devoted six pages of the Board's 1922 report to the Wake family, including a chart that summarized the family's transgressions and their cost to taxpayers (see figure 5.2). Her staff argued that the Board's annual appropriation of $20,000, which funded preventive work, put taxpayer money to more constructive use than the approximately $20,000 that the state had "heedlessly poured out on this family."[38]

Board staff used their findings to create the exhibit that they showed at the 1922 state fair, and after the fair the exhibit took on a new life. The Board added pictures of "disgraceful episodes" in the family's history as well as charts showing the expense to the state of the family's offspring, presumably without permission from the beleaguered Wakes, whose remaining shreds of anonymity were destroyed. The exhibit was quite popular over the next several years, being "in almost constant use." Staff took it to meetings of women's clubs and the Conference for Social Service. Parts of it were published in the *Survey*, perhaps the leading journal for social workers, after which requests came to borrow the exhibit from as far away as Chicago, Minnesota, and Iowa. In 1924 the Board purchased new projection equipment, "an entertaining little machine" that could be used to show pictures and charts from the Wake family project. With the new display methods enhancing their appeal, the charts were "the center of attraction" at the state Congress of Parents and Teachers.[39] Their proud creator, the Board's publicity agent in the 1920s, even took copies of the charts with her to her new job in Florida, where she hung them on her wall for years and used them for talks.[40] The materials circulated as late as 1927, when the Illinois Children's Home and Aid Society borrowed them for its annual meeting. They appeared again at the Conference for Social Services, and three college classes came to the Board's Raleigh offices to see the exhibit. By then, newspapers reported, the family's total cost to the state had been $32,000.[41]

The Board studied one more family in the 1920s: the "Fehler" family, whose sobriquet referred to the German word for "defect." The Fehler study most closely followed the methods of other eugenic family studies, with particular attention to tracing how defects were inherited between generations. The family had come to the attention of a state welfare official when he met Nancy

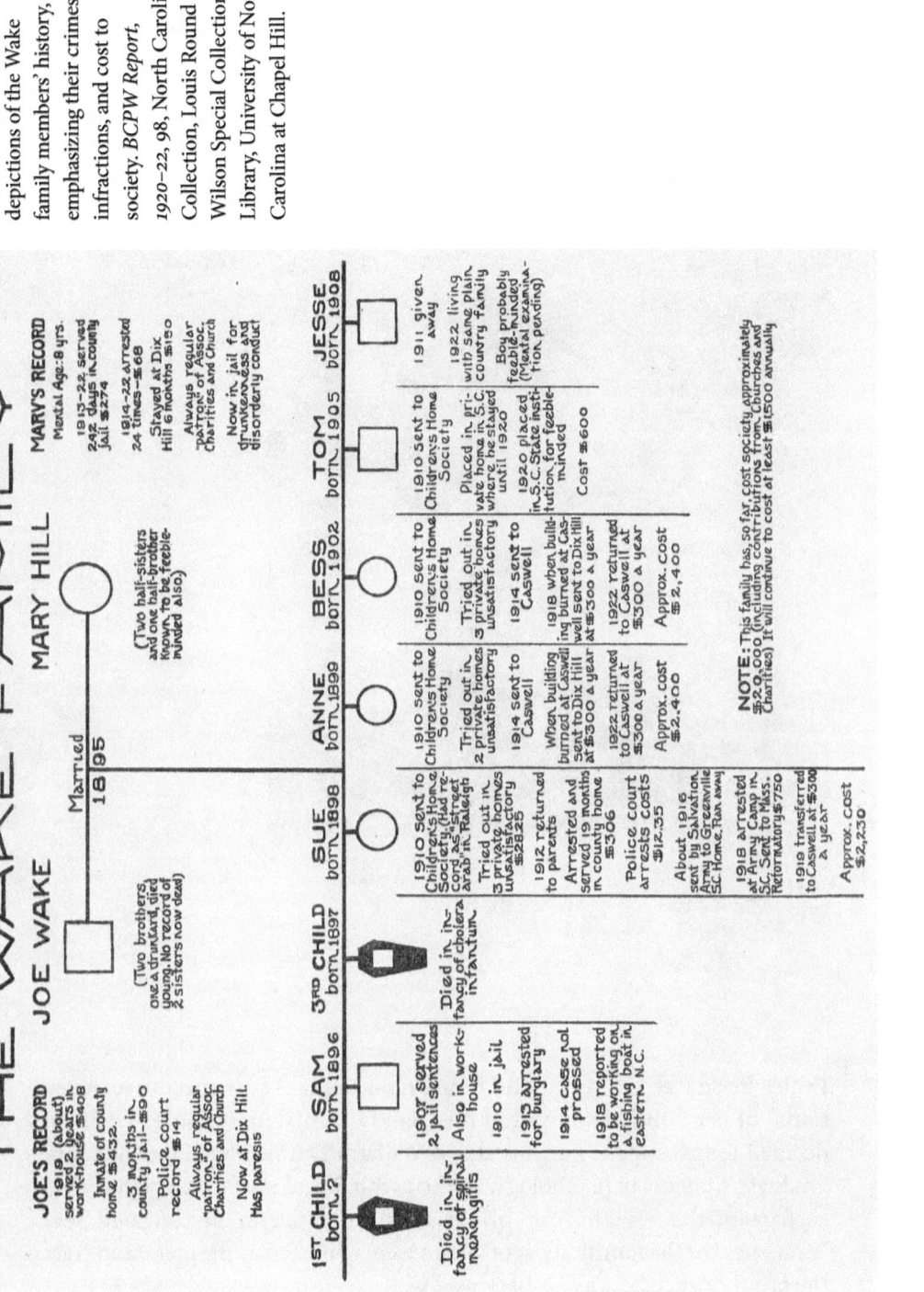

Figure 5.2 One of the boards depictions of the Wake family members' history, emphasizing their crimes, infractions, and cost to society. *BCPW Report, 1920–22*, 98, North Carolina Collection, Louis Round Wilson Special Collections Library, University of North Carolina at Chapel Hill.

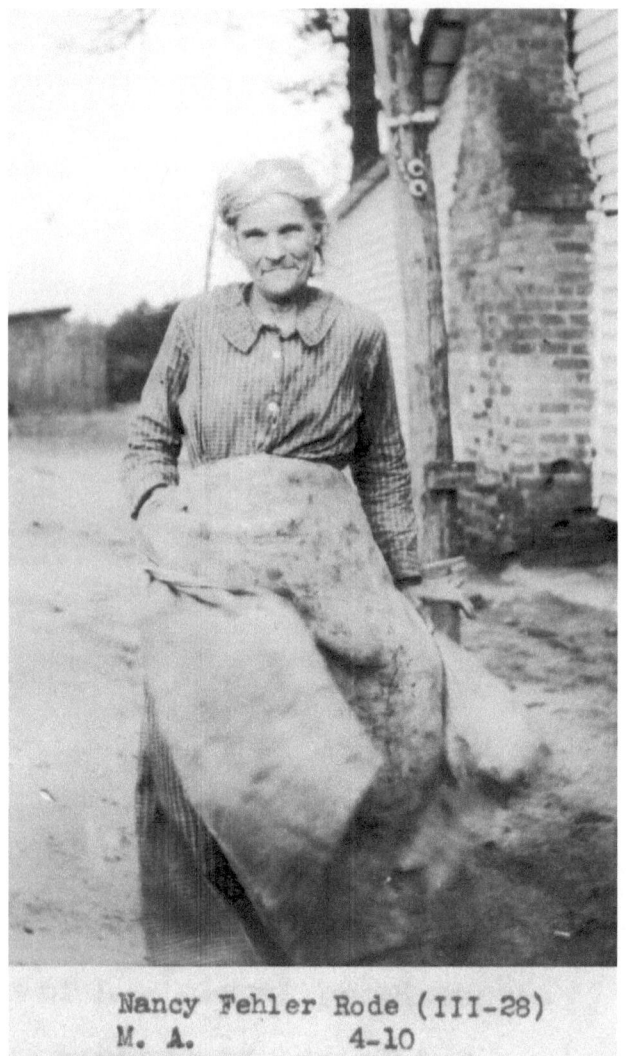

Figure 5.3 Nancy Fehler Rode, the member of the family who first drew Glenn's attention. Based on IQ tests he administered, Glenn listed her IQ as 30 and her mental age as four years and ten months old. Glenn, "The Fehlers," 111.

Fehler Rode (see figure 5.3) and heard reports that "four successive generations" of her family had lived in the "Sand County" poorhouse. The Board decided to investigate. For this study, William Darby Glenn, one of Crane's graduate students in psychology, worked with Board staff to study the Fehlers as part of the research for his dissertation.[42] Glenn investigated seven "branches" of the family, most of whom were white tenant farmers, and traced the family's ancestors as far back as 1815.

Between 1922 and 1926, Glenn spent nine months doing fieldwork. He interviewed as many members of the family as he could but refused to trust their accounts, looking also at court records, institutional records, and "verified information from responsible individuals," such as physicians or landlords. He gave mental exams to 114 people, including "consorts" of the Fehler family. Some resisted; in at least one case, a child was "hidden away" when the tests were given, probably under the assumption that testing would lead the authorities to institutionalize him. Glenn found nobody over the mental age of eleven. For almost 250 other living and dead family members, he gathered "various evidences" of their intelligence, suggesting that much of this evidence was hearsay. He presented detailed descriptions of each family member he could identify, noting factors such as the number of stillborn children, sexual promiscuity, cousin marriages, venereal disease, education levels, and racial mixing. For a few people, he described how social factors "operat[ed] to introduce a superior strain" into the family.[43]

Whenever possible, Glenn took a photograph of living subjects, apparently to document their social context. More practically, his subjects were suspicious of him, and sometimes promising a copy of a photograph was "successful in overcoming their hostility." Most of the photographs show small groups of family members in the dirt yards outside their homes, some in their Sunday best, others in worn work clothes. Each subject was captioned with their name, the alphanumeric code Glenn used to denote their place in the family tree, their "mental age," their chronological age, and their IQ as determined by his testing. Nearby pages described whatever details of their life Glenn saw as relevant. Don Fehler (see figure 5.4), for example, who was pictured with his three children and his second wife, was identified merely as an unsuccessful tenant farmer with an IQ of 55 whose first wife had been "taciturn and slatternly from the hard work in the fields and from childbirth." Glenn's descriptions tend to lack sympathy or to ignore the humanity of his subjects, but his photographs evoke their hard lives and sometimes—as with Lina Fehler Eck (see figure 5.5)—their barely concealed ire at Glenn's intrusion into their lives.[44]

Although his research was at the behest of and funded by the Board, Glenn also used his findings for his doctoral dissertation. His academic research aim was to investigate the heritability of mental defects, particularly whether the "degree of defect" was inherited. He compiled multipage charts linking family members and charting results of intelligence tests (see figure 5.6). From this mountain of descriptive data, he attempted to extrapolate findings. He presented statistical analysis about several topics, including the hypothesis that "the degree of defect in offspring is determined to a great extent" by the parents' intelligence and that "defective individuals" had more children. He also

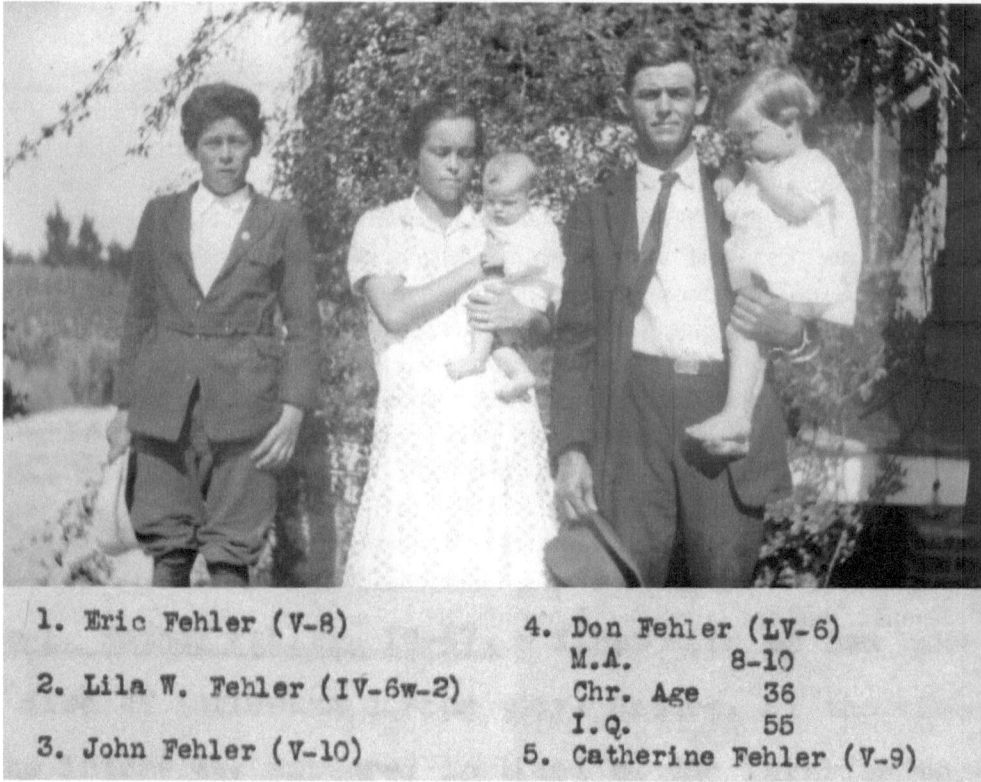

1. Eric Fehler (V-8)
2. Lila W. Fehler (IV-6w-2)
3. John Fehler (V-10)
4. Don Fehler (LV-6)
   M.A.   8-10
   Chr. Age 36
   I.Q.   55
5. Catherine Fehler (V-9)

Figure 5.4 Don Fehler and his family. Glenn assigned Don Fehler an IQ of 55 and a mental age of eight years and ten months. Glenn, "The Fehlers," 18.

found that mental defects were associated with illegitimacy, delinquency, sexual offenses, and institutional cases. He found a correlation between low "economic adjustment" and low IQs, and he assumed that lack of measurable intelligence led to poverty, rather than the inverse.[45]

While Glenn was conducting his research, the Board reported with gusto on his initial findings. His work, they said, laid out in a "forceful manner the necessity for preventing propagation in such families" and controlling "cacogenic strains." In a markedly different tone than the sober and cold account in his dissertation, Glenn's public reports on the Fehlers appealed to financial considerations and moral outrage. He highlighted the cost of the antisocial behavior of the family's 380 current members, describing how they "lived their nonproductive lives in misery, poverty, and ignorance." The family was full of illegitimate children, racial mixing, bad tempers, prostitution, murder, cruelty, "immorality," "depravity," and "general social crimes." He also selected—from among the hundreds of family members—Fehlers who had

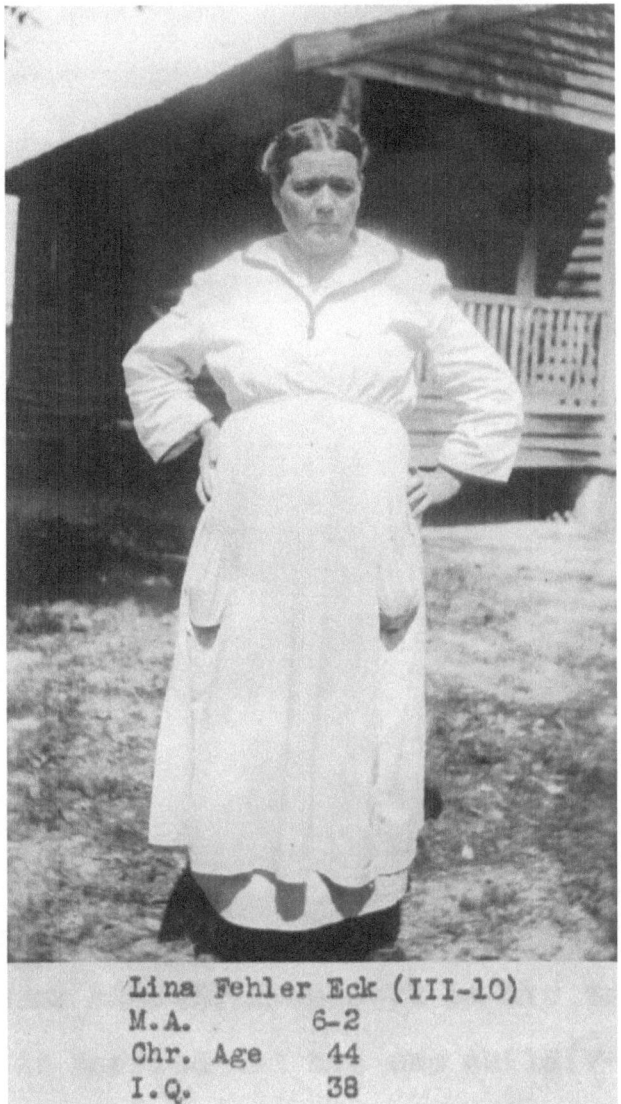

Figure 5.5 Lina Fehler Eck, whom Glenn judged as having an IQ of 38 and a mental age of six years and two months. Glenn, "The Fehlers," 61.

"outstanding records in crime and degeneracy," and he assaulted readers with their "sordid histories": Nancy Fehler prostituted herself for a can of snuff, and Lizzie Fehler was convicted of the murder of three of her stepchildren and bore two illegitimate children of her own. Often Glenn emphasized their animalistic nature. Red Fehler "roved the woods and climbed trees from which he yelled for hours like an animal," and had cut off all his toes with an axe.

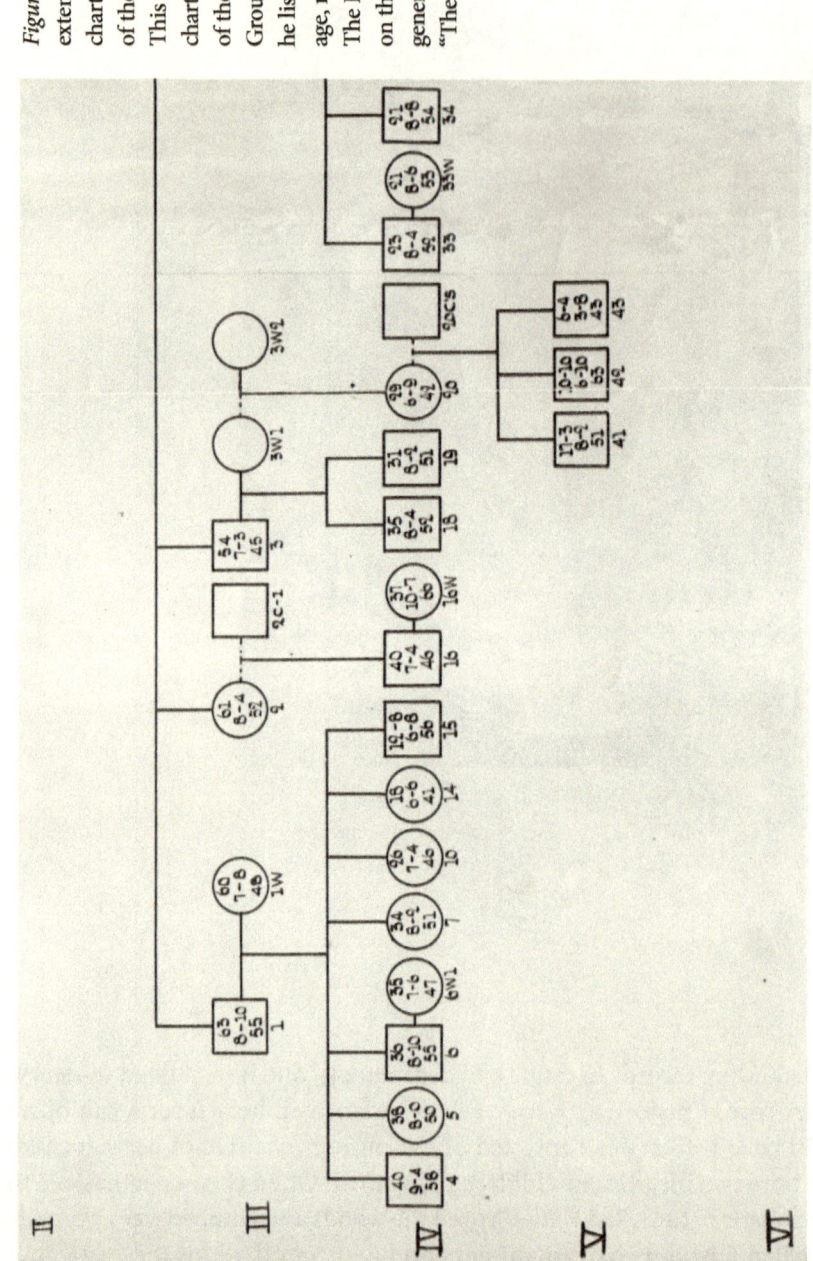

Figure 5.6 Glenn created extensive genealogical charts for the members of the family he tested. This is an excerpt of a chart titled "Presentation of the Data on the Tested Group." For each subject he listed chronological age, mental age, and IQ. The Roman numerals on the left indicate generations. Glenn, "The Fehlers," 206.

Gerty Fehler "was as mean and low as a dog. She was a regular terror after men," and had two illegitimate children fathered by Black men, as did many of the women Glenn described. "And so the murky details go in case after case," Glenn concluded his nearly two-page list. Kate Burr Johnson used material on the Fehler family in lectures, but the Board apparently never created educational displays about the Fehlers as they did for the Wake family, despite Glenn's abundant material, perhaps because he took so long to finish his research. He defended his dissertation in May 1930, at which point the lack of funds "greatly cramped" the Board's publicity efforts.[46]

These family studies, as a group, reveal how the Board hoped to quantify the social and economic costs of mental defects. All three studies were about predominantly white families, and in describing all three the Board used the rhetorical strategy of long lists of social offenses, including violence, petty crime, sexual deviance, and mixed-race children. Each study, however, had a slightly different focus. The Swamp Island study highlighted the importance of social workers in preserving children from immoral or isolated environments, bringing them into the fold of modern civilization. The other studies focused more on the dangers of mental defects. The Wake family charts hammered home the financial costs of ignoring feeblemindedness, and the study of the Fehler family's six generations showed the supposedly high degree of heritability of mental defects and the rapid propagation of people with mental defects. Together, these family studies were powerful illustrations of how "cacogenic" families extracted costs from upstanding citizens.

Educating the Public

The Board used the wealth of evidence that Crane and his associates produced, as well as stories they gathered from county welfare workers, in a relentless public campaign to convince North Carolinians about the menace of feeblemindedness and to promote eugenics principles as a possible solution. State welfare officials declared that their "prime object" was to reduce social problems, namely "delinquency, crime, dependency, and mental defectiveness." A critical component of their strategy was to educate the public about "the extent of mental defectiveness in North Carolina; its menace as a factor in race deterioration, and the imperative necessity for its control." These educational efforts were part and parcel of their broader goal of increasing public support for the work and funding of the welfare office. Johnson created a publicity bureau that oversaw education efforts including talks, exhibits, and print publications.[47] In each of these forums, the Board's staff emphasized the importance of preventive action (whether in the field of mental hygiene or elsewhere), fostered political support for eugenic segregation and sterilization, and pushed individual North Carolinians to carefully select their mates.

In print publications, the Board shaped its message depending on the audience. Staff produced dense biennial reports for legislators, filled with statistical summaries as evidence that public funds were well spent, and special bulletins for social workers dedicated to particular subjects such as juvenile court laws. To reach a broader audience, the Board also published a four-page monthly newsletter, *Public Welfare Progress*, which was "designed to elicit public attention." By 1926 its circulation exceeded six thousand. Nearly every issue contained some item about eugenics or mental hygiene, including both the state's eugenics initiatives and innovations in other states.[48]

In *Public Welfare Progress*, readers learned about current ideas and practices regarding eugenics, mental illness, and feeblemindedness. Articles that described Crane's work examining people across the state functioned as implicit advertisements for his services. Readers were routinely updated about goings-on at Caswell, including the latest training methods there, as well as fluff pieces about field day events. Guest articles by heads of the state's institutions advocated sterilization, outlined the mental hygiene movement, or described how mentally defective white children were "clogging" the public school system and should instead be sent to Caswell.[49] Other articles reported the content of addresses by local leaders at medical meetings or social welfare conferences, such as Johnson's statement at the National Conference of Social Work that "the segregation and prevention of increase of the mentally defective is absolutely essential to the purification of our blood stream," which editor Nell Battle Lewis highlighted in a special issue distributed at the state fair.[50]

The newsletter also frequently included material from national leaders. The editor often summarized new publications or developments elsewhere, or threw in pithy quotes by leading thinkers, visually highlighted in stand-alone boxes. Almost all of these short quotes addressed some aspect of eugenics or mental hygiene. In 1924 Lewis published a quote by Dr. Martin Barr, the expert who had tested Lydia Spruill. He condemned the birth of "mental or moral cripples" and hoped for "the day when men and women shall realize that parenthood is not a right, but a vocation to which all are not called; and that the grasping of it by the victims, the diseased and the defective is practically the crime of touching the sacred Ark of the Covenant, for which the penalty was death." Other articles or features encapsulated key principles for the uninformed reader, such as "Reproduction of Unfit Costly," which cited research on the Jukes family. Similarly, in 1926 the newsletter used material from the National Committee for Mental Hygiene to clarify the differences between feeblemindedness and insanity, although its own articles often blurred the distinctions in practice.[51]

Some articles seem intended merely to feed fears about the menace of the feebleminded. In 1923 the editor warned that without action, in another four generations the "lower mental and physical types" could constitute 90 percent of the population. One of the strangest articles is a brief piece from 1924, entitled "Suppos'n." Suppose, it posited, two couples of different intelligence levels married and reproduced. After five generations, the prolific feebleminded couple would have produced 1,024 offspring, while the "honor graduate of Harvard" and "honor graduate of Bryn Mawr" would have produced thirty-two people with "superior intelligence." The article ended, "Query: 32 is to 1,024 as civilization is to what? This is a little joke at which people of the twenty-first century will probably laugh heartily."[52] By the twenty-first century, the editor assumed, eugenics programs would have had such complete success in improving the quality of the population and of civilization itself that denizens of the future would find humor in the specter of disaster averted.

Other pieces along the lines of editorial commentary aimed to build political support for the Board's goals, particularly for expanding space at Caswell or exploring other avenues to limit the reproduction of the feebleminded. Many items circled a familiar theme, telling the pitiful story of some feebleminded young woman, describing her offspring—or future offspring—then asking what might be done to prevent the spread of her condition. One front-page feature described a nameless, hypothetical feebleminded woman who was "wandering from place to place" with her three "mentally defective" children while pregnant once more. The article outlined the way she "[bred] defectives" who "sap[ped] the health of State's population," with an almost chant-like refrain punctuating each paragraph: "And there is no room at the Caswell Training School!" The article concluded, "It is a fact, a *fact*, a FACT that the mentally inferior are reproducing themselves five times more swiftly at present than the superior," and ended with one last chorus of its lament.[53]

In some cases, Johnson and her publicity staff opened up the question of what should be done when segregation efforts fell short. In a brief piece in 1926, editor Lucy F. Lay reprinted the text of two letters that had arrived in the same morning's mail, both about feebleminded women who had "presented puzzling problems" to social workers. Both women had multiple children and were reportedly incompetent to raise them. Both had some past history with a county home or other institution, and in each case the institution seemed like an insufficient solution. Lay commented that these women's cases indicated "only a small part of the difficulties in handling those who are mentally deficient" and concluded by saying, "Just two letters out of one day's mail. What would you suggest as a solution?" Her rhetorical question reveals officials' frustration as they dealt with complex cases where poverty, mental problems, and extramarital sex were intertwined. Lay's prompt also put the burden of solving the problem on her readers. As they considered these two cases, readers might also consider the larger problem. On the very same page they were presented a solution: an article by W. H. Dixon, the new superintendent of Caswell, offered "Some Suggestions in Regard to State's Mental Defectives." Dixon advocated marriage restrictions and sterilization as preventive measures.[54]

The Board's publicity bureau also produced exhibits along the lines of the Wake family exhibit at the state fair. Another eugenics-themed exhibit took the form of a contest. At the 1926 Conference for Social Service, staff of the Division of Mental Health and Hygiene selected photographs of five girls from one institution (probably Samarcand) whom Harry Crane had tested for intelligence.[55] He decided that two were normal and three were feebleminded, and he assigned IQs to each. The staff presented each picture on a large piece of cardboard and asked conference attendees to rank the children "from brightest to dullest," based simply on their appearance. The point was to discredit "an idea that is still somewhat prevalent—that it is possible to 'pick out' a feeble-minded child by looking at him." Rather, conference-goers should understand the importance of having a mental exam done by a trained professional. This point may have been lost on the two dozen conference attendees who submitted answers to the "guessing contest," since the staff shared the answers only in *Public Welfare Progress* four months later. At that point, they reprinted the five photographs, giving readers a chance to play at home. This time, they did a better job of driving home the message that social workers should "have a mental exam made" (see figure 5.7). This print "exhibit" was later reproduced in *The Nation's Health*, indicating its popularity among readers.[56]

The Board staff frequently gave lectures, which allowed them to tailor their message to specific audiences and benefit from subsequent newspaper coverage. The Conference for Social Service, of course, regularly heard about Crane's work and conditions at Caswell. Johnson, Crane, McNairy, and others in their network talked in many other forums as well: at Rotary Club lunches, Lions Club gatherings, college orientations, women's club meetings, and conferences of teachers. They talked about family studies, eugenic marriages and the duty to marry well, the social costs of mental defects, the overflowing dorms at Caswell, and the need for a stronger sterilization law.[57] In some of these lectures, Crane used new technology to his advantage. On at least one of his regular visits to Caswell to administer psychological tests, he brought equipment to make a "moving picture" of the inmates and their surroundings. He put together a film that he used in lectures, including to a group of UNC psychology students and to a

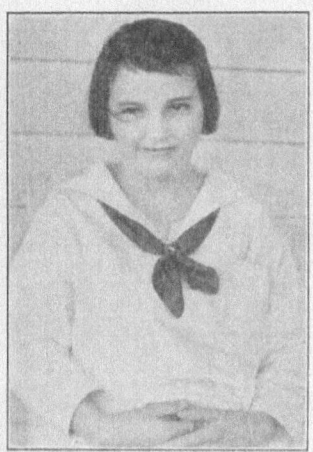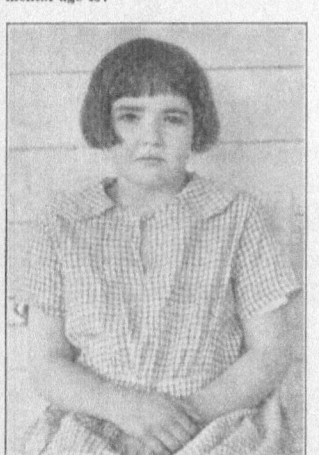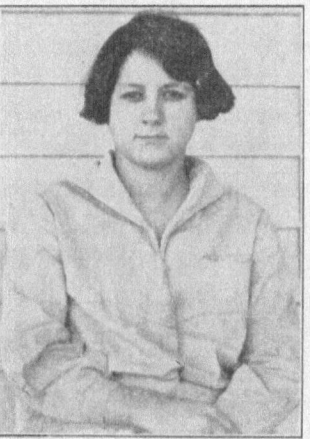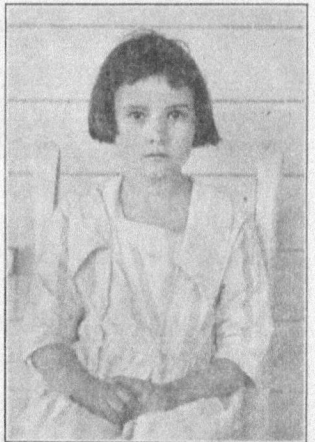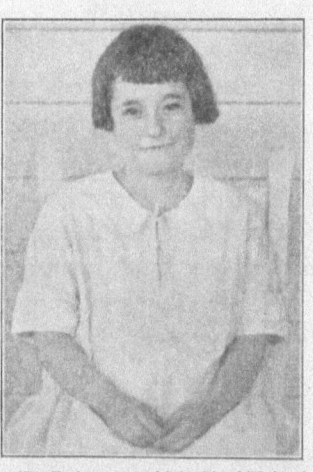

Figure 5.7 The Board used this collection of images of five young girls to illustrate the necessity of mental testing. "Which One Would You Choose for the Brightest?" *Public Welfare Progress* 7, no. 7 (July 1926): 4, North Carolina Collection, Louis Round Wilson Special Collections Library, University of North Carolina at Chapel Hill.

parent–teacher association. As he showed the film, he talked about the "nature and classification" of feeblemindedness.[58]

Seeking a "Really Effective Instrument": Attempts to Pass Sterilization Laws

By the early 1920s, there was consensus among many social welfare officials and doctors that the state needed a more effective sterilization law, and during the 1920s they tried several times to make the law more "workable." The problem, in their view, was that the sterilization law passed in 1919 in the wake of the fires at Caswell set up too many bureaucratic barriers. That law required the approval of the governor, the secretary of the state Board of Health, and a "board of consultation" comprising heads of state institutions.[59] After passing the law, the legislature did not bother to set up such a board. Historians and contemporary observers alike have assumed that because of these obstacles, the 1919 law did not lead to any sterilizations.[60]

There is some reason, however, to believe that at least a few sterilizations did take place as a result of the 1919 law, thanks to Caswell superintendent C. Banks McNairy's machinations. When the legislature did not convene a board to review cases, McNairy stepped into the vacuum. In September 1919, he gathered the heads of other institutions in Raleigh to form what he called a "State Board of Mental Hygiene," which he claimed was the official body to "confer and act" on sterilization cases before passing them on to the governor.[61] Then on April 13, 1920, at McNairy's request, the joint board of directors of all the state hospitals adopted a motion that allowed superintendents of each institution to sterilize inmates, requiring only the approval of two other physicians who examined the patient and "the State Board of Mental Hygiene, as the law directs." The motion made no mention of the law's requirement that operations be "affirmed" by the governor and the secretary of the state Board of Health.[62]

McNairy, then, had created an administrative pathway for heads of institutions to sterilize their patients with approval from only a handful of doctors. In line with national trends at the time, he hoped to sterilize and then parole inmates for whom Caswell could provide no more training. He might have also had in mind a question he raised at the April 13 meeting: what to do with a handful of male inmates who exhibited "a great deal of animalism and at times are insane and violent."[63] As the board continued its meeting the following day, they instructed McNairy to work with the superintendent of the Raleigh mental hospital to "place" two boys there temporarily "for an operation"—a necessary move because Caswell lacked surgical facilities and trained medical staff.[64] With this instruction, McNairy might have felt he had all the authority he needed to have the boys sterilized. Several months later,

McNairy reported that the boys had been moved promptly to Dix Hill, although he did not confirm that they had been sterilized.[65]

McNairy also offered at least once to have noninstitutional residents admitted temporarily for sterilization. In the fall of 1919, J. R. McCracken, the Haywood County health officer and president of the state Health Officers' Association, tried to obtain approval to castrate two troublesome white teenage boys at the county home. One of the boys had been caught several times having sex with a "mentally defective" girl. McCracken was an advocate of sterilization and other eugenics policies, and in this case he thought castration was "the best solution of the problem." In his September 1919 letter about the two boys, he tried to get the state health officer and the governor to sign off on the castration operations. His letter landed on the desk of McNairy, as the head of the semiofficial Board of Mental Hygiene. Even though the boys were not at one of the state institutions authorized to perform sterilizations, McNairy offered to have the board consider their cases. He also proposed, at least in cases of "urgent necessity," to admit "all such persons who are a menace to society" to a state institution "long enough for such treatment as may be deemed advisable." That is, McNairy wanted to admit people to institutions temporarily, for just enough time for a surgical sterilization procedure, since the law made no provision for noninstitutional sterilization. He advised McCracken to try to get the boys admitted to Caswell or the Raleigh mental hospital.[66] No record exists concerning the fate of these two Haywood County boys. Perhaps, facing bureaucratic hurdles, McCracken dropped his efforts to castrate them. Or perhaps the boys were castrated, either after being admitted to an institution or because McCracken took McNairy's willingness to bend other parts of the law as a wink and a nod toward extralegal action.

Whether or not the Haywood County boys were among them, dozens of inmates of the Raleigh mental hospital were sterilized during the 1920s, sometimes in an attempt at psychiatric treatment. Hubert Royster, one of the hospital's advisory board of surgeons, reported on the operations that he and other doctors had performed at Dix Hill between 1922 and 1932. Those surgeries included thirty-six "therapeutic sterilizations," fourteen "asexualizations," and seventy-seven hysterectomies or salpingectomies performed ostensibly for other reasons, including fibroids, ovarian cysts, pelvic inflammatory disease, or uterine prolapse.[67] Such sterilizations were not uncommon for psychiatric institutions; many medical doctors believed that sterilization would help alleviate patients' suffering. For women, the effects were thought to be social and psychological, while some doctors argued that men could be physically as well as mentally "rejuvenated" by a vasectomy.[68] In his description of the sterilizations at Dix Hill, Royster was not clear about surgeons'

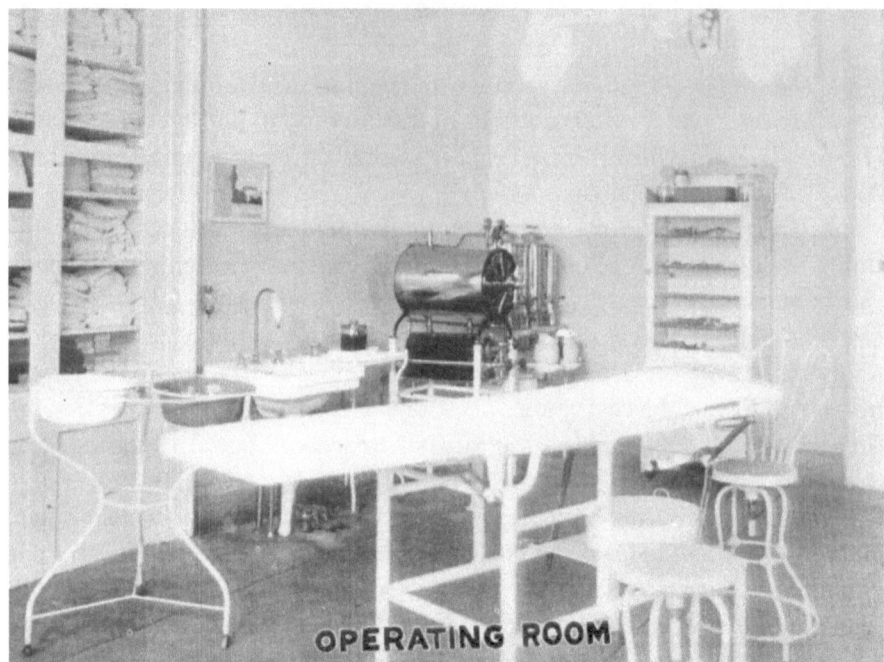

Figure 5.8 The operating room at the State Hospital at Raleigh, where institutional officials performed dozens of sterilization surgeries in the 1920s. *Report of the State Hospital for the Insane at Raleigh, N.C., 1920–22,* 22a, North Carolina Collection, Louis Round Wilson Special Collections Library, University of North Carolina at Chapel Hill.

rationales, although he did not mention the 1919 law and seemed to assume that surgeons had the right to operate on patients as part of their treatment strategy. He reported that some patients became "more cooperative" after surgery, particularly in cases such as complete uterine prolapse where they had been in physical distress. Still, Royster seemed skeptical about the necessity of all of these operations, arguing that they had minimal value as psychiatric treatment and were the result of "ambitious operators who cut into anybody who will lie still long enough."[69]

Regardless of whether any sterilizations were the direct result of the law, it was clear to McNairy and his allies that following the letter of the 1919 law was cumbersome. They continued to push for changes. In 1922 McNairy suggested that he, as superintendent, should have sole discretion in deciding when to sterilize an inmate. Commissioner Kate Burr Johnson and her staff agreed that neither the governor nor a statewide board should be involved. Unlike McNairy, however, they wanted to "provide a safeguard" to both institutions and inmates by requiring the approval of two other physicians. They included both ideas in their report to the legislature. Either plan would substantially reduce red tape and let McNairy enact plans to sterilize inmates before sending them out on "parole."[70]

In early 1923, one longtime supporter of Caswell tried to put these plans into action. John R. Baggett, a state senator from the small eastern town of Lillington, had been a trustee of Caswell since its founding in 1911 and was at the April 1920 meeting when the board of directors approved McNairy's plan for institutional heads to sterilize inmates on their own authority. In his work with Hardy, McNairy, and the other trustees, Baggett had become convinced that eugenic principles could prevent future generations of children like Caswell's inmates and save the state "a million dollars." On January 17, 1923, Baggett introduced two bills in the Senate. The first, which passed into law, rescinded the age limit at Caswell so that people over thirty could be admitted. (The legislature also appropriated $500,000 for new buildings at Caswell, although this fell short of the amount a legislative committee requested in order to expand the school's capacity to a thousand inmates.)[71] The second of Baggett's bills, which did not pass, laid out a plan for sterilization similar to Johnson's. It would have left decisions about sterilization to superintendents, trustees, and physicians of institutions, eliminating the requirement for approval of higher authorities. The Senate passed Baggett's bill and sent it to the House, where it got a favorable committee report. On February 26, however, "in a tabling mood," the House killed the sterilization bill along with several others, all "by sweeping majorities." It is not clear why the bill failed, although it might have been because some legislators objected that it did not require inmates' families to be consulted before sterilization.[72] The divergent outcomes of Baggett's two bills indicate that support for custodial institutions outstripped support for sterilization.

Undeterred by the failure of Baggett's 1923 sterilization bill, other reformers joined the chorus of state officials calling for a revised sterilization law. In his 1924 report, state psychologist Harry Crane asked the legislature to modify the 1919 sterilization law "to make it really an effective instrument for the preventing of the continuation of defective mental strains." *Public Welfare Progress* reprinted several articles, mostly from physicians, along these lines. In 1924, the white Federation of Women's Clubs went "on record as approving a workable sterilization law." Several months later, members of the state League of Women Voters passed a similar resolution at their annual convention in Raleigh, arguing that the "increase of the mentally unfit" was a "serious menace." Custodial institutions, they believed, could never be adequate to "segregate and train this class of people," and, like the Federation of Women's Clubs, they went "on record as approving a workable sterilization law."[73]

Clubwomen's interest in sterilization may have been influenced by recent legislative developments in Virginia. On a single day in March 1924,

Virginia passed two related laws, the Racial Integrity Act and the Eugenical Sterilization Act. The state's Anglo-Saxon Clubs, formed in 1922 as a genteel alternative to the Ku Klux Klan, lobbied for both, as did a small group of doctors and lawyers. The sterilization law, based on Harry Laughlin's "Model Eugenical Sterilization Law," would be upheld by the Supreme Court in *Buck v. Bell* in 1927. In 1924, North Carolina's reformers knew only that Virginia had passed a law more likely than North Carolina's to be used, since it placed sole responsibility for decisions about individual cases in the hands of special boards at each institution, with a nominal appeals process.[74]

When the legislature convened in 1925, Democratic representative James Cornelius Braswell introduced another sterilization bill. A physician and farmer, Braswell was a member of the Nash County health board and had already served two terms in the state legislature. Braswell sponsored a sterilization bill out of his belief that "if there is one immutable law of nature, it is that life begets life" and that "if some curb is not placed by the State we will have a multiplication of what we have at the school for the feeble-minded." His bill allowed heads of institutions to perform sterilizations with approval from only their boards of trustees, similar to Baggett's 1923 bill. The House sent the bill to the Senate, where the public health committee quickly returned it with a favorable report.[75]

Then, however, the end-of-session rush stymied Braswell's bill. It sat on the calendar for almost a week while the legislature plowed through its final business. On the last day of the session, as the Senate tried to move quickly through its full calendar, Braswell's sterilization bill was among those they tabled with little debate. Even given more time, however, the Senate may have killed the bill. Under the headline "Senators Horrified," one newspaper reported that "the senate would have none of it." One senator "declared that the bill was the 'most horrible' presented at the session," although he did not say why. Another later remembered his opposition as stemming from his belief that the sterilization operation would deprive its targets of sexual pleasure. This belief was not uncommon, especially since sterilization programs in some states arose from experimental programs in castrating criminals. On this topic, medical and welfare professionals often went on the offensive, arguing that sterilization operations in no way harmed patients.[76]

None of the public pushback to sterilization came from a concern about evolutionary science, although the state was in the midst of a massive debate about it. Less than a week before Braswell introduced his bill, the state was engulfed in political and religious turmoil over a bill that would have banned the teaching of evolution in public schools. North Carolina's battle over the

"Poole bill" prefigured the Scopes trial in Tennessee a few months later, a battle between fundamentalists and modernists over the very heart and soul of Christianity. Although the Poole bill failed in the House, it unleashed a firestorm of concern about Darwinism and, more generally, about what fundamentalists saw as secular modernism. Yet even fundamentalists who feared the corrupting influences of evolutionary theories apparently were unfazed by eugenics, despite its roots in distorted Darwinian theories. The House of Representatives had a knock-down, drag-out fight about the teaching of evolution, but House members easily passed Braswell's sterilization bill. And Braswell himself had voted *for* the Poole bill, thus supporting calls to end the teaching of evolution.[77]

Why did the mid-1920s religious furor over evolution apparently ignore eugenics? Perhaps this lack of concern was due to how North Carolina's reformers discussed the topic: in their depiction, eugenics depended not on a Darwinian belief in evolution but only on a belief in divinely sanctioned Mendelian processes of breeding, or even Lamarckian ideas of modification. Over the previous decade, pleas for eugenics had taken the form of religious or moral admonishments more often than scientific screeds. William Louis Poteat, the Wake Forest professor, is a telling example. In many articles and speeches, he promoted eugenics in religious terms, as the "projection of Golden Rule down the stream of protoplasm" or as part of the project of creating the ideal citizen "for the work of the Kingdom" of God. But while his liberal theology and teaching about evolution made him a target of fundamentalist attacks, his framing of eugenics in religious terms did not generate vocal dissent.[78] In any case, the swing toward fundamentalism in the 1920s did not dampen the growing support for eugenics.

"A Special Remedy": The Report on Caswell and the Problem of the Feebleminded

Despite the lack of sufficient support to pass two sterilization bills, many legislators still considered the problem of the feebleminded to merit their attention. As in 1919, Caswell Training School became a prism for officials' concern. In 1925, the Caswell board fired superintendent C. Banks McNairy amid charges of abuse and mismanagement.[79] The firing drew attention to questions of institutional management, and the Caswell board felt forced to reconsider the fundamental purpose of Caswell. Noting that Caswell's "scope" had always been in question, with disagreement about what types and ages of feebleminded people the school should admit, Governor Angus W. MacLean created a committee to study Caswell and "its relation to the problem of the feebleminded." To head the committee, he appointed Watson Smith

Rankin, the outgoing state health officer and one of the founders of the Conference for Social Service. The committee included two other doctors, the state superintendent of public instruction, and business and professional leaders.[80]

The committee studied the issue for almost a year and ultimately recommended greater use of sterilization. Rankin assigned them over one hundred hours of reading—their final report included a bibliography—and members met with welfare officials Kate Burr Johnson, Harry Crane, and Emeth Tuttle to hear their expert opinions. The committee also consulted with specialists outside the state, including several authorities from New York. The final report, released to the public in September 1926, surveyed "the latest findings" about feeblemindedness and treatment approaches. Rankin seems to have written the main body of the report, with lawyer James O. Carr of Wilmington contributing a section on existing legal provisions for "dealing with the feebleminded in North Carolina." The committee made seven policy recommendations, including increasing Caswell's capacity from around four hundred to two thousand and creating special classes within the public school system for children who were slightly "retarded in mental development," which might ease the pressure on Caswell. But the major recommendation, according to the *Greensboro Record*, was "legislation permitting sterilization in certain cases." Like McNairy and Johnson, the committee recommended loosening the restrictions on sterilization set forth in the 1919 law: institutional heads should get approval from the heads of the state health and welfare boards, but not the governor.[81]

At the same time, the committee argued that "sterilization cannot be considered as of any value as a *general* remedy for the problem of feeblemindedness," although it was valuable "as a special remedy for certain individual cases." This new note of caution was the product of recent studies that questioned assumptions about the heritability of feeblemindedness. The committee pinpointed a shift in expert opinion around 1920, after which some specialists argued that feeblemindedness was a product of heredity only half the time, compared to earlier estimates of around 90 percent.[82] Moreover, experts began to regard feeblemindedness not as a single, inheritable trait with a biological definition, but as a legal or sociological term that could encompass multiple combinations of traits and a variety of conditions. Rankin recognized that "the problem is a vastly more complex one than the popular heredity chart of not long ago made it."[83] North Carolina's committee concluded not only that it would be impossible to sterilize everyone who exhibited signs of feeblemindedness, but also that this plan would fail to stem feeblemindedness. To them, large-scale sterilization efforts were not the solution.

Despite revising their ideas about the causes of feeblemindedness, the committee followed national leaders in continuing to fear the unrestricted reproduction of feebleminded people, whatever the genesis of their condition. While the issue was far more complicated than black-and-white boxes on a family chart, the crux of the problem remained selecting people whose sterilization would have the greatest impact. The committee estimated that 2 percent of the population, or 55,000 people in North Carolina, were feebleminded. They commented sardonically that most of these people "blended with [the population] so completely that it would be most enlightening if those who prescribe sterilization would accompany their prescriptions, like a careful and wise physician, with directions for taking."[84] That is, how were state officials to determine who should be sterilized?

The committee's policy recommendations indicate that they believed heads of the state's prisons, hospitals, and Caswell were the best judges of candidates of sterilization. Despite their reservations about the value of sterilization as a "general remedy," their plan would have cleared legal and logistical barriers between institutional heads and quick sterilizations. Their guideline was that the decision to sterilize should be "in the interest of the general welfare," language that actually eliminated the 1919 law's insistence that sterilization be for the mental, moral, or physical improvement of the patient.[85]

This discrepancy between theory and policy marks a transitional moment. By 1926, some medical professionals questioned the scientific legitimacy and efficacy of eugenic sterilization, but the wider public, including many doctors, continued to see sterilization and other eugenic measures as useful tools of social policy, thanks in part to the success of welfare officials in painting mental defect as a social problem and eugenics as the solution. The committee's report itself mirrors this divide between theory and policy. The main body of the report, probably written by Watson Smith Rankin, grappled with medical professionals' new, more cautious views. Lawyer James Carr's contributions on the "relation of the problem of feeblemindedness to the courts," on the other hand, focused on the phrase in Caswell's charter about its duty to work toward the "ultimate eradication" of mental deficiency. For Carr, "no responsibility resting on the school is greater than this." The problem was complicated, he argued, by the fact that some training was a dangerous thing; when Caswell students with some training were turned "out on society," "we are sending out into the world a somewhat improved human being, whose power and tendency to reproduce his kind is as great, if not even greater, than if he had never been admitted to these institutions." Carr believed the state needed "more drastic methods than any now proposed by the law" in order to eradicate feeblemindedness.[86] Carr and other members of this committee, fully exposed to up-to-date medical views that were skeptical of sterilization as a fix-all solution for feeblemindedness, were also immersed in social views that, in the end, trumped scientific caution.

The 1927 Supreme Court decision in *Buck v. Bell* signaled the triumph of this line of thought. The court's decision affirmed the legality of Virginia's 1924 sterilization statute, with Justice Oliver Wendell Holmes's now infamous declaration that "three generations of imbeciles are enough." The nation took note. Virginia's law had been based on the Eugenics Record Office's model statute, which was designed to pass tests of constitutionality. *Buck v. Bell* lit a clear path forward through the dark maze of legal questions, and interest in passing state sterilization laws, already growing in the mid-1920s, reached new heights. In North Carolina, Commissioner Kate Burr Johnson called the decision "most significant." She contrasted Virginia's statute with North's Carolina's law, which was "barely if ever enforced" because it was "not workable." She lamented the futility of the welfare board's repeated efforts to get the legislature to "untie some of this red tape." But she was hopeful: she felt that the Supreme Court decision had "greatly strengthened" the Board's position that sterilization was "the only way" to reduce the "crop of mental defectives."[87]

Legislative Success: Millner's 1929 Bill

Calls for a "more workable sterilization law" finally came to fruition in 1929. Although various groups had lobbied intermittently during the previous decade, none of these groups played a decisive role in the passage of the 1929 law. The proximate cause was neither the Conference for Social Service, the Federation of Women's Clubs, nor a medical society. Still, their years of lobbying laid the groundwork for the easy passage of the bill. The influence of this network of pro-eugenics activists is manifest in the discussion of the bill as well as the career of the legislator who ultimately sponsored it.

That man was Republican Henry L. Millner, a New York native and a first-time legislator in 1929. His long career as a civil engineer had taken him to Europe and Australia, but by 1917 he had settled in Morganton. There he ran an electrical company, attended a Methodist church, and became involved in local politics. Millner's long tenure on the Burke County welfare board, from 1919 to 1933, indicates his commitment to welfare. In many years on the board, he would also have learned about state officials' theories through monthly copies of *Public Welfare Progress* and through correspondence with state officials. He was particularly interested in studying the problem of how to protect society from the "mentally defective."[88] In addition, Millner may have had a personal connection with Commissioner Kate Burr Johnson, since Johnson had deep family ties to Morganton.[89]

On January 21, 1929, Millner introduced a bill "to provide for the sterilization of the mentally defective and feeble-minded inmates of charitable and penal institutions of the State of North Carolina." The basic intent of the bill was the same as the 1919 law, but it granted institutional heads the leeway McNairy had requested in the past.[90] Instead of requiring the signature of the governor, sterilizations required approval from a group of professionals: the commissioner of public welfare, the secretary of the state Board of Health, and the chief medical officers of two institutions for the feebleminded or insane. In addition, the bill specified that no one could be held criminally or civilly liable for performing sterilizations in accordance with the law. Finally, Millner's plans opened the possibility of sterilization for men and women who were not housed in institutions. In those cases, when relatives or legal guardians petitioned for the sterilization of feebleminded or mentally defective people who were not institutionalized, a panel of four reviewers would sign off on the case, and county commissioners would pay for the operation.[91] In making the case for the bill, Millner pointed to California, Delaware, and Pennsylvania's "successful" sterilization laws.[92]

The Senate debate and eventual unanimous approval demonstrate the success of reformers' campaigns to educate the public about eugenics as "in line with advanced thought of the day." After a favorable report from the committee on public welfare, of which Millner was a member, the almost singular voice of opposition belonged to Democratic Senator Thomas Coleman Galloway, a lawyer and Baptist from Brevard. Galloway believed the bill allowed "a practice that had been tried and proven false by Asiatics in the days of eunuchs." Thomas Lester Johnson, who had *opposed* the 1925 sterilization bill, stepped in to defend the bill, explaining that based on his conversations with "doctors and welfare experts," he understood that "the bill would not deprive the sterilized person of sex life, only stopping possible propagation."[93] The only other objection reported in the News and Observer came from William Grimes Clark of Edgecombe. Clark, perhaps concerned about abuse of the bill's provisions, moved to send it to the committee on public health for further review. He withdrew his motion when he learned that state health officials had already approved of the bill in an appearance before the public welfare committee.[94]

A far larger number of senators took the floor to urge passage of the bill, without reservations. Millner spoke first, reminding the senators of Governor Gardner's "plea for pure bred seed and pure bred stock in this State," and arguing that "North Carolina also needed better bred people." Other supporters' backgrounds reaffirm the influence of medical and welfare professionals in directly or indirectly assuring the bill's success. The Senate's only physician, Henry B. Ivey, emphasized the difference between sterilization and castration and argued that sterilization was a safe, simple operation with no effects on "natural desires." Other vocal proponents included Democrats John T. Alderman of Vance County, Lloyd L. Gravely of Nash County, and Marvin K. Blount of Pitt County, all three members of the committee on public welfare that had reported favorably on the bill. Their committee assignment meant they had heard the pro-sterilization testimony of state health officer Charles Laughinghouse and perhaps read recent pro-eugenics publications of the state welfare board.[95]

But just as the House took up the bill, a veteran of the state's welfare office intervened to denounce the whole affair in the Raleigh *News and Observer*. According to former Commissioner Roland F. Beasley, who had returned to his North Carolina newspaper career after working for an oil company in Texas, the bill was "foolish" and "not worth the paper that it is written on." The 1919 sterilization law was useless, he charged, and a new law would be no better, serving only to "further clutter up the statute books." People already segregated in institutions would not reproduce, and so many thousands of feebleminded people lived outside institutions that authorities could never hope to sterilize them all. Moreover, Beasley quoted the superintendent of one of the nation's largest mental institutions to argue that caring for "dependents" was a social responsibility whose fulfillment resulted in "a better and more humane society." According to this logic, eliminating the feebleminded, criminals, or the insane would deprive society of an opportunity for humanitarian action and moral development. Beasley thus objected to sterilization on both scientific and moral grounds, but his most damning conclusion was simply that the magnitude of the problem of feeblemindedness made sterilization futile.[96]

Beasley's objections made no impression in the House. After a favorable report from the committee on public welfare and explanations of the bill's "safeguards," there was no real opposition. The assembly suspended the rules to push the bill through almost immediately on Saturday, February 16, with the only protests (from Republican representatives) focused on procedural matters, not the bill's substance. Newspapers reported that the bill for "cutting off racial defectives before their conception" "had a walk-over and nobody thought to take a record vote." The tone of that day's proceedings was indecorous, even playful, as legislators "made mighty merry over the bill." With low attendance and empty lobbies, the lawmakers "took the fiercest joy in razzing each other." The next item on the agenda was debate about a federal highway system, during which the House adopted a satirical amendment that "the U.S. government shall in conjunction with the celestial powers construct a system of highways connecting the sun and planets, and all the stars of the universe."[97] Two days later, on February 18, 1929, the sterilization bill became law.[98]

The passage of a second sterilization law in 1929 was the product of pro-eugenic activists' persistence. For over two decades, medical and social welfare professionals and Progressive reformers had discussed principles of eugenics and debated possible policies. During the 1920s, Crane and his allies worked to provide evidence of supposedly rampant mental defects and the horrifying social costs of cacogenic families. State welfare officials and their allies, in turn, spent years educating the public about these problems at state fairs, in classes, and in club meetings. Although in 1923 and 1925 sterilization lacked enough supporters, the debates over these bills allowed advocates of sterilization in the legislature chances to break down opposition among their colleagues through exposure to the gospel of eugenics or emphasis on the financial costs of feeblemindedness. By 1929—in the wake of *Buck v. Bell* and renewed calls for sterilization from Rankin's committee—little opposition surfaced. The 1929 law seemed, to reformers, to be the "workable" law they had been seeking, one they hoped would finally allow them to eradicate feeblemindedness and mental illness.

On a national level, one aspect of North Carolina's new law drew particular attention. Sterilization laws in other states allowed institutional officials to operate on their inmates. North Carolina's law went further in allowing noninstitutional residents to be sterilized. The Eugenics Record Office's *Eugenical News* praised this "unique feature" of allowing operations on noninmates as one that must be developed in other states if sterilization was truly to work. The editors of *Eugenical News* framed North Carolina's law as part of the "gradual [improvement] in the newer sterilization statutes."[99]

Of course, most of North Carolina's reformers cared little about whether they pleased national eugenics organizations. Fervent champions of eugenic sterilization—McNairy, Johnson, and a few other well-placed allies—were the exception rather than the rule. Rather, most reformers' and legislators' willingness to accept sterilization grew out of the past two decades of debate about social problems in their state and reformers' long education in the language and principles of eugenics. In the 1920s, advocates of sterilization painted compelling portraits of problems that most white North Carolinians cared about—widespread poverty, racial mixing, and other problems highlighted so effectively in the welfare board's publicity efforts about cacogenic families. They promised that eugenic sterilization could erase all these problems. And by 1929, they had convinced a critical mass of believers.

Chapter 6

Brewer v. Valk

   Legal Strategies in Addressing Female Delinquency and Feeblemindedness

In 1920, a sixteen-year-old white girl named Mary left her parents' home to marry June Brewer, an older white man who picked up work as a waiter, painter, or factory hand. Settling in Winston-Salem, the couple struggled to make ends meet as their family grew. Soon after their first child was born they began to receive help from local charities. As the family became more desperate, they and their five children also drew negative attention from social workers for begging in the streets, disturbing the neighborhood, and the children's behavior at school. By 1932, when Mary was twenty-eight, local authorities had taken away all five children and decided that Mary should be sterilized under the eugenic sterilization law passed in 1929. When Winston-Salem officials ordered her sterilization in August 1932, county welfare superintendents and institutional officials across the state had already sterilized over forty people.

But unlike these other people, Mary Brewer became both a plaintiff and a pawn in a state Supreme Court case, *Brewer v. Valk*. The decision in this case overturned the 1929 sterilization law and paved the way for the passage of a new sterilization law in 1933, the creation of the Eugenics Board, and four decades of well-organized, state-sponsored sterilization. This case is thus pivotal in the development of North Carolina's eugenics programs. Other accounts of *Brewer v. Valk* characterize it as a straightforward case of a wronged woman seeking to protect her rights, but the remaining evidence suggests that the case is far more complex.[1] *Brewer v. Valk* was a conspiracy—the product of a group of political elites attempting to save a law that they suspected was unconstitutional by reframing it before it could be challenged, and doing so on their own terms. By 1932, a group of welfare officials, medical doctors, and lawyers had realized that the 1929 law had inadequate protections for due process. Worried about this weakness, they wanted to improve the law before it could be overturned. Their challenge was not a response to grassroots concerns about equal protection, but an attempt to create a more efficient system of sterilization. To do so, they manipulated the court system, a foundational institution in American democracy. The case bears remarkable similarity to *Buck v. Bell*, the infamous 1927 Supreme Court case that condoned sterilization in

Virginia: in both, lawyers for plaintiff and defense colluded to create a test case that left untouched the core principles of the sterilization program.

The case also allows us to examine the development of eugenics policy as the Great Depression enveloped the country. To the extent that social workers saw Brewer as an ideal target of sterilization, her case reveals social workers' continuing association of white poverty with feeblemindedness and their willing use of eugenics-based policies to address social problems. As poverty, hunger, and social unrest grew in the 1930s, social workers did not reexamine their assumptions about the root causes of social dysfunction. Rather, they continued to choose hereditarian explanations even though many of these problems were caused or exacerbated by economic forces beyond individual control. The story of Mary Brewer highlights the limits of the state's vision of welfare, and the consequences for people whom officials saw as unfit, on the cusp of the New Deal.

"The Practical Application of the Law": Sterilization in the Great Depression, 1929–1933

In 1929, the Great Depression engulfed the country and revealed the weakness inherent in a decentralized welfare system: the response to widespread economic ravages was in the hands of local officials who relied on small revenues to fund county welfare programs. Coming after a series of agricultural crises, the Depression had particularly crippling effects on the South's farmers and rural areas. North Carolina started the Depression ranked forty-fifth in the nation in per capita income, and farmers could only watch as crop prices dropped. Prices for tobacco, the major crop in the eastern half of the state, dropped from a norm of 20 cents a pound to a low of 8.4 cents in 1931. In one county dominated by tobacco growing, two-thirds of farms were foreclosed in 1930. North Carolina's light industry, particularly cigarette production, mitigated some of the shocks, but by December 1930 as many as 70,000 wage earners were unemployed—in a state with 209,000 industrial workers at the time of the crash. A study in 1929–30 found that of 140,000 school children examined, 23,000 were malnourished. Local governments' inability to collect property taxes even led thirty-four counties and towns to default. As farmers lost their land and children went hungry, the traditional sources of support—local relief budgets and charity organizations—were quickly overwhelmed by demand.[2]

The state's initial response was paltry. After advocating a "live-at-home" program whose main focus was encouraging farmers to grow food crops instead of cash crops, Governor O. Max Gardner appointed a thirteen-member Council on Unemployment and Relief in December 1930. The governor's council used the State Emergency Fund to pay Board of Charities and Public Welfare staff to coordinate relief efforts in eighty-two counties. They organized local councils, which mobilized civic and religious groups to provide free food and clothing for children, temporary sleeping quarters, and sometimes free medical care. But relief funds themselves still came from their usual source, namely county funds set aside for "outdoor relief," augmented in some urban areas by Associated Charities or other private funds. While the county-unit system increased officials' ability to train social workers and oversee social services, the state welfare board's charter did not include direct distribution of relief, which remained the domain of local boards. The state legislature spent no money on unemployment relief. Likewise, the state welfare board provided little direct assistance to the indigent and unemployed. The state provided direct assistance only to a select few families through the Mother's Aid program, which attempted to support "worthy" mothers, and starting in 1929 also provided emergency funds to needy families of prisoners.[3]

As the Depression took hold and state welfare officials tried to help organize local relief efforts, they were also implementing the new sterilization law, passed in February 1929. The major responsibility fell to R. Eugene Brown. Brown was a graduate of UNC, where he had worked with Odum's Institute for Research in the Social Sciences. He then worked for the state Salary and Wage Commission until 1925, when he joined the Board of Charities and Public Welfare. He led the Division of Institutions, which had constitutional authority to "investigate and supervise" charitable and penal institutions. When the sterilization law was passed, Brown and his two staff members took on the responsibility of facilitating the process. They created a petition form to collect information the law required about the person's medical and family history (see figure 6.1). They received petitions from institutional heads, county officials, or families, then distributed the petitions to a board composed of the heads the state welfare and health boards and the chief medical officers of two state institutions. Assuming the board approved the case, staff notified the proper authorities that the sterilization could proceed, and they recorded key statistics about the cases. They worked closely with the Division of Mental Health and Hygiene, which actually got increased funding in 1931 to hire an assistant psychologist and part-time fieldworker, allowing them to triple the number of examinations they did (and to increase their index card collection by 64 percent).[4] Even in the midst of the Depression, the legislature apparently saw value in offering mental testing services and educating the state about mental defects.

Brown, Johnson, and their colleagues in the state welfare office wanted county social workers to use the new sterilization law, and they started an educational campaign to spread awareness about it, building on the past

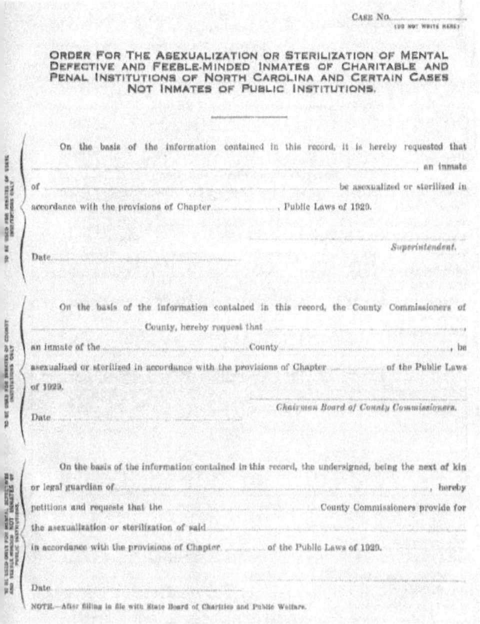

Case No. ____ (DO NOT WRITE HERE)

ORDER FOR THE ASEXUALIZATION OR STERILIZATION OF MENTAL DEFECTIVE AND FEEBLE-MINDED INMATES OF CHARITABLE AND PENAL INSTITUTIONS OF NORTH CAROLINA AND CERTAIN CASES NOT INMATES OF PUBLIC INSTITUTIONS.

On the basis of the information contained in this record, it is hereby requested that ____, an inmate of ____ be asexualized or sterilized in accordance with the provisions of Chapter ____, Public Laws of 1929.

____ *Superintendent.*

Date ____

On the basis of the information contained in this record, the County Commissioners of ____ County, hereby request that ____, an inmate of the ____ County ____, be asexualized or sterilized in accordance with the provisions of Chapter ____ of the Public Laws of 1929.

____ *Chairman Board of County Commissioners.*

Date ____

On the basis of the information contained in this record, the undersigned, being the next of kin or legal guardian of ____, hereby petitions and requests that the ____ County Commissioners provide for the asexualization or sterilization of said ____ in accordance with the provisions of Chapter ____ of the Public Laws of 1929.

Date ____

NOTE.—After filling in file with State Board of Charities and Public Welfare.

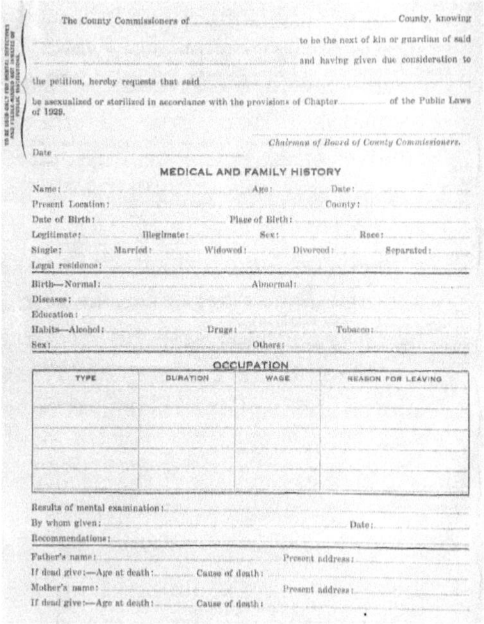

The County Commissioners of ____ County, knowing ____ to be the next of kin or guardian of said ____ and having given due consideration to the petition, hereby requests that said ____ be asexualized or sterilized in accordance with the provisions of Chapter ____ of the Public Laws of 1929.

____ *Chairman of Board of County Commissioners.*

Date ____

MEDICAL AND FAMILY HISTORY

Name: ____ Age: ____ Date: ____
Present Location: ____ County: ____
Date of Birth: ____ Place of Birth: ____
Legitimate: ____ Illegimate: ____ Sex: ____ Race: ____
Single: ____ Married: ____ Widowed: ____ Divorced: ____ Separated: ____
Legal residence: ____
Birth—Normal: ____ Abnormal: ____
Diseases: ____
Education: ____
Habits—Alcohol: ____ Drugs: ____ Tobacco: ____
Sex: ____ Others: ____

OCCUPATION

TYPE	DURATION	WAGE	REASON FOR LEAVING

Results of mental examination: ____
By whom given: ____ Date: ____
Recommendations: ____
Father's name: ____ Present address: ____
If dead give:—Age at death: ____ Cause of death: ____
Mother's name: ____ Present address: ____
If dead give:—Age at death: ____ Cause of death: ____

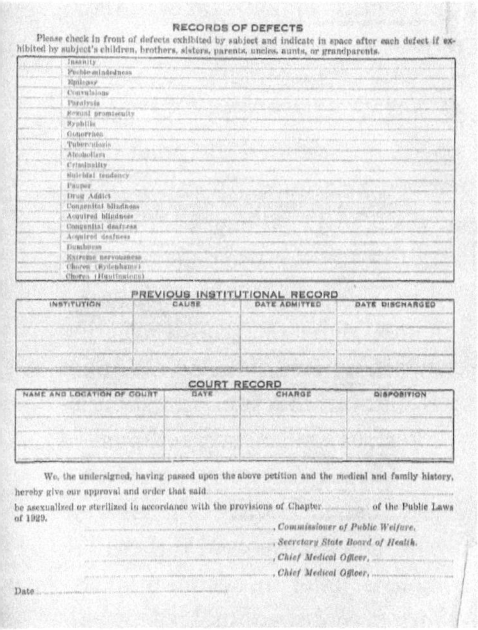

RECORDS OF DEFECTS

Please check in front of defects exhibited by subject and indicate in space after each defect if exhibited by subject's children, brothers, sisters, parents, uncles, aunts, or grandparents.

	Insanity	
	Feeble-mindedness	
	Epilepsy	
	Convulsions	
	Paralysis	
	Sexual promiscuity	
	Syphilis	
	Gonorrhea	
	Tuberculosis	
	Alcoholism	
	Criminality	
	Suicidal tendency	
	Pauper	
	Drug Addict	
	Congenital blindness	
	Acquired blindness	
	Congenital deafness	
	Acquired deafness	
	Dumbness	
	Extreme nervousness	
	Chorea (Sydenhams)	
	Chorea (Huntingtons)	

PREVIOUS INSTITUTIONAL RECORD

INSTITUTION	CAUSE	DATE ADMITTED	DATE DISCHARGED

COURT RECORD

NAME AND LOCATION OF COURT	DATE	CHARGE	DISPOSITION

We, the undersigned, having passed upon the above petition and the medical and family history, hereby give our approval and order that said ____ be asexualized or sterilized in accordance with the provisions of Chapter ____ of the Public Laws of 1929.

____, *Commissioner of Public Welfare.*
____, *Secretary State Board of Health.*
____, *Chief Medical Officer,* ____
____, *Chief Medical Officer,* ____

Date ____

Figure 6.1 Excerpt of a blank form for officials to record rationales and approval for sterilization under the 1929 law. "Order for the Asexualization or Sterilization of Mental Defective and Feeble-Minded Inmates of Charitable and Penal Institutions of North Carolina and Certain Cases Not Inmates of Public Institutions," in "Documents Concerning Amendments of N.C. Public Laws of 1929," chapter 34: "Sterilization of Persons Mentally Defective." This image is in the custody of the Kathrine R. Everett Law Library Rare Book Collection at the University of North Carolina School of Law, Chapel Hill, North Carolina.

decade's campaigns about feeblemindedness.[5] As soon as the law was passed, they used the front page of *Public Welfare Progress* to proclaim, "State Adopts Usable Law for Sterilization of Defectives." Here and in other messages, they framed sterilization in social rather than purely hereditarian terms, as a "'preventive' measure that will lighten the burden of the socially useless." State psychologist Harry Crane argued that the goal was not to create a superior type but to prevent the procreation of "one particularly undesirable type," such as feebleminded residents of county homes who had lots of illegitimate children. State officials sought to educate social workers about how to recognize feeblemindedness, underscored the importance of mental testing, argued for the importance of "eugenical social work" as part of broader social reform efforts, and explained sterilization procedures, such as how to request blank case forms.[6]

The messages about the need for sterilization at one session in 1929 were typical. In the wake of the new law, the Board put a special emphasis on mental hygiene in that year's summer training institute; the 125 attendees spent half a week learning about mental hygiene. In response to multiple requests for information from county superintendents, the state board arranged to have Raleigh surgeon Hubert Royster discuss "the practical application of the law." Royster, who had performed most of the surgeries at the Raleigh mental hospital for the last decade, told welfare workers that "the problem is to eradicate poor inheritance to start with. We must not breed from our worst." Aware that sterilization was not universally accepted, he defended the practice on several counts. It was not a radical new practice, he argued. Over half of the states in the country had sterilization laws, with most challenges arising not because of a law's intent but because of its wording. Royster also defended sterilization as a better alternative than institutional segregation, which he argued was "a more serious deprivation of individual rights than the destruction of reproductive powers." The Board published a summary of his points under the title "Sterilization Is a Way of Guiding Evolution" in a subsequent bulletin, so they reached all the state's welfare workers, as well as several thousand other subscribers.[7]

As Royster's defense of sterilization indicates, some county officials were reluctant to use the law, most often because of the cost involved rather than because of ethical concerns. The Board tried to counter this economic concern directly. In one edition of *Public Welfare Progress*, editor Lisbeth Parrott used the case of a woman whom she labeled "feebleminded, a pauper, an inmate of a county home," and "abnormally sexed, practicing incest and miscegenation." She included a blurry photograph (see figure 6.2). Welfare officials had long made the case that eugenics programs would ultimately save money by preventing the birth of "additional defective offspring [who] would

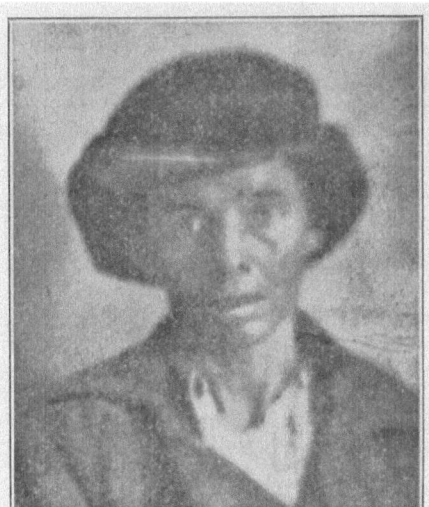

Figure 6.2 In this photograph and accompanying text published in their monthly bulletin, welfare officials made a case that sterilizations operations would ultimately save money. "$100 Now vs. Thousands for Future Care!" *Public Welfare Progress* 11, no. 1 (January 1930): 2, North Carolina Collection, Louis Round Wilson Special Collections Library, University of North Carolina at Chapel Hill.

$100 NOW VS. THOUSANDS FOR FUTURE CARE!

The woman above is the mother of two little boys, both feebleminded.

One child is the son of his mother's father. The other is the child of a county home inmate.

Their mother is feebleminded, a pauper, an inmate of a county home. She is abnormally sexed, practicing incest and miscegenation. It is difficult to restrain her from indulging in sexual promiscuity with male inmates at the county home.

An application is now being made to have this woman sterilized so that she will not produce any more children.

The operation will probably cost around $100.

Is it not worth this small investment now to prevent additional defective offspring that would be burdens to the state during their generation and that would carry the defective strain into the bloodstream of the future?

$100 Now Vs. Thousands for Future Care!

be burdens to the state ... and would carry the defective strain into the bloodstreams of the future." Parrott used a similar logic as she ridiculed any county official who would refuse to come up with the $100 for a sterilization operation in a case like this. In a tone echoing one of the new advertising firms springing up around the country, Parrott's headline argued for "$100 Now vs. Thousands for Future Care!" From the perspective of county officials, however, $100 was a large investment. At the time, a mother lucky enough to get Mothers' Aid from the state could expect eighteen to twenty dollars to support herself and four children for a month, on average.[8]

Table 6.1 Sterilization operations by year, location, and type of operation, 1929–32

Year	Location	Male (vasectomy)	Male (castration)	Female (salpingectomy)	Female (ovariectomy)	Total
1929	State institution	—	—	—	—	3
	County home	—	1	—	1	
	Noninstitutional	1	—	—	—	
1930	State institution	—	1	4	4	17
	County home	—	1	2	—	
	Noninstitutional	—	—	4	1	
1931	State institution	—	—	3	—	11
	County home	—	—	3	1	
	Noninstitutional	—	—	4	—	
1932	State institution	—	9	5	1	18
	County home	—	—	—	—	
	Noninstitutional	—	—	2	1	
Total		1	12	27	9	49

Source: Information compiled from several sets of statistics that refer to different time periods, each with slightly different information. See R. Eugene Brown, "Sterilization Law Is Being Used," *Public Welfare Progress* 11, no. 4 (April 1930): 5; *BCPW Report, 1930–32*, 76; Brown, *Eugenical Sterilization in North Carolina* (1935), 13, 16–20; and *First Biennial Report of the Eugenics Board, 1934–36*, 13–15.

In the first four years of the program, the state sterilized forty-nine people (see table 6.1). In this same time period, the state reviewed at least seventy-one cases, denying at least sixteen sterilization petitions for unspecified reasons and approving at least six petitions for which the operation did not happen. Often there was a backlog between cases approved and operations performed, because of the number of parties involved in administering cases. Brown received the first sterilization case in August 1929. By December the state board had received and approved five more cases, but they had not gotten confirmation that any of the operations had actually taken place. One year after the law was passed, twenty-one cases had been approved but only fourteen sterilizations performed.[9]

Spotty surviving records make it difficult to trace particulars about the people sterilized, but published aggregate statistics provide some insight into the state's aims. Although various tallies conflict in some details, some consistent patterns nevertheless emerge about the people who were sterilized. Almost all of the people sterilized were diagnosed as feebleminded, sometimes in addition to problems like psychosis or epilepsy. All twenty-one of the people sterilized in the program's first year were reported to be "sexually promiscuous." About three-quarters were women, and three-quarters were white. Just over half were residents of state institutions, and the rest were evenly split between residing in county homes and on their own, in eleven counties. Most were unmarried, but about half of the women were already mothers, including one white woman whom officials noted had given birth to a child with a Black father (signaling, to them, that she was feebleminded). Some were teenagers, as young as fourteen, and at least one girl who had her ovaries removed lived in an orphanage. At least six were Black men or boys who were castrated at the state mental hospital for African Americans at Goldsboro.[10]

One early case drew attention from the press and allows a fuller picture of the state's typical targets, although key information is still missing. First reported in *Public Welfare Progress* in November 1929 under the heading "Let's Use the Law" and picked up by the *Winston-Salem Journal*, the story functioned as a cautionary tale and highlighted what state officials saw as an opportunity to redress past failures. At the center of the story were a white husband and wife, both reportedly feebleminded. The husband had been an inmate at the Macon County poorhouse before he ran away to marry his wife, who was several decades his junior. Still "public charges," they lived in dire poverty in a one-room "mountain hovel" with their four children. The father could not find work at the local sawmill, and when a field agent from the state board found them, all six were "huddled in rags" in a "room indescribably filthy," two corners occupied by "broken down beds with filthy bedclothes."[11]

Lois Dosher, the field agent, tried to convince the county commissioners to have the couple sterilized, and the *Winston-Salem Journal* reported that "the first sterilization under the Millner sterilization law ... will take place soon" if they accepted her recommendation. In addition to sterilizing both parents "so that they cannot bring any more useless progeny into the world," Dosher proposed sending two of the children to Caswell and the oldest, only eight years old, to the ward for epileptics at the state hospital for the insane in Raleigh. The Board opined that "cases like this show that North Carolina was wise in passing the Millner sterilization law. No effort to put this law into effect should be spared if it means that this low grade of human stock will not be allowed to multiply."[12]

Fires at Samarcand: White Female Delinquency and Feeblemindedness

As welfare officials began to use the sterilization law, a high-stakes arson trial drew public attention to the intersection of female delinquency, sexual deviance, and feeblemindedness. The trial, which focused on sixteen white teenage inmates at Samarcand, is a revealing snapshot of the public's conflicted feelings about the role of state institutions, the exact nature of feeblemindedness,

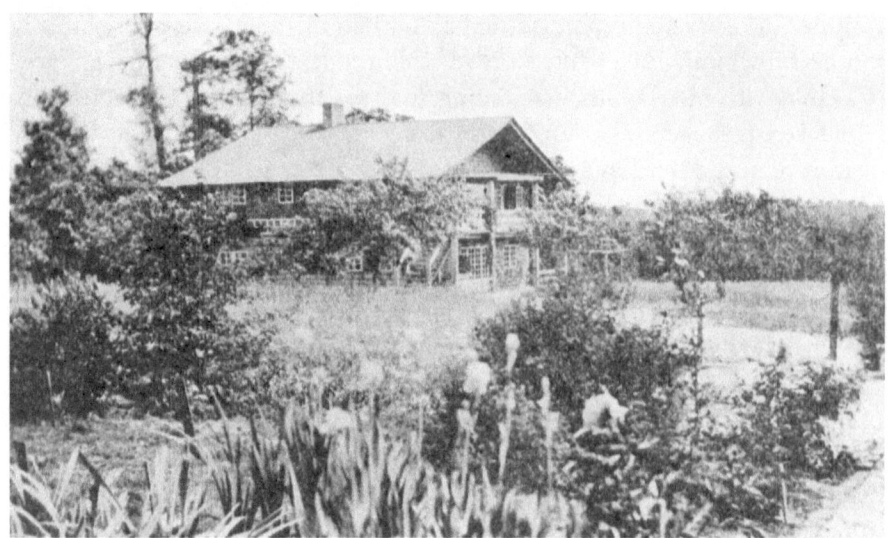

Figure 6.3 A photograph of a residential "cottage" at Samarcand Manor, where state officials hoped the girls would learn the value of "wholesomeness and honesty." *BCPW Bulletin* 1, no. 3 (July–September 1918): 3, 16, North Carolina Collection, Louis Round Wilson Special Collections Library, University of North Carolina at Chapel Hill.

and changing sexual norms for white teenagers. At the same time, the ultimate outcomes show that by 1931, public sentiment mattered less than the legal powers already bestowed on state officials to decide the fate of the sixteen girls.[13]

By 1931, Samarcand had been open for a decade under the supervision of the original superintendent, Agnes MacNaughton. The institution usually had about 215 residents, mostly working-class girls there on charges of vagrancy or immorality. Most were committed for at least a year, but the institution could keep them for up to three years. While there, the girls received a minimum amount of schooling but a great deal of "vocational training," since their labor doing laundry or cleaning helped the institution to function. An "honor" system rewarded the most compliant girls with privileges like field day, white dresses, and residence in the "honor cottage." Girls who talked back or tried to escape were punished with relegation to a "disciplinary cottage," solitary confinement, or whippings at the hands of staff or even peers.[14]

To the outside world, Samarcand continued to present itself as a benevolent home where mother-like figures redeemed white girls from degradation, as its founders had intended (see figure 6.3). Yet in painting this picture, officials were actively trying to counter the "popular impression" that the school was "a social sink full of scarlet women"—an idea linked in part to the school's origins in the anti-vice campaigns of World War I. In 1931, roughly a third of girls at the school had some kind of venereal disease, but the public thought the number was much higher.[15]

On March 12, 1931, a group of girls set fire to two dorms. In the immediate aftermath of the fire, Samarcand's staff questioned them and got some to confess. The girls were taken to local jails, where some acted "like raving maniacs." They smashed windows, ran around "perfectly nude," lit their beds on fire, and attacked firefighters who came to rescue them. According to the girls, they had been promised a chance to listen to the Victrola and dance, and they thought a fire would at least bring someone to them. Although the girls got some sympathetic newspaper coverage, a grand jury charged the girls with arson, a capital crime in North Carolina. Most of them were juveniles, but angry legislators passed a special bill to remove their juvenile status and allow prosecution as adults.[16]

The girls soon had a champion. Nell Battle Lewis, a career journalist who had worked as the state welfare board's publicity agent in the 1920s, had recently gotten a law degree and opened her own law practice in Raleigh. The case immediately captured her attention. She had long been interested in questions of women's rights, penal reform, and teenage delinquency, having covered these topics in her weekly column for the *News and Observer* and in articles she wrote for *Public Welfare Progress*. She described herself as "very favorably disposed" toward Samarcand. She had even written a glowing feature about the institution in 1926 that praised it as one of the state's best-run institutions and described its pervasive "good spirit" and the "well-mannered, nice-looking little girls."[17]

At the request of someone who knew one of the girls, Lewis took on arguments for the girls' legal defense.[18] Lewis met with the girls, and her interviews pushed her toward a two-pronged defense strategy. The first thrust of her defense was to cast the alleged arsonists as "victims of negligence." The girls had leveled accusations of abuse and negligence at Samarcand. Punishments, they said, included solitary confinement for up to three months in bedbug-infested rooms or whippings of up to one hundred lashes with leather straps while lying prone on the carpet. Their accusations sparked public outcry and even an investigation by state welfare officials. Officials' report acknowledged that staff used harsh punishments and recommended some changes, such as setting bounds on punishments and standardizing the parole process.[19] When Lewis visited Samarcand to gather evidence for her defense, she was more disturbed by what she saw. She believed that "a small ring" of staff ran a "petty dictatorship." Superintendent MacNaughton told Lewis that she was not even sure that any of the defendants were guilty. The only evidence was that one nurse, the leader of the "petty dictatorship," claimed the girls had confessed to her. Wanting more information, Lewis wrote to several women who had worked there, and she received replies detailing abuses. Lewis tried to capitalize on the public's outrage about whippings and other harsh punishments at the institution. Although they were "problem children" and should be wards of the state, she argued, they did not deserve punishments such as they had received at Samarcand.[20]

Lewis's second, and main, strategy was to demonstrate that the girls were mentally defective. The day after she first met with some of the girls in the Moore County jail, she wrote to Harry Crane, the state's part-time psychologist, whom she knew from her time working for the state welfare board. Based on her visit with them, she told Crane she was "satisfied that some of those girls are mentally defective." Lewis asked Crane to examine the girls, "as their mental condition, of course, is of great importance in their defense"—that is, she hoped to argue that their mental status as children meant they were unable to understand their actions. Lewis thought at least half of the girls might be mentally defective, but there were four in particular for whom she thought an examination was "highly important." Crane traveled to interview and test those girls, finding that their "mental ages" ranged from nine to eleven years old.[21]

When the girls went to trial, the judge did not buy Lewis's primary argument: that these girls were children whose heredity and environment had shaped them. Lewis argued in an impassioned speech that "some of them were born mentally defective, others came from broken homes, from homes where parents were handicapped. They are the products of subtle forces that have played on them since their birth." Crane also testified that the girls could not distinguish between good and bad behavior. The judge, however, told the girls that he thought they could understand their social offenses. He sentenced twelve of the girls to terms ranging from eighteen months (if they "behaved") to five years (if they did not). The girls were sent straight to the state prison, where they were placed above death row, the only fireproof wing in the prison.[22]

Despite Lewis's courtroom loss, public opinion leaned toward the girls. In their first reports, some newspapers questioned why the girls had gone to such drastic lengths, implying that their treatment at a state institution justified their actions at least in part. Although one person who attended the trial said they deserved the maximum sentence of ten years, most were more lenient. Newspapers reported on the "bright-faced" girls dressed in "attractive silk and cotton prints," partly thanks to the efforts of Lewis, who had requested help from sympathetic women who lived near the jails to dress them "neatly and modestly" so they would "make a good impression." Local observers commented that the girls "have already been punished twice over" and that they needed "help, not punishment." As historian Susan Cahn has observed, the trial was "a moment of reckoning" about juvenile delinquency in white girls, part of the continuing debate about how to manage the "girl problem" and determine the bounds of normal female adolescence in a moment when youthful behavior challenged tradition. The result was that many members of the public "attempted to incorporate modern definitions of adolescent sexuality into a charitable embrace of white delinquent girls."[23]

Similarly, the meaning of white feeblemindedness once again was up for discussion in this trial. One of Lewis's central arguments was that the girls were the mental age of children. Her depiction of the girls' mental defects made them victims rather than criminals, a notable contrast to the usual depictions of feebleminded girls as a "menace." Some newspapers followed her lead, describing the girls' mental defects as one way in which they were "victims of circumstances." More commonly, however, newspapers simply did not mention the girls' mental status, focusing instead on other aspects of their behavior, whether sensational or pitiable. But neither did anyone take issue with her argument that they were the mental age of children. In the aftermath of the verdict, one editorial generally sympathetic toward the girls—it argued for an investigation into Samarcand—described its inmates in two ways: "young women whose slant is becoming a menace to society" and "underbrained females."[24] Perhaps many onlookers similarly assumed that deviance and feeblemindedness were naturally linked.

The public attention from the trial brought some reforms to Samarcand and led to a changing of the guard. Lewis's charges of mistreatment at Samarcand drew public attention, and continued scrutiny led to both specific changes in institutional policy and Superintendent MacNaughton's resignation. Her replacement was Grace Robson, the former superintendent of a New Jersey institution for feebleminded women. While MacNaughton had overseen at least two sterilization operations under the 1929 law, Robson saw sterilization as an important tool to be used as girls were paroled. In her first four years, she worked with county officials to have twenty-eight former inmates sterilized.[25]

The ultimate lesson of the Samarcand arson trial is that it highlights a divergence in public opinion and official policy. As Cahn argues, while many citizens viewed the girls sympathetically, the state itself "opted for a far harsher approach that treated female delinquents as sexually immoral, physically degenerate criminals subject to severely punitive measures."[26] The Samarcand arson trial did not lead directly to sterilizations elsewhere, and the trial did not include public discussion of sterilization. Feebleminded white women and girls, including teenagers, were already the focal point of sterilization. But in an ironic twist, pressure from a sympathetic public led to a change in leadership at Samarcand, which in turn led to more sterilizations. The whole episode also increased skepticism about the institution's ability to reform girls, echoing past shifts in views about other institutions. Just as officials and the public had previously had high hopes for Caswell's ability to manage the feebleminded population and in the late 1910s had turned to sterilization as a more efficient preventive mechanism, so by 1931 public opinion shifted away from optimistic hopes that Samarcand could meaningfully reform wayward girls. Yet in 1931 public opinion mattered little: institutional officials already had the legal power to commit inmates and sterilize them.

In the midst of the trial, a new girl arrived at Samarcand, probably unnoticed amid the turmoil. Margaret Brewer was only eight years old—young to be committed to Samarcand, but not the youngest. Some of the girls were as young as five. Brewer was from Winston-Salem, where she had been a "nuisance" in school and had been found begging and far from her home.[27] Although Margaret's arrival at Samarcand went unheralded, her mother Mary was soon to become the center of a pivotal Supreme Court case.

Brewer v. Valk

As welfare officials began to apply the sterilization law, they became aware of its shortcomings. State psychologist Harry Crane worried that the law did not place enough emphasis on the family history of the patient, allowing for sterilizations beyond those "quite clearly established to be hereditary in type." Other onlookers had legal concerns: while the 1929 law gave officials much more power to act, it did so at the expense of due process protections for the people nominated for sterilization, making the law vulnerable to legal challenges. Mere months after it passed, UNC law professor Robert Wettach commented that the lack of provision for hearing or appeal made the act "of doubtful constitutionality in its procedure, however much we may approve of its purpose." R. Eugene Brown, the head of the welfare board's division of institutions, echoed these concerns in the ERO's *Eugenical News*, a frequent forum for discussions about how to refine eugenic laws. And at least one county attorney advised his county's commissioners not to sign a sterilization petition because he thought the law was unconstitutional. These concerns were not unfounded; a 1931 review of three state sterilization laws that had been overturned without replacements indicated that two were because of due process. For comparison, North Carolina officials had examples of laws that seemed more likely to withstand scrutiny, both model statutes produced by the ERO and laws on the books in twenty-six other states, including the Virginia law that the Supreme Court had allowed to stand in *Buck v. Bell* in 1927.[28]

The historical record is not conclusive, but the remaining evidence surrounding Mary Brewer's sterilization case suggests that by 1932 key reformers and officials, concerned the law might be challenged, were looking for a test case. When Mary Brewer of Winston-Salem appeared, she likely seemed perfect because she closely resembled the image of an "unfit" person that welfare officials had promulgated over the past decade. She was a supposedly feebleminded white woman who had repeatedly demonstrated her unwillingness to cooperate with welfare officials; she had several children judged to be delinquent or feebleminded; and observers characterized her as an incompetent mother. In the eyes of officials, she was passing on her defects to another generation through both inherited traits and poor environment. Many of the state's white elites would have seen her in terms similar to the Wake family, as a drain on public resources. Her gender was also likely a factor. Although officials could have targeted her husband for sterilization, they more frequently sterilized women because of sexual double standards, the importance of maintaining images of white womanhood, and some public reluctance to "unsex" men. Although Mary's diagnosis of feeblemindedness sufficed as a legal basis for sterilization, social workers' consistent concern about her mothering may have also been a reason, in their minds, to sterilize her. To officials, Brewer thus seemed an ideal fit for the law's requirements: a "mentally defective or feeble-minded" woman for whom sterilization was in the "public good." By using her for their test case, the reformers behind the legal challenge might hope to avoid discussion of the merits of sterilization itself.[29]

Mary was born in 1904 in Greensboro, North Carolina.[30] By 1920, she was the oldest of nine children, living in Broadbay, a small township a few miles away from Winston-Salem. Her father, Webster Oldham, was a machinist at a chair factory, and their neighbors labored at the tobacco and furniture factories that punctuated the rural Piedmont landscape. The family seemed to make ends meet: they were able to buy a home, and the older children had attended enough school to read and write. As in many other working-class families, however, the older children also worked. Mary started working as early as the age of ten, with experience in a hosiery mill and a cigarette factory. By fifteen, she earned wages in a knitting mill as a "seamstress machinist."[31]

In September 1920, at age sixteen, Mary left her parents and married Junius Brewer, a native of Winston-Salem a decade her senior. June, as he was known, waited tables in his brother-in-law's café, although he had also worked since he was a teenager in various factory or manual labor jobs, and later he worked as a painter. Mary had their first child in 1921 or 1922, and in the next seven years she had four more children. Consumed with taking care of her children, Mary was unable to earn wages. June's jobs barely paid the rent, and he drank and gambled away much of his earnings. He may also have left his wife and children for periods of time, since he wound up in municipal court at least once for not supporting his family. The family moved frequently; every time they showed up in the city directory it was in a different location.³²

The Brewer family's poverty attracted the attention of local officials and charitable groups. Soon after their first child was born, the Brewers began to receive help from the city's Associated Charities. Welfare workers who visited the family noted that they were "often hungry," and they "tried to reinstate the family and tried to get Mr. Brewer to work," apparently to no avail. The Brewers had run-ins with authorities because of a "neighborhood disturbance" and reports that the Brewers let their children play near the highway. When their oldest daughter Margaret began school in 1929, she was immediately marked as a "problem child" for her tardiness and irregular attendance, and for stealing other children's lunches because she was hungry.³³

Mary often took her children through the streets to beg for scraps or spare change, and there were reports of her daughter Margaret "fishing into garbage cans for anything she could find." One snowy day in the fall of 1930, Mary was out begging with her baby Sadie in her arms, and she wandered into a neighborhood filled with the spacious dwellings of industrialists. One of these was the home of Lucy Hodgins Hanes Chatham and her husband Thurmond, a textile manufacturing magnate. The Chathams or one of their neighbors, probably upset that Mary had disturbed the quiet peace of their wealthy sanctuary, reported her to the city welfare department. Welfare officials once again visited the family, promised that Associated Charities would provide aid, and warned them not to beg.³⁴

From there, the family's situation spiraled downward. In early 1931, the police repeatedly hauled home eight-year-old Margaret, who spent nights begging and sleeping in cars or in a bathroom at nearby Salem College. One night the police found her two miles from home. After a failed attempt to send Margaret to a foster home, officials arranged for a "physical and psychiatric examination" of the girl and her mother Mary. On March 2, 1931, a psychology professor at Salem College declared Mary "feeble-minded"; although she had "no evidence of disorder or derangement," she had an IQ of only 51. Margaret was sent to Samarcand for delinquency. Soon Mary and June's other children were taken away from them: two children were shipped off to a juvenile relief home and the other two were sent to live with their grandparents. Repeated childbirth had taken a toll on Mary's health, and in July 1931 she had an abortion because she was too "frail" to carry the pregnancy to term. She may have also contracted tuberculosis.³⁵

Throughout their interactions with the family, social workers and neighbors viewed Mary Brewer mostly with disdain and frustration. They commented that the Brewers' home "was dirty, unkempt, the children in bad condition, undernourished." They condemned Mary's behavior, noting her "dirty language" and her "horrible temper tantrums." They criticized her for her lack of "proper attitude toward her children" and for not "keeping a home like a mother should."[36] Mary Brewer's situation was, of course, complicated by her poverty. Tied to home by her young children's needs and married to a man who seemed unable or unwilling to work to feed his children, Mary had few options. Taking her children begging on the streets gave her some control over her income, even if it was not a steady source of funds. Judging by welfare officials' testimony, however, they saw Mary Brewer as ungrateful and obstreperous. In the minds of professional social workers as well as the wider public, Mary Brewer was a clear example of a feebleminded woman who was not fit to be a mother and who had likely passed on her feeblemindedness to her children. In 1932, when Brewer was twenty-eight years old, officials decided to sterilize her.

Mary Brewer's sterilization case seems to have been constructed from the beginning as a test case of the law. The lawyers and officials involved in the case acted with an unusual level of coordination and attention to detail, and the timing of some of their activities indicates even more behind-the-scenes collusion. We have no record of how the case began, but five of the men who soon played leading roles in the case worked within a single block of each other in downtown Winston-Salem, clustered around the Forsyth County courthouse. One of the men was Forsyth County welfare superintendent Alvin W. Cline, who first became aware of the Brewer family around 1929. He worked in the basement of the county courthouse. On the west corner of the courthouse was the O'Hanlon building, which held the law offices of William T. Wilson, a respected lawyer who went on to become a judge and then mayor of the city.[37] On the south corner was the Wachovia Bank and Trust building, where young lawyer Jerry Hester had an office on the eighth floor. Down the hall from Hester was lawyer Fred Hutchins, and on the fourth floor was Arthur Valk, a surgeon.[38] Each of them was soon involved in the case. To be sure, the O'Hanlon and Wachovia buildings contained a number of lawyers and doctors. Still, the geographic proximity of these key figures is a physical manifestation of the ways people with social, professional, and political power moved in the same circles. It is easy to imagine that at least some of these men knew each other from church or civic groups, where they might have talked about their difficult cases or frustrations with "source[s] of trouble" like the Brewers.

The case began on April 16, 1932, when lawyer William T. Wilson filed a petition to be appointed as Mary Brewer's legal guardian, on the grounds that she was so "devoid of . . . mental capacity" that she could not manage her affairs. The sheriff delivered a copy of the petition to Mary Brewer, notifying her that there would be a hearing on April 28 to decide on her mental competence. Whether because she did not understand the paperwork, did not care, or could not leave her children, Brewer did not attend the hearing. But Wilson and county welfare superintendent Cline had organized a full event that stretched over two days. Lengthy testimony came from at least five witnesses, including Cline, two other social workers, a neighbor, and the psychology professor who had examined Brewer and her daughter a year before. The hearing took place before a jury of twelve members. Although the jurors never met Brewer, instead hearing only witness testimony, they agreed that Brewer was "incompetent to manage her affairs." The court granted Wilson's petition to act as her guardian.[39] It was not out of the ordinary to appoint a legal guardian for a feebleminded person, but it *was* unusual for the initial hearing on guardianship to take place before a jury, which the law on appointing guardians did not require. And although the court was supposed to research the case and hold a hearing, the amount of testimony and documentation in this case seems excessive. It is reasonable to see this unusually involved guardianship hearing as a preliminary move in constructing a test case.

Equally odd, Mary Brewer soon had a lawyer, despite the lack of any ongoing legal proceedings. Hanselle "Jerry" Hester was a vivacious young man who had recently graduated from Duke's law school and established a successful practice in Winston-Salem. He first appeared in the case *not* on Brewer's side, but representing Wilson at the April 28–29 hearing. Several weeks later, however, he filed papers with the court noting that he intended to represent her.[40] As with many aspects of this case, it is hard to know whether Brewer initiated this action; the legal battles over Brewer's potential sterilization render her opinions invisible even as they offer most of the evidence that remains about her life and her family. It is possible that Brewer finally grew tired of the state's interference with her family and sought legal assistance. This scenario seems highly unlikely, given her general disregard of instructions from authorities and the fact that Hester had already appeared on the opposing side. The more likely scenario is that Wilson, Hester, and their allies within a tight network of reform-minded professionals in Winston-Salem realized that Brewer would need legal representation if she was to be part of a test case of the sterilization law.

Although the case saw little public action over the summer, the speed with which the case moved in the fall indicates that, in fact, significant things were happening behind the scenes. Namely, it was likely over the summer that the groundwork was laid for the Winston-Salem–based group of lawyers to work with another group of lawyers eighty miles away in Durham. Here, a group of law students and lawyers in Duke University's new Legal Aid Clinic were working on *both* sides of the case by the fall. The founder of the clinic was John S. Bradway, an avid social reformer who had relocated to Duke from a law school in California in 1931.

John S. Bradway was born in Swarthmore, Pennsylvania, in 1890. He attended Haverford, a Pennsylvania school with Quaker ties, then law school at the University of Pennsylvania. After graduating in 1914, he worked for three years both at law firms and in legal aid, then served in the Navy during World War I. On his return, he became increasingly involved in legal aid, including becoming an officer in the National Association of Legal Aid Societies in 1922. He also moved toward teaching, beginning with part-time roles at his alma maters. In 1929, Justin Miller, dean of the University of Southern California Law School, offered Bradway a faculty position to start a legal aid clinic there. A year later, Miller left to head Duke University's Law School, and the following year Miller recruited Bradway to once more found a legal aid clinic, this time at Duke.[41]

Bradway's interest in legal aid overlapped with an interest in social reform that probably made him unusually receptive to discussions surrounding sterilization. His colleague Justin Miller was a founding trustee of the Human Betterment Foundation, an influential eugenics organization founded in 1928 in California. Miller may have introduced Bradway to leading figures there, including Rufus B. von KleinSmid, the president of the University of Southern California and one of the founders of the Human Betterment Foundation. By the time he arrived in North Carolina, Bradway seems to have been interested in the overlap of law and social reform. In the fall of 1932, Bradway began to organize what became the Durham Crime Study Club, for which he served as president. In March 1933, the club invited UNC faculty member and state psychologist Harry Crane to speak about the relationship between "mental abnormality" and crime. By 1934, Bradway was one of a handful of contributing members to the North Carolina Conference for Social Service, and he later served as president of the CSS. He was also a committed member of the local mental hygiene society and eventually served as president of the state's Mental Hygiene Society. He remained in favor of sterilization through at least the early 1950s, when he published an article defending the legality of the state's statute.[42]

In the 1930s, Bradway's Legal Aid Clinic at Duke was at the forefront of legal education. Law schools had avoided practical training, using only case studies in class rather than interactions with real clients. Bradway believed practical training was important, however, to decrease the "cold shock" a new lawyer felt on meeting his first client. Because the local bar feared the Duke clinic would take away business, Bradway worked closely with local lawyers and set strict eligibility requirements for clients, turning away those

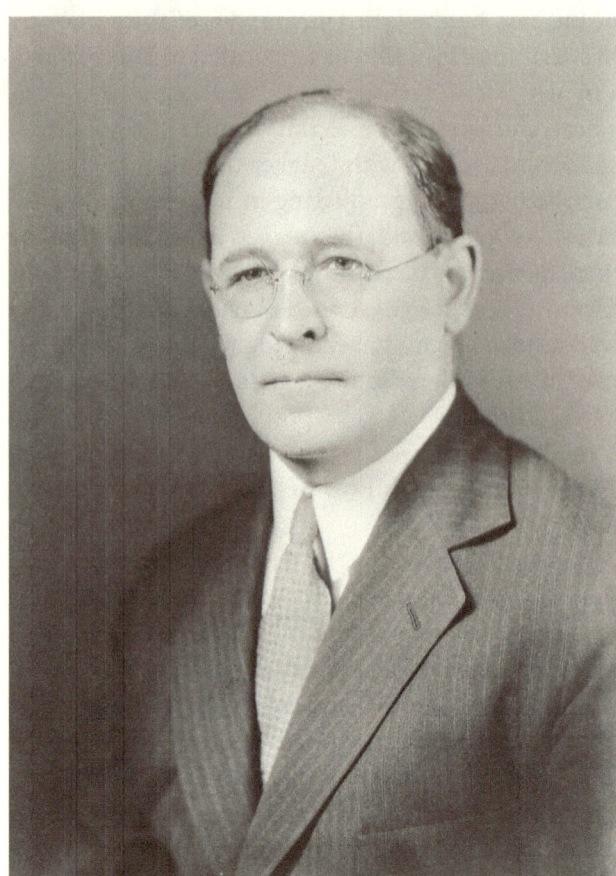

Figure 6.4 John S. Bradway, the founder of Duke's Legal Aid Clinic and one of the architects of the 1933 sterilization law. Bradway, John Saeger [Law], People Series, University Archives Photography Collection, UA.01.15.0009, 1961–2011, Box 4, David M. Rubenstein Rare Book and Manuscript Library, Duke University.

who had the ability to pay. He also developed impressive materials for helping his students learn the routines of legal work, such as how to interview clients, how to document their findings, and how to write briefs. He set high standards for his students, opposing any "procedure which short-changed the client" or made the client think their problem was unimportant. To ensure that students were adequately supervised, he organized the clinic as a "law partnership with myself as a senior partner," and he took care to spend social time with the students as well. He also wrangled funding for two staff attorneys, two secretaries, and a part-time lawyer. The clinic course ran for the full academic year, and in 1932 it was required for all third-year students. Each student was expected to spend 100 to 160 hours during the year working on their assigned cases. In 1932–33, the group of sixteen students handled around thirty cases, mostly contract law, criminal matters, and property cases.[43]

It is unclear exactly how Brewer's case wound up in the Duke Legal Aid Clinic, although there are several possibilities. Bradway usually found cases for the clinic either through his network of legal contacts or when he was interested in an article he saw in the newspaper. Jerry Hester, Brewer's lawyer, got his law degree from Duke in 1931 and may have maintained connections there. Fred S. Hutchins, a well-established Winston-Salem lawyer and public attorney who eventually represented Wilson, had been involved in Winston-Salem's efforts in 1929 to establish a legal aid clinic there. As part of those efforts he corresponded with John Bradway, who was then in California.[44] Perhaps Hester and Hutchins—who worked on the same floor of the Wachovia Building—talked about the case during the summer of 1932 and came up with the idea of bringing in Bradway's students.

In the fall of 1932, the Brewer case moved quickly. On August 1, Brewer's court-appointed guardian Wilson filed a request with the Forsyth County commissioners to have Brewer sterilized. The county commissioners approved the request that same day. On August 2, Wilson ordered Arthur Valk, an experienced physician and surgeon whose offices were in Wilson's building, to perform the operation.[45] Here, the legal record informs us, Hester (on Brewer's behalf) sought a restraining order against both Wilson and Valk, who became codefendants in the case.[46] In a hearing before the Superior Court on October 8, Hester argued that the state's sterilization statute violated due process. This argument merits emphasis: Hester shaped Brewer's plea to question only a narrow sliver of the sterilization law—the lack of a right to notice and a hearing, not more fundamental medical or social arguments for sterilization.[47] The judge agreed and issued an injunction restraining Wilson and Valk from sterilizing her.[48] Once again, it is impossible to know how Mary Brewer reacted: Did she celebrate, or was she more concerned with regaining custody of her five children? Was she even present at the hearing?

The response to the injunction in October 1932 is another signal that this case was unusual. First, Wilson and Valk, now represented by Fred Hutchins, decided not to protest the injunction. Instead, they allowed it to become permanent but on October 10, only two days later, appealed the entire case to the state supreme court, suggesting that they were privy to larger plans in the making.[49] Moreover, on the same day they filed the appeal, counsel for the two sides—representing both appellant and appellee—jointly filed a twenty-seven-page record of the facts in the case. It is possible that Hutchins, Wilson, and Valk decided that the supreme court would be amenable to their appeal and hoped to bring Mary Brewer to the operating room that way. But the rapid response by both appellant and appellee makes it more likely that the lawyers on both sides of the case were collaborating with a goal in mind from at least early October.

Certainly, by the time the case was filed with the state supreme court, the array of lawyers was suspiciously linked. On the plaintiff's team, Jerry Hester was joined by two people affiliated with Duke. "Freckled and friendly," Gordon E. Dean had taken his JD in California but had taught at Duke since earning his LLM in criminal law there in the spring of 1932. Dean's illustrious career eventually landed him at the head of the Atomic Energy Commission and a position as an aide to President Harry Truman. William C. Lassiter, the final member of Brewer's team, was a third-year law student at Duke with "tremendous energy and considerable ability." Bradway remarked, however, that Lassiter was also "temperamental" and "impatient." As a third-year law student at Duke, he was a classmate of his counterparts on the defense team. Hutchins's partners on the team defending Valk and Wilson were Edward C. Bryson and T. Spruill Thornton. Thornton was a third-year law student at Duke University and was required to participate in Bradway's Legal Aid Clinic. He was the lowest-performing member of the group, spending only thirty-two hours on clinic cases by the beginning of February, compared to his classmate Lassiter's eighty-nine hours. Bryson, who also enrolled as a law student, had helped run the clinic since its founding in 1931 and later became a member of Duke's faculty.[50] At one point, Bryson and Hester, representing the two sides, even filed a *joint* brief to address one of the supreme court justices' questions about whether the plaintiff had standing to file a suit against a court-appointed guardian.[51]

On February 8, 1933, the state supreme court upheld the lower court's decision, rejecting the appellants' arguments that the state's police powers justified their intervention. Because Hester, ostensibly on behalf of Brewer, had framed his legal challenge only around the questions of whether notice and hearing were necessary, the court ruled on those same questions. They found that the state sterilization law violated the Fourteenth Amendment and similar clauses in the state constitution.[52] With this decision, the court threw out North Carolina's sterilization law, less than four years old. But thanks to the nature of the legal challenge, the fundamental principles of the sterilization program remained untouched. In their decision, the seven justices took no issue with the idea of sterilization, noting that "the record discloses harrowing things in regard to this woman" and that "we always have had and always will have people of low mentality without normal intelligence. It has been since the beginning of time." Since they believed that the causes of mental defects included "heredity" and "the sins of the fathers," they hinted that sterilization was an apt solution for these problems, although they left decisions about "the dangerous and seriousness of an operation of this kind" to physicians.[53]

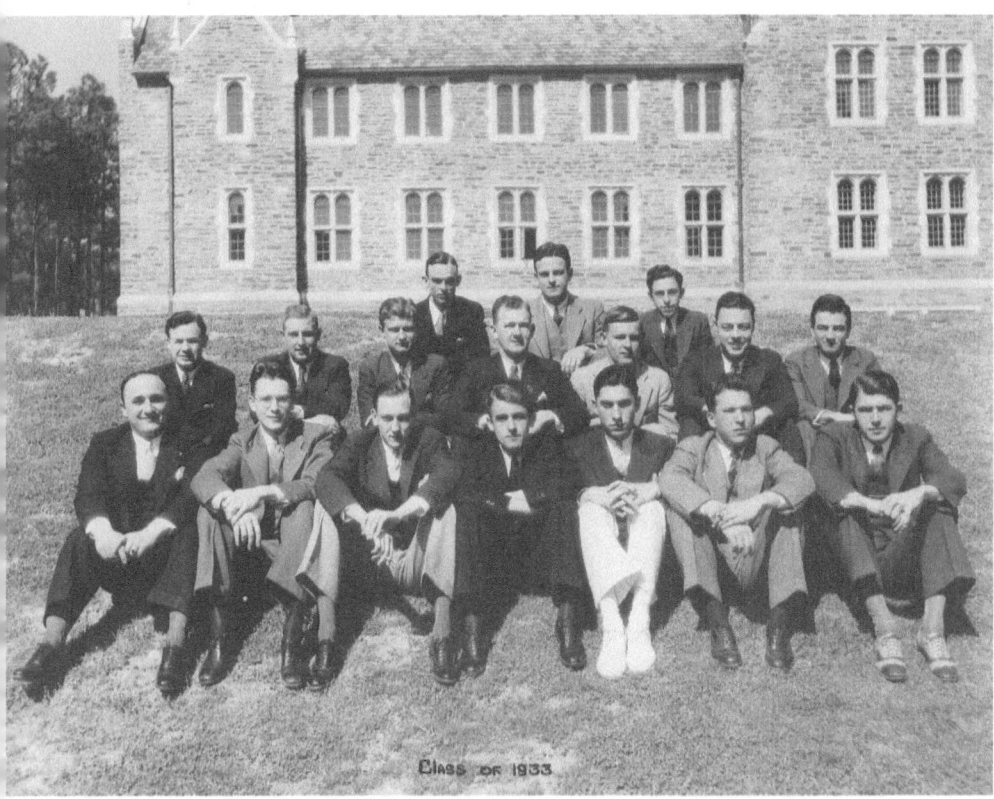

Figure 6.5 The graduating class of Duke Law School, 1933. William C. Lassiter, a member of Mary Brewer's defense team through his participation in Duke's Legal Aid Clinic, is at the right end of the second row. Duke University School of Law Class and Alumni Photograph Collection, Goodson Law Library, Duke University.

Plugging the Holes: The 1933 Sterilization Law and the Eugenics Board

Almost immediately, advocates of sterilization began to draft a new law. Bradway and his Duke students were among the first to try to "plug the hole which our case punched" in the sterilization law—a strong indication that this had been their intention all along.[54] Within three days after the supreme court decision, Bradway drafted a new sterilization bill based on Virginia's and California's statutes and gathered the students who had worked on the case. Edward Bryson, Gordon Dean, William Lassiter, and T. Spruill Thornton—two students from each side of the supreme court arguments—spent a long Saturday in mid-February together working through the various sections of Bradway's draft. They suggested creating a "central board for the state" modeled after Idaho's State Board of Eugenics, which would travel around the state to hear both institutional and noninstitutional cases. Bradway forwarded their suggestions to Robert Wettach, the UNC law professor who had raised concerns about the old law's constitutionality back in 1929, and the group continued to work on the bill.[55]

Bradway and his students were not the only ones drafting a bill. A subcommittee from the North Carolina Conference of Social Service that included Harry W. Crane, the UNC psychology professor who served as the director of mental hygiene for the state welfare board, and R. Eugene Brown, the state welfare official who had overseen sterilizations so far, drafted a list of recommendations for amending the bill. They wanted to ease some of the law's restrictions, such as lowering the number of case reviewers from four to three. At the same time, on February 22, Representative William A. Thompson, who two decades before had introduced the bill to create Caswell and was a longtime member of the Caswell board of directors, was working on his own version of the bill, perhaps in correspondence with Caswell superintendent W. H. Dixon. Thompson's proposal, the simplest and least patient-friendly of the alternatives, merely added a clause to the 1929 law that required five days' notice to the next of kin or legal guardian and provided for the right of appeal through the court system, presumably during that five-day window, without offering a chance for a hearing.[56]

John Bradway was aware that Thompson introduced his bill in the House on February 22, but he pressed on. He believed that his draft bill "clarifi[ed] the situation considerably," and would cost no more than the current system. With help from Wettach at UNC and state welfare board staffers R. Eugene Brown and Harry Crane, he worked through at least six drafts of his bill, honing the ideas and language to be legally unassailable.[57]

On March 20, 1933, Representative Thompson introduced a second sterilization bill in the House, this one based verbatim on the text that Bradway and his group had produced.[58] Although Thompson's first bill had been quickly sent to the Senate, the Senate tabled it when he introduced the second bill, perhaps at his request. The new Bradway version moved as quickly as possible through the legislative machinery, with final passage by the Senate just two weeks after Thompson introduced it in the House. The "Act to Amend Chapter 34 of the Public Laws of 1929 of North Carolina, Relating to the Sterilization of Persons Mentally Defective" was enacted on April 5, 1933.[59]

Where the 1929 sterilization law lacked specifics, the 1933 law went to the other extreme, with instructions for what seems like every possible scenario. Its principal innovation was to create a permanent five-member Eugenics Board that would hear all sterilization petitions based on feeblemindedness, mental disease, or epilepsy, regardless of whether the petitions came from institutional heads, welfare workers, or relatives. The 1929 law had required that four reviewers sign off on sterilizations but had not required that the reviewers meet to discuss the case or hold a hearing. The Eugenics Board included these four members—the heads of the state welfare and health boards, the chief medical officers of two of the state's institutions for the feebleminded or mentally ill—as well as the attorney general, for good measure.

Although the new law gave its targets the protection of fifteen days' notice, a hearing, and a clear appeals process, it also expanded the rationales for sterilization and widened the umbrella of legal protection for state officials and doctors. The new law retained two of the prior reasons for sterilization: when the operation was for the "public good" or would be in the "best interest of the mental, moral, or physical improvement of the patient." It added several other scenarios, such as cases in which doctors believed the patient "would be likely, unless operated upon, to procreate a child or children who would have a tendency to serious physical, mental, or nervous disease or deficiency." Moreover, the law required institutional heads to consider every patient for sterilization before being discharged or paroled.[60]

R. Eugene Brown wrote later that North Carolina's sterilization law was based on "considerable study" of the model statutes prepared by the Eugenics Record Office.[61] Although Brown, Bradway, and others may have considered the legal principles of the ERO's model laws, they used markedly different language. A comparison of the North Carolina law with the ERO's "model statute" for "voluntary sexual sterilization of certain natural classes" reveals the divergence between "pure" eugenic principles and their interpretation by social workers and lawyers. The ERO's law was littered with eugenics-laden terms such as "cacogenic" and "human pedigree analysis" that might have seemed like unnecessary jargon to Bradway and company. None of the extant drafts of the North Carolina bill contain such terms. Instead, the lawyers and welfare officials who drafted the bill translated these specialists' terms into phrases more familiar to the average ear. "A tendency to serious physical, mental, or nervous disease or deficiency" replaced "cacogenic," and "a complete medical history [and] an adequate social case history" stood in for "human pedigree analysis."[62] This language also reflected social workers' focus on solving real problems rather than debating academic points about eugenic theories. The only appearance of the word "eugenics" was in the name of the board. On one hand, the phrasing of North Carolina's law might indicate that Bradway and company believed that North Carolina's lawmakers or the public at large were unfamiliar with more arcane eugenic terminology. On the other hand, the law's easy use of the phrase "Eugenics Board," with no further explanation, shows that North Carolinians grasped the essentials.

Bradway was not content to let the 1933 sterilization law rest. He helped draft the forms that the Eugenics Board used for its petitions and hearings.

To make sure the board's procedures would pass muster, he wrote to officials with experience in running eugenics programs in other states, including Ezra S. Gosney of California's Human Betterment Foundation, for their recommendations about the mechanics of their hearings. As he told a Michigan official, "I feel certain that somebody is going to attack the Board because the findings are insufficient and I would like to advise them in advance how they can spare themselves in this embarrassment." He passed this information on to the Eugenics Board's secretary, R. Eugene Brown. He also pestered Brown about finding another case "we could use . . . to test out the constitutionality of the act," as lawyers in Virginia had done with Carrie Buck, although Brown seems to have ignored his pleas.[63]

As for Mary Brewer, we know little about her family's life after the case, when the document trail thins. We do know that in 1940, at age sixteen, her son Junius was an inmate at Jackson Training School. Her daughter Margaret, who had been sent to Samarcand in 1931 at age eight, had left the institution by 1940 at age seventeen—although Margaret could easily have been among the 115 girls whom Samarcand officials had sterilized by then. Mary, her husband June, and the rest of her children disappear from Winston-Salem city directories and census records. Given social workers' suspicion that she had tuberculosis, perhaps Mary died soon after the case, leaving her children to be raised by their widowed father or in the foster homes where social workers had placed them. Or perhaps she and June packed up their family and left the city or state, as some families did in a desperate move to avoid further interactions with officials.[64]

Brewer v. Valk inverted the path of *Buck v. Bell* in Virginia, where from the beginning a small group of elite white men planned an ideal test case to *affirm* Virginia's sterilization law. In *Buck v. Bell*, they selected their plaintiff with care, represented both Carrie Buck and the doctors who wished to sterilize her, and shepherded the case through to the Supreme Court, which affirmed the constitutionality of the law.[65] In *Brewer v. Valk*, Bradway and his allies were aware that North Carolina's law lacked necessary provisions for consent and hearing and was thus vulnerable to challenge. They seem to have set up an ideal scenario in which to strike down potentially problematic sections of the law while leaving its fundamental principles untouched.

The grand irony of *Brewer* is that it is cited in case law as precedent for the expansion of procedural due process, particularly the right to notice and a hearing.[66] Yet the same opinion ruled that sterilization did *not* violate *substantive* due process. The irony increases because this case for due process rights was pursued ostensibly on behalf of a woman whose own court-appointed guardian pushed for her to be sterilized. Her voice has been nearly erased from the historical record, but it seems that Mary Brewer was at best a willing accomplice in plans that extended far beyond her own. At worst, Brewer was a woman whose encounters with officialdom were fraught and who became an unknowing instrument of a small group of elite men. Although Mary Brewer's case is unique, the apparent disregard for her opinion or even her well-being is indicative of the assumptions that undergirded the entire eugenic sterilization program. Mary Brewer's poverty, her lack of education, and her failure to be a good mother in the eyes of her neighbors meant that she had very little say in a case that was a key step in expanding North Carolina's eugenics programs.

The passage of a robust sterilization law in 1933 capped more than a decade of lobbying and education aimed at adding sterilization as a potential weapon in social workers' arsenal against the purported spread of feeblemindedness. It also built on reformers' success in building a welfare apparatus. Unlike the debates surrounding sterilization proposals in 1919, 1923, 1925, and 1929, the push for the 1933 sterilization law faced no resistance. It was the logical, although not necessary, outcome of a campaign that had begun three decades before when medical and social welfare professionals sought to interest reformers in principles of eugenics. That campaign had continued throughout the 1920s as reform-minded legislators broke down the remaining opposition among their colleagues through exposure to the principles of eugenics, appeals to Christian charity, or analyses of the costs of social problems.

By the time Mary Brewer's lawyer challenged the law in 1932, eugenic sterilization was more firmly entrenched than ever. Her lawsuit, apparently engineered in backroom deals, opened the door for a resolution of the remaining legal questions. Indeed, by the time the General Assembly met in the spring of 1933, the questions that remained about eugenic sterilization were purely legal. The passage of the law opened new possibilities for policymakers and welfare officials. As economic depression simultaneously burdened and invigorated the state's welfare system, the state began an active sterilization program, reinforced by research and training that continued to assert the legitimacy of eugenics principles for social welfare work.

Chapter 7

The Human Element in the Modern Welfare State

One day in the mid-1930s, Orange County welfare superintendent George H. Lawrence and his staff received a call from Mrs. Oscar Chambers of Hillsborough, the county seat. Chambers had taken in a young white girl named Pearl because of her troubled past: two years earlier, when she lived with her sister, Pearl had borne a child out of wedlock. The father was a mill hand named Tink, probably one of the many young men who worked at the cotton mill outside town. Pearl had no money, and her brother-in-law forced her to leave. Although Chambers was apparently not related to the teenage girl, she took in Pearl and her toddler Peggy, paying her two dollars a week as a housekeeper and presumably intending to keep her busy enough to stay away from men. But now, on the phone with the caseworker from the Orange County welfare department, Chambers asked for a private interview and said that Pearl was "in trouble" again, pregnant this time from an affair with an older man who had promised to marry her and then disappeared. At first, Chambers wanted to keep the toddler and send Pearl away, but when welfare workers pointed out that no one else would be likely to take in a pregnant sixteen-year-old, Chambers relented.

Welfare officials suggested, instead, that they seek sterilization for Pearl. They gave her a mental test that indicated her IQ was 35, which was sufficient grounds for sterilization. Later, doctors recommended an abortion on physical grounds after an examination at Duke Hospital showed her to be anemic and "physically unfit for childbirth." Probably accompanied by welfare officials, Pearl was taken to Duke Hospital, where doctors performed both operations.[1]

Pearl's case is one of a handful for which we have any details, but in many respects her case mirrors the profile of dozens of others in the 1930s. After 1933, the creation of the Eugenics Board streamlined the approval process for sterilization, and with the growth of social work because of New Deal relief programs, social workers' increased interaction with poor people sometimes led them to decide that sterilization, rather than a benefit check or job assistance, was the response that best served the state's needs. Like Pearl, most of the people sterilized in the 1930s and 1940s were poor white girls or women whose behavior in some way undermined images of white Southern womanhood.

As North Carolina moved into the long years of the Great Depression, federal funds reshaped life for many citizens, particularly white men and their families. The New Deal provided an unprecedented degree of relief from poverty and hardship, and it also wrought momentous changes in Southern state government. As one state official wrote, the widespread suffering of the Depression underscored as never before "the human element in government. The security of every man, woman, and child in America is now recognized as the main governmental objective."[2] Welfare officials framed their spending on social programs as more than temporary relief, but rather as a way to help "unfortunate citizens" become men and women who could "buil[d] great civilizations." They even promised that the state would gradually and responsibly expand welfare support "until as many of its citizens receive its benefits as possible."[3] Across the South, state participation in federal programs dramatically expanded public welfare spending. In 1929, Southern states spent $21 million on welfare, and by 1937–38 they spent more than $74 million.[4] Similarly, the growth of relief programs created new functions for state government, continuing Progressive-Era trends of expanding state services. In the two decades after 1929, state expenditures in the South quadrupled, mirroring the growth in welfare spending.[5]

State politicians secured New Deal funds by complying with new federal requirements, but in some cases they layered programs over existing institutions and programs. Social Security programs ultimately were the domain of the state's existing welfare bureaucracy, forcing federal officials to contend with local structures and politics.[6] At the same time, with the infusion of federal funds, North Carolina's welfare departments grew in number and size, fulfilling Alexander McAlister's vision of a strong network of county departments with centralized supervision. Social workers found themselves in the limelight, suddenly charged with distributing millions of dollars in relief checks and assigning government-funded jobs to hundreds of thousands of people. The sheer volume of work forced the state to recruit hundreds more social workers, most entirely new to the field of social work. The task of training these social workers fell to state Board of Charities and Public Welfare, in collaboration with UNC. Even at moments when the Board's viability was threatened by budget cuts or political maneuvering, a handful of state welfare officials and faculty at UNC were responsible for inculcating standards of professionalism into a new generation of welfare workers.

Training in eugenics ideology continued to be a part of the welfare board's standard instruction for new social workers. As in the 1920s, the principles undergirding the state's social worker training were based on both ideologies of "fitness" and widely accepted principles of casework. Social workers were supposed to investigate every recipient of relief. As gatekeepers to the only road to meaningful economic security for many families, they wielded enormous power to deny relief when families did not meet their definition of deserving. Even in a decade when poverty became a normal way of life, social workers were trained to see some families as *abnormally* poor, penurious not because of the widespread economic devastation alone but because of some underlying flaw in mind, character, or skin color.

While social workers provided jobs, relief checks, or government foodstuffs for "normal" families, they sought to identify "unfit" people and sometimes denied them those benefits, or sought to contain them in institutions or sterilize them. The head of the state's Eugenics Board regarded sterilization as "one among many indispensable procedures in any modern program of social welfare," useful for people "unable to meet unaided the responsibilities of citizenship in a highly competitive society."[7] The tight institutional linkage of eugenics and welfare programs created a smooth path to sterilization, one that broadened over time. By the end of the 1930s, over 850 people had been sterilized, mostly poor white women. The practices of the 1930s were a continuing manifestation of the long-standing belief among state welfare officials that feebleminded or delinquent white people were a threat to the body politic.

The New Deal and the Politics of Relief in North Carolina

As the Depression unfolded, the state's welfare office had a new leader. Kate Burr Johnson left North Carolina in 1930 to become the head of New Jersey's State Home for Delinquent Girls in Trenton, where she remained for nineteen years. Her successor as commissioner of public welfare was Annie Kizer Bost, who, like Johnson, was a dedicated clubwoman and reformer. Born in 1883, Bost grew up in Piedmont North Carolina. After graduating from the State Normal School at Greensboro, she taught school for six years. In 1909 she married W. Thomas Bost, the Raleigh correspondent for the *Greensboro Daily News*. They raised their two sons in Raleigh, where she became a fixture in the community, involved in many organizations and her Lutheran church. She also served as president of the Raleigh Woman's Club, and for three years she was the executive secretary of the state Federation of Women's Clubs. Observers noted her "sparkle and warm geniality," as well as her "endless vitality and brilliance." Before she became commissioner, however, she had no notable social work training. Rather, her appointment was likely due more to her husband's friendship with Governor O. Max Gardner. After she was appointed, she spent six weeks observing welfare work in other states to prepare for the job.[8]

Once in office, Bost proved to be an effective administrator, but as the Depression strained the capacity of state and local welfare programs, she had few options. Bost's agency was often undermined as state politicians played politics with federal money. Governors and legislators created new agencies and tried to sideline the welfare board, which had often been a thorn in their side because of its attempts at prison reform, occasional charges of misconduct against institutional officials, and ongoing efforts to gain control of county welfare superintendents. Nevertheless, during all the political battles over the agency's standing, Bost and her staff remained responsible for training social workers, giving state welfare officials a significant way to shape the provision of relief on the ground.

After the state's minimally funded attempts to organize local relief efforts through the Governor's Council (1930–32), the amount of money available for relief increased drastically in July 1932, when Congress gave the Reconstruction Finance Corporation (RFC) $300 million to loan to states and cities. In September, Gardner created the Governor's Office of Relief (GOR) to receive the RFC funds. By November 1932, the state was using federal funds to support over 87,000 people via direct relief (cash payments)—the first time that anything besides county or private funds directly supported North Carolinians en masse. In January 1933, a work relief program began that employed over 97,000 people in its first month. At the program's peak in February 1933, the case load included over a quarter of the state's population. By the end of the spring in 1933, North Carolina had received almost $6 million in RFC funds, among the highest amounts in the South.[9]

As federal relief efforts increased in 1932 and 1933, the Board of Charities and Public Welfare found itself sidelined, its main function training the social workers who staffed the new agencies. Bost played a nominal role as "administrative assistant" to the GOR director. Some current and former Board staff members also provided expertise: Lois Dosher became one of ten field supervisors at the GOR after several years' service at the welfare board as director of the Division of County Organization, and Roy M. Brown, who had worked for the Board in the 1920s and was currently working at UNC's School of Public Administration, became the technical supervisor for the GOR.[10] The Board's most significant contribution to the GOR's work was training the hundreds of new social workers who distributed relief funds.

Meanwhile, the state welfare board faced multiple funding cuts, staff shortages, and outright attacks. The staff struggled to carry on their normal work. They did continue most of their key functions—supervising institutions, overseeing Mothers' Aid work, and providing mental testing—but with Dosher spending almost all her time elsewhere and federal relief funds controlled by other agencies, the Board had to scale back its fieldwork program. By January 1933, the state faced a dire revenue shortage, with insufficient funds to pay appropriations. Many state agencies had already faced cuts, including a 17 percent cut for the Board of Charities and Public Welfare in 1932–33. Then in March 1933, the Board was almost gutted. The legislature proposed to drastically reduce the Board's appropriation to $4,250, which would have covered salaries for only a couple of staff members, likely eliminating all of the Board's work save its constitutional mandate to inspect institutions. The bill would have terminated funding for Mothers' Aid, the one cash benefit that the state had provided before the Depression. The welfare board called an emergency meeting, and its well-connected members were able to avert disaster: the bill was killed, the Board maintained its staff with only a 13.5 percent cut to the administrative budget, and Mothers' Aid was funded at roughly three-quarters of the previous year's level. Still, by June 1933, the combined appropriations and donations for the state welfare board were less than 60 percent of the pre-crisis amount.[11]

In the spring of 1933, the country was optimistic that President-Elect Franklin Delano Roosevelt's promised "New Deal" would lighten their burdens. RFC funds had been welcome showers on a parched landscape, but were far from enough to meet the level of need in North Carolina. FDR's New Deal, an exercise in rapid-fire experimentation, tackled the country's economic woes from a variety of angles, at first seeking to shore up industry, provide relief for the unemployed, and address the banking crisis. Some of FDR's earliest attempts targeted the agricultural sector, which had suffered from low crop prices and droughts even before the Depression began. For example, the Agricultural Adjustment Act established price controls in an attempt to stabilize production. Ultimately, New Deal agricultural programs benefited landowners more than tenant farmers or other agricultural laborers, and they did little for Black farmers. New labor regulations in the National Industrial Recovery Act had little effect in North Carolina before they were declared unconstitutional, and other labor bills offered meager help to North Carolina's underpaid and mostly nonunionized laborers.[12]

Programs to provide relief to the unemployed had more immediate impact on North Carolinians, although they still fell short of meeting the needs of many families. The Federal Emergency Relief Administration (FERA), created on May 12, 1933, sent grants to state governments, mostly for direct relief payments, but with attached standards on spending.[13] In North Carolina, Governor John Ehringhaus continued Gardner's decision to administer federal grants via a relief agency separate from the Board of Charities and Public Welfare.[14] To head this new agency, the North Carolina Emergency Relief Administration (NC ERA), Ehringhaus appointed Annie Land O'Berry. A Goldsboro resident, O'Berry had long been a leader of the state's white clubwomen with an interest in social welfare, including conducting a survey on conditions for women working in industry and taking a course on social work at Columbia. She had tried to use her political connections to Governor

Gardner to be appointed as Kate Burr Johnson's replacement as welfare commissioner in 1930, but concerns about her health cost her the position. When the Depression began, she helped raise $5,000 for white-collar workers who did not qualify for regular poor relief, and she got a job as a field supervisor administering RFC funds. In 1933, O'Berry's recent experience in relief efforts—as well as her work to elect Ehringhaus as governor in 1932 and her husband's recent election as a state legislator—made her a logical choice to head the NC ERA. By all accounts she was a competent administrator who resisted political interference in the agency's work.[15]

In two years, the ERA distributed $40.8 million in relief payments. Funds were mostly in the form of direct payments, to an average of more than 300,000 recipients each month. The agency also ran camps for transient workers, made loans to farmers, and used over $800,000 in Civil Works Administration funds to hire 70,000 people for building and infrastructure projects. At its peak, ERA staff included 220 employees in the state office and around 2,000 local workers who monitored relief cases. Although approximately 10 percent of the state's population received some kind of relief, ERA programs were not enough to meet families' needs. North Carolina received less in per capita FERA grants than every other Southern state except Virginia. A family of five who did receive relief benefits could expect $133 a year in 1933— at a time when Harry Crane paid sixty dollars a *month* to rent his Durham house, and when the mean annual income for a five-person family in North Carolina was $1,015. Many families did not get help or lost their benefits because of funding shortages. By one estimate, ten thousand displaced tenant farmers sought help from relief offices in Eastern North Carolina.[16]

The creation of NC ERA further undermined the state welfare board, although the Board continued to train social workers. With control over relief funds that were 0.2 percent the size of ERA-controlled federal relief funds, the Board's staff were underpaid and demoralized. They also had to deal with county welfare officers pulled into new roles at the ERA. The Board's main relevance quickly became its training efforts.[17] The NC ERA, like the Governor's Office of Relief before it, needed to hire hundreds of fieldworkers on short notice, but had few in-house staff with experience. The ERA capitalized first on the Board's existing structure, using each county's Board-approved superintendent of public welfare as a local administrator.[18] This assignment made it hard for welfare superintendents to complete Mothers' Aid casework or be in regular contact with Board staff, but it did mean that ERA staff were familiar with the Board's approach to case work. The Board of Charities and Public Welfare also collaborated with UNC's Schools of Public Welfare and Public Administration to train new relief workers, aiming to "standardiz[e] social work throughout the state."

They continued to offer segregated summer institutes for white and Black social workers. In response to the increased need for training, in 1933 the Board increased the duration of the white institute from one week of training to four in order to prepare over a hundred workers for administering federal programs, with training in "case work methods and administration, especially office organization." The Board also continued to hold regional meetings to educate both social workers and interested citizens. In the fall of 1933, attendance at the six meetings reached 800, up from 347 in 1930.[19]

Another organizational upheaval came at the end of 1935 as federal work relief programs began to replace federal direct relief programs (like the ERA), ultimately to the benefit of the Board of Charities and Public Welfare. O'Berry had tried to position NC ERA to take over North Carolina's homegrown welfare programs, arguing that the Board was duplicating her efforts. Although she had some support from federal officials, she failed, and in February 1935, in preparation for Social Security programs on the horizon, relief cases of "unemployables" went back to county welfare departments under the Board. In December 1935, the federal government ended grants for direct relief, and state leaders liquidated NC ERA. Work relief programs went to the new Works Progress Administration, headed by a political appointee.[20] For the next four and a half years, the WPA employed an average of 27,700 people annually.[21] Most of the ERA's other functions went to the Board of Charities and Public Welfare. To ease the transition, the federal government gave the Board an eighteen-month, $225,000 grant beginning in January 1936. The Board reclaimed the responsibility of overseeing local welfare work, with grant funds supporting a new Division of Field Social Work. The Board also became responsible for administering all federal benefits through county welfare offices, including distributing surplus commodities, referring people to the WPA, and assigning people to Civilian Conservation Corps (CCC) projects.[22]

Around the same time, the Social Security Act of 1935 put in motion even greater changes. Although the state initially refused to match federal funds for some programs, the Board of Charities and Public Welfare was able to take immediate advantage of programs that did not require state funding, such as Child Welfare Services.[23] Eventually North Carolina restructured welfare offices to meet federal requirements, primarily the centralization of some functions at the state level. In 1937, at the Board's urging, the legislature made the state welfare board responsible for Old Age Assistance (OAA) and Aid to Dependent Children (ADC), bringing state policies into line with federal requirements for administering the various arms of Social Security.[24] That year they appropriated $1 million for old-age assistance and half a million dollars for dependent children. To administer Social Security programs, the state added a Division of Public Assistance to the Board of Charities and Public

Welfare in July 1937.[25] The Board did not gain this new power without a fight. Bost and her allies had to accede to provisions in the new laws that required the governor's approval for the appointment of the commissioner and the head of the new Division of Public Assistance, as well as the reappointment of all county welfare boards and superintendents. They did successfully fight a provision that would have scrapped the existing welfare advisory board and allowed the governor to appoint new members friendly to him. While some allies of the Board remained concerned about whether the Board could maintain its political independence, the Board had survived the most tenuous moments of its existence yet and come out stronger.[26]

The ERA transition grant, the Social Security Act, and North Carolina's supporting 1937 legislation injected new life in the Board of Public Welfare after several years of shrinking budgets and political uncertainty. With these new funds and new mandate, the Board jumped into action. State staff more than doubled because of federal grants, and new fieldwork supervisors provided greater oversight of local programs. One of the Board's first steps was to place a trained caseworker in each county, which required at least twenty-five counties to organize a welfare department. In addition, thirty-one counties replaced their part-time superintendents of public welfare with a full-time social worker. These caseworkers certified people's eligibility for existing federal programs such as surplus commodity distribution and relief jobs. Beginning in 1937, they also took on administration of Old Age Assistance, Aid to Dependent Children, and "general relief." By June 1940, hundreds of social workers had distributed over $3 million in ADC benefits to children and their families, with an average monthly grant around sixteen dollars per family, similar to the amounts the state had provided to Mothers' Aid families.[27] The slate of Social Security laws in 1937 finally provided the funding and legal powers that completed the scheme McAlister envisioned in 1917: a fully staffed county-unit system overseen by a powerful central office.

The clear losers in this transition were Black North Carolinians, who had benefited in the 1920s and early 1930s from North Carolina's unique support of Black social work.[28] North Carolina had staked new territory with its Division of Work Among Negroes, which trained Black social workers and coordinated their public and private efforts. Raleigh was home to the Bishop Tuttle School, one of the South's two programs for Black social workers, and through the early years of the Depression these newly minted professionals easily found jobs. In 1932, twenty-six trained Black workers were employed in public and private agencies, and by 1934 that number had jumped to eighty-two. Early in the Depression, division director Lawrence Oxley was partly successful in pushing white officials to include Black people in relief programs. While he was temporarily assigned to the Governor's Council in 1930, Oxley used data to show that Black unemployment was serious, particularly because as the economy worsened white people were more willing to take the low-wage, low-status jobs that Black people had held. Black people constituted about a quarter of the state's population but two-thirds of relief cases, meaning a Black person was almost three times more likely to seek relief. Because of Oxley's advocacy, Governor Gardner created a Black advisory committee, and the state paid around a hundred Black workers, including farm agents, health workers, and welfare workers, to organize private relief efforts. The state also took over responsibility for funding the Division of Work Among Negroes in 1931, after years of support from the Laura Spelman Rockefeller Memorial. Still, under the Governor's Council, relief channels were racially segregated, with separate state advisory committees and district relief committees. North Carolina's segregated parallel approach influenced the federal model; Oxley was part of a Black advisory committee to Hoover's planning committee, which recommended the "North Carolina Plan" to other states with large Black populations.[29]

Black welfare programs were always a second-tier priority for white officials. To win even small victories, Oxley had to tread a fine line in making a case for using public funds to help Black people. Oxley stressed that Black communities first maximized private efforts, that Black attitudes were cooperative, and that "self-help activities" were part of teaching "individual responsibility." Oxley and other state welfare officials built on the long-standing Progressive attitude that interracial cooperation was necessary because the economic vitality and social stability of the state depended on it, but their goal was never equality.[30] When the state liquidated NC ERA, Black social workers were the first to lose their jobs. By June 1936, only eight or nine remained employed with county welfare departments. By 1940, that number had risen to about thirty workers, but only two of the state board's eighty-one staff members worked in the Division of Work Among Negroes, "consulting" with other divisions "whenever problems arise affecting the life of the Negro citizenry," helping to place Black social workers, and providing the annual public welfare institute for Black workers.[31] In addition, African Americans were less likely to receive support than white people. Although the state did not publish rates of payment or denial of benefits, the overall trend is clear: in 1937–38, only 22 percent of ADC relief went to Black people in a state where they made up 27.5 percent of the population—and were far more likely to live in poverty. Black applicants for relief were more often labeled "undeserving" or were registered only after white applicants' claims were filled. The mass dismissal of Black social workers because of shifts in federal funding and the clear bias in ADC payments fit neatly within the context of New Deal programs, which did little to protect the rights of minorities and women.[32]

"Preventive" Social Work and Mental Hygiene in the 1930s

Despite the uncertain future the welfare board faced in the first half of the 1930s, it continued to train social workers and provide mental testing services to the state. Among legislators and state officials, support remained strong for sterilization, with a governor's commission in 1937 calling for increased use of sterilization. Against this backdrop, state welfare officials organized the training of hundreds of new social workers, who were instructed to investigate families' eligibility for new federal benefits and wherever possible to help families become self-sustaining. Constantly needing to defend public welfare spending on an unprecedented scale, welfare officials painted the average recipient of public assistance as a trustworthy and deserving person, who had simply fallen on hard times. They increased their emphasis on saving children, focusing on retraining juvenile delinquents and redeeming neglected children through a change of environment. At the same time, they quietly but consistently reported on eugenic sterilizations, implicitly making the point that targets of sterilization were different—not citizens to be rehabilitated or supported, but a group whose future offspring should be removed from the pool of potential welfare recipients if the system of public assistance was to deserve the public trust.

The work of Harry Crane's Division of Mental Hygiene actually expanded during the Board of Charities and Public Welfare's tenuous period. A full-time assistant psychologist was added in 1931, and while the rest of the Board was hit with funding cuts in 1933, federal funds from FERA and the Civil Works Administration added workers to Crane's staff. In 1936 they added a second full-time psychologist using federal funds allotted to the Division of Child Welfare. With these staff, they created more case files and committed to studying all white children who entered the Eastern Carolina Training School and Samarcand, where they continued to find a close association between delinquency and feeblemindedness. They also studied children at Efland and Morison, the Black institutions for delinquent children, aiming to make a case for expanding those institutions. They continued to offer mental testing services to the state, examining 1,150 cases in one biennial period. They also began to coordinate their efforts more closely with the state's Department of Public Instruction. As they fielded more requests for testing of individual pupils in public schools, a staff psychologist worked with the department to do a complete survey of all 1,188 white children in one public school, finding that 4.1 percent of them were mentally defective and another 5.0 percent were borderline cases. Crane and his staff also continued their educational mission. Crane presented to Boy Scout leaders, the Durham Crime Study Club, local mental hygiene societies, and district welfare conferences. In one period of two years, he and his staff gave sixty-five talks on mental hygiene topics, including two extensive lecture series.[33]

The new Eugenics Board, formed in February 1933, functioned as part of the state welfare board. Beginning in October 1933 and continuing for four decades, the Eugenics Board met monthly to review cases and order sterilizations. Bost led the Eugenics Board as the commissioner of public welfare, joined by the attorney general, two heads of state mental hospitals, and the state health officer.[34] R. Eugene Brown, who had informally overseen sterilization petitions since 1929, became secretary of the Eugenics Board. Brown continued efforts to educate the public about the need for sterilization as an "important" part of "any broad and constructive welfare program," publishing newspaper articles and a handbook that explained the program's legal foundations and procedures. The Wake family of 1920s infamy made an appearance in his publications, with Brown estimating that they had now cost the state at least $40,000.[35]

An extensive study of mental health in the state commissioned by the governor praised the way "mental health implications" permeated the work of all the welfare board's divisions. That pattern was evident in physical space, as well. Over the years, the Board of Charities and Public Welfare's growing staff had splintered to at least three separate locations. In 1938 they moved to a single floor in a new building in Raleigh, and they established a central file room where they could systematically store files from all divisions. Staff from Mental Hygiene, Child Welfare, Public Assistance, the Eugenics Board, and other divisions could now work "in much closer coordination," including by cross-referencing their case files. These files now included index cards Crane and his staff had compiled on thousands of North Carolinians they deemed to be mentally defective, including 70,195 cards they reported adding between 1934 and 1936. By 1938, their files included information on around 175,000 people, almost 5 percent of the entire state population. The state office also attempted to gradually collect files on every single relief case across the state. State officials thus had at their fingertips a powerful means of finding people who were both impoverished and judged to have mental defects.[36]

By 1937, state welfare officials oversaw hundreds of local social workers who investigated families and certified their eligibility for public assistance. Most of these county staff were new to social work, with backgrounds in teaching or clerical work, and the state's first task was to train them.[37] The Board of Charities and Public Welfare and UNC cooperated in these trainings, as they had for nearly two decades; by 1941, 61 percent of county social workers were trained at UNC's School of Public Welfare, with senior caseworkers receiving over thirty semester hours of social work training, on average.[38] UNC offered college-level coursework, and the Board hosted racially segregated summer institutes with hundreds of attendees. The Board also divided the state into ten districts, and every six weeks they hosted a daylong conference for county superintendents in each district. In 1938, they reported that 350 white social workers attended the five-day summer institute, and over 1,800 people attended these district conferences. They also hosted daylong training sessions focused on casework procedures and how to interview potential recipients. With federal funding to hire more state-level staff, the state board increased its scrutiny of these local workers. Fieldwork supervisors made multiple visits per month to each county to consult with county workers on "difficult situations" and presumably to make sure they were following guidelines for recordkeeping and funding eligibility.[39]

With Commissioner Bost an avid supporter of sterilization, eugenics principles continued to be a part of the state welfare board's standard instruction. At the public welfare institutes of 1934 and 1935, for example, students heard presentations from Eugenics Board secretary R. Eugene Brown about his work.[40] Any student who took a course at UNC's School of Public Welfare also would have encountered the basic principles of eugenics and learned that such principles were integral to the "care" of certain groups of people. According to syllabi collected by Roy M. Brown, the director of the public welfare program at UNC, nearly all social work courses contained substantial sections on eugenics, feeblemindedness, intelligence testing, and sterilization. Brown's own course on "Social Laws" dealt with three topics under "care of the feebleminded": "Caswell Training School," "sterilization," and "birth control." Wiley Sanders, who had worked for the Board of Charities and Public Welfare in the 1920s, began his 1938 "Introduction to Social Work" course by surveying the "major problems attacked by social work," which in his definition included poverty, mental deficiency, and mental diseases. Harry Crane taught a class called "Mental Hygiene" that focused on "feeble-mindedness, psychoses, and minor mental aberrations in relation to social work; and ways in which a social worker may be a factor in mental hygiene." A course on "Population" studied "quality and quantity," including problems of "race, immigration, and eugenics." Other professors routinely assigned standard eugenics texts: family studies such as *The Jukes* and *The Kallikak Family*, as well as theoretical treatises such as Guyer's *Being Well Born*, Goddard's *Sterilization and Segregation*, and Landman's *Human Sterilization*.[41]

As in the 1920s, the Board encouraged social workers to consider "preventive" social work and distinguish between different types of families. On one hand, state officials continued to hold up Mothers' Aid recipients as model families. The purpose of Mothers' Aid was allowing an eligible woman to stay home to "guide the development of the personalities of her children as only a good mother can." The new Aid to Dependent Children program allowed welfare officials to vastly expand the program with the same aims. As they planned in 1936 for the transition, they encouraged lawmakers to incorporate "the methods of administration" of the Mothers' Aid law into legislation that enabled the cost-sharing required by ADC. Although the ADC-enabling law was less specific than Mothers' Aid about the "kind of mother eligible," it still required that a child's relative maintain "a safe and proper home" for the child in order to receive ADC funds. Officials painted male participants in Civilian Conservation Corps programs similarly, as the ideal recipient of government aid, emphasizing that these young men were selected for "purpose, ambition, and character." Board reports argued that the program allowed these young men to develop new skills and good habits, including "increased ability to adjust to economic conditions, broadened knowledge of current events, understanding the value of health and sanitation . . . and improved employability." This new knowledge, in turn, would allow them to contribute to society in the future.[42]

In the eyes of state officials, not every family qualified for these programs, and they trained caseworkers accordingly. They worried that social workers might focus only on distributing relief funds and forget that "there will always be families and individuals whose personal maladjustments have little direct relationship to economic distress." Other messages focused on the need to be alert for mental defects or other signs that a family's poverty was not "normal." Eligibility guidelines required that recipients be residents of the state for at least a year before receiving aid—but if the social worker decided that the person was a "pauper," that requirement went up to three years. In one sample period in 1938, social workers denied 21 percent of the applications for general relief, although the statistics do not indicate their grounds for denial. The standards for ADC were even higher, at 31 percent of cases denied in that same time period. As under Mothers' Aid, families were sometimes denied assistance for not meeting eligibility criteria or for "not cooperating."[43]

Social workers put this training into practice as they applied intense scrutiny to recipients of federal benefits. Relief funds came with close supervision: every person applying for federal benefits underwent screening at their local welfare office, where trained social workers questioned them about their personal lives. Their investigations included a home visit and questions about "savings, debts, relatives, health, and diet." They also interviewed community members who knew the needy families, posing questions "to clergymen, to school teachers, to public nurses or to whatever society might possibly assist them." For some families, scrutiny involved tests by Crane and his staff. In one two-year period, about 43 percent of people they tested came to them from county welfare staff (with others coming from state institutions or teachers). State officials felt that if they could create several traveling mental hygiene clinics, many more county officials would bring people for testing.[44]

Table 7.1 Sterilization operations by year and type of operation, 1929–44

Year	Male		Female		Total
	Vasectomy	Castration	Salpingectomy	Ovariectomy	
1929	1	1	—	1	3
1930	—	2	10	5	17
1931	—	—	10	1	11
1932	—	9	7	2	18
1933	1	—	3	—	4
1934	7	8	45	1	61
1935	17	7	152	2	178
1936	11	1	86	—	98
1937	18	3	105	2	128
1938	53	3	144	2	202
1939	34	2	102	—	138
1940	45	2	112	—	159
1941	45	4	132	—	181
1942	32	4	112	—	148
1943	29	4	119	0	152
1944 (to June 30)	4	—	38	—	42
Total	297	50	1,177	16	1,540

Source: Biennial Report of the North Carolina Eugenics Board, 1942–44, 10.

The state's hundreds of new social workers also approached their work with assumptions based on their own backgrounds. County social workers were predominantly white, middle-class women with some work experience but little previous social work training. Most held a college degree, and many had experience as teachers or clerical workers. The average caseworker in 1941 made $1,210 to $1,360 a year, solidly within the range of the average income nationwide. Their salary alone would have set them apart from their clients.[45]

Sterilization in Practice

For about 175 people every year in the late 1930s, social workers or institutional officials decided that the public good necessitated sterilization.[46] The remaining records of the Eugenics Board make clear that the state welfare board's rhetoric about fitness resonated with many social workers. The demographic patterns of the people sterilized match the Board of Charities and Public Welfare's long-standing depiction of the "unfit"—a poor white girl or woman, ostensibly feebleminded, who likely had children out of wedlock or fathered by a Black man. By the time Commissioner Bost left her post in 1944, the state had sterilized 1,540 people (see table 7.1). About half of the operations were on

Table 7.2 Sterilization operations performed before and after the creation of the Eugenics Board, by origin of petition

Origin of petition	1929–32	1933–44	Total (1929–44)
State institutions	27	909	936
County institutions	9	57	66
Noninstitutional	13	525	538
Total	49	1,491	1,540

Source: Information compiled from several sets of statistics that refer to different time periods, each with slightly different information. See R. Eugene Brown, "Sterilization Law Is Being Used," *Public Welfare Progress* 11, no. 4 (April 1930): 5; *BCPW Report, 1930–32*, 76; Brown, *Eugenical Sterilization in North Carolina* (1935), 13, 16–20; *First Biennial Report of the Eugenics Board, 1934–36*; and *Biennial Report of the Eugenics Board, 1942–44*, 9–11.

children or teenagers under nineteen, three-quarters were on girls or women, and about three-quarters were on white people. By far the most common reason indicated for sterilization was feeblemindedness (almost two-thirds of cases), with epilepsy, dementia praecox, and manic depressive psychosis also common diagnoses.[47]

Eugenics Board secretary R. Eugene Brown developed a process intended to streamline approvals as much as the law allowed. Any institutional head or county welfare superintendent could complete a petition to have someone sterilized on the basis that they were feebleminded, epileptic, or mentally diseased, or that the sterilization was good for the patient or the public. Brown collected petitions and presented a summary of cases before the Eugenics Board each month, highlighting details that he believed were salient.[48] In most cases, the Eugenics Board obtained the "consent" of the person's guardian, but sometimes family members refused to consent and instead appeared at the Eugenic Board's meeting to argue against the operation. The Eugenics Board almost always approved an operation; in its first eleven years of operation, it denied only forty-five petitions, less than 3 percent of the cases. Once the operation was approved, a nearby surgeon would carry out the order. Brown and his staff carefully tracked whether operations had been performed; in about 15 percent of cases, the operation was not performed.[49]

Until the early 1950s, the majority of petitions came from heads of institutions seeking to sterilize their residents (see table 7.2). In particular, they hoped to sterilize people before they released them back to their homes. Grace Robson, who took over as the head of Samarcand Manor in late 1933, worked with county superintendents to sterilize twenty-eight former inmates in 1935.[50] Brown wanted to sterilize all Caswell inmates except for the few "normal children" who had been "committed through error." Caswell, Samarcand, Jackson, and the other correctional facilities did not have surgical facilities to do sterilizations, so their inmates had to be sent to one of the mental hospitals that did. After 1935, Caswell was more able to sterilize its inmates because the legislature appropriated $1,500 annually to cover sterilization costs.[51] By 1944, 140 Caswell inmates and 208 Samarcand inmates had been sterilized. Still, during Bost's tenure, the Raleigh mental hospital was responsible for the most institutional sterilizations. About fifty inmates there were sterilized each year, a notable increase over the roughly dozen sterilizations the mental hospital had averaged during the 1920s and early 1930s, before the Eugenics Board gave officials more legal protection for their work.[52] The second most active institution was the mental hospital for Black people at Goldsboro, which was also designated as the state institution for feebleminded Black people. Of the Black people sterilized in this period, more than half were at Goldsboro. It was the one place in the state where more men were sterilized than women, perhaps a product of white fears about Black men's sexuality.[53]

North Carolina stood out in the nation for permitting the sterilization of people who lived *outside* of institutions, allowing a rare chance to explore ways in which social work professionals responded to eugenics programs.[54] Eugenic sterilization patterns during Bost's tenure illuminate how social workers negotiated the divide between urban and rural areas and between their own middle-class background and communities of poor, often illiterate people. Social workers were mostly natives of the state whose professional training provided them with a new perspective on the problems of their state. Eugenic-derived messages about "fit" and "unfit" people permeated their professional landscape. In addressing local problems, they drew on theoretical models from their training that prompted them to view the state's social problems as residing in individuals and families rather than in the larger economic, education, or class systems.

Between 1933 and 1944, 525 petitions (35 percent of total petitions) originated outside institutions. These petitions were concentrated in a few counties, demonstrating the eagerness with which certain social workers embraced eugenic sterilization as a pragmatic solution to widespread poverty in the context of underfunded welfare departments, while others did not submit a single petition. Predictably, counties with the highest numbers of sterilizations contained urban centers: Mecklenburg (Charlotte), Wake (Raleigh), Forsyth (Winston-Salem), Guilford (Greensboro), and Durham (Durham). But these figures look different if they are adjusted for population size. Between 1933 and 1945, several counties significantly exceeded the average sterilization rate of 1.725 per 10,000 people (see table 7.3). Most of these counties share two qualities: first, they were rural. Their population densities fell below the state's average population density of seventy-three persons per square mile. Second, many of these counties are close to the state capital in Raleigh,

Table 7.3 Noninstitutional sterilization petition rates in selected North Carolina counties (counties with highest per capita sterilization petition rates), 1934–44

County	Petitions submitted	Population density in 1940 (people per square mile)	Population in 1940	Sterilization petitions per 10,000 people
State (total or mean)	607	72.7	3,571,623	1.70
Orange	31	58.0	23,072	13.44
Moore	31	46.1	30,969	10.01
Transylvania	12	32.3	12,241	9.80
Avery	11	54.9	13,561	8.11
Lee	12	73.5	18,743	6.40
Chatham	15	35.0	24,726	6.07
Anson	15	53.4	28,443	5.27
Durham	42	268.4	80,244	5.23
Vance	15	111.4	29,961	5.01
Onslow	7	23.7	17,939	3.90
Cherokee	7	40.3	18,813	3.72
Northampton	10	52.4	28,299	3.53
Caldwell	11	75.2	35,795	3.07
Montgomery	5	33.4	16,280	3.07
Warren	7	52.0	23,145	3.02
Nash	16	100.7	55,608	2.88
Burke	11	76.3	38,615	2.85
Davie	4	56.5	14,909	2.68
Sampson	11	49.3	47,440	2.32
Edgecombe	11	96.2	49,162	2.24
Watauga	4	56.6	18,114	2.21
Wake	24	126.5	109,544	2.19
Wilkes	9	56.2	43,003	2.09
Wayne	12	105.1	58,328	2.06
Cabarrus	12	165.0	59,393	2.02
Duplin	8	48.3	39,739	2.01

Source: This tally differs slightly from the figures in Table 7.2 because the data sources are different. The Eugenics Board did not publish a breakdown by county. Instead, data here are compiled from a database created by Johanna Schoen of petitions submitted to sterilize noninstitutional residents and residents of county homes, by county, 1934–44. Data from 1934–37 are less complete. I am very grateful to Schoen for sharing this information with me. Population totals and population density data are from the *1940 U.S. Census of Population*, vol. 1: *Number of Inhabitants*, 773–74.

the headquarters of the state welfare board, and to the state university at Chapel Hill (see map 7.1). All of the counties that participated in the four-county welfare demonstration in the 1920s (Chatham, Cherokee, Durham, and Orange) had high rates. Equally telling, all twenty-three counties that submitted zero petitions between 1933 and 1944 were on the far east and west edges of the state, the farthest from the capital and the university.

Proximity, in fact, was key. In the 1930s, North Carolina's roads were abysmal. Although state fieldwork supervisors visited each county office two to three times per month, county caseworkers' ability to travel was restricted by small county travel budgets during the Depression and by gasoline rationing and tire shortages during the subsequent war. Travel difficulties hampered rural social workers' ability not only to deal with their caseloads, but also to attend UNC training programs or district meetings. Repeated exposure to training was more feasible for social workers who worked close to Chapel Hill, and this training was likely one factor that led social workers to submit sterilization petitions at higher rates.[55]

We have invaluable evidence about noninstitutional sterilizations and social workers' decisions from two contemporary studies, including one statewide analysis and one in-depth study of a county with a high sterilization rate. For her master's degree in social work, Eleanor Welborn analyzed 229 noninstitutional sterilization cases statewide from 1933 to 1938. J. McLean Benson, a sociology student at UNC, wrote a master's thesis in 1936 on sterilization in Orange County.[56]

Orange County was likely state officials' ideal of a sterilization program because its welfare department was interested in "securing a better generation, both mentally and physically." Orange County had the highest per capita sterilization rate in this time period, largely because the superintendent of public welfare was George H. Lawrence. Lawrence had been a student at UNC, where his academic work included research in the early 1920s on a feebleminded family, a study of Mothers' Aid families, and a study of boys at Jackson Training School. He also oversaw Orange County's participation in the four-county welfare demonstration and wrote his thesis about that effort. He and Benson's thesis adviser Ernest Groves were both members of the Conference for Social Service committee that worked on revising the state's sterilization law in the wake of *Brewer v. Valk*. Starting in 1932, Lawrence taught social work at UNC, supervising students' fieldwork training and simultaneously overseeing Orange County's welfare program.[57]

In his thesis, Benson examined twenty-one sterilization cases that Lawrence submitted, including eighteen noninstitutional cases. These case studies provide insight into Lawrence's thought processes, suggesting that he saw eugenic sterilization as a solution to many social problems beyond hereditary

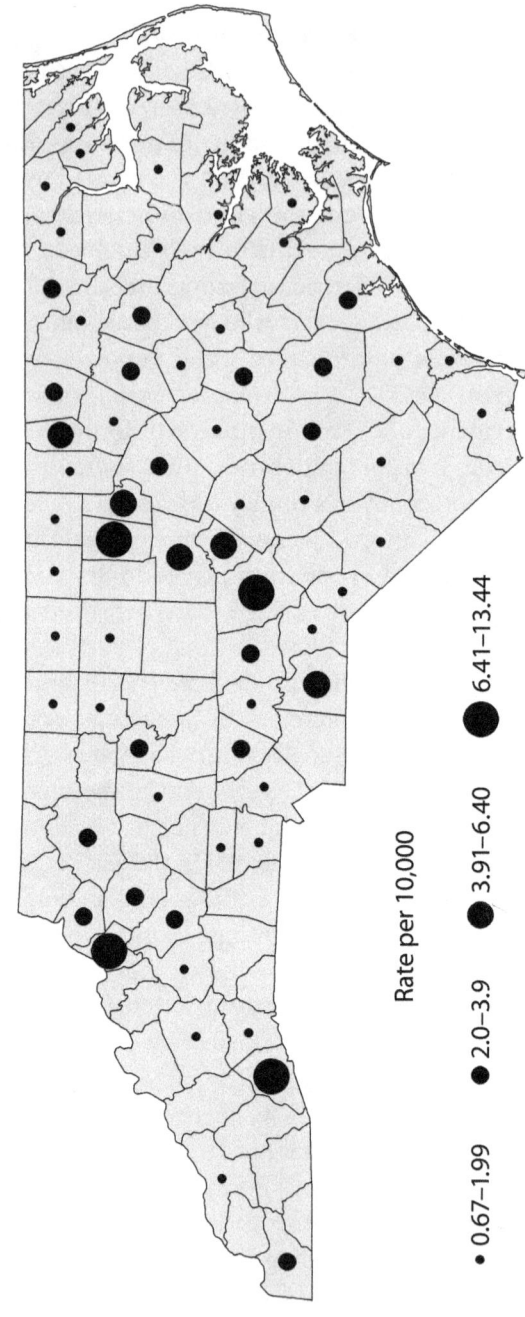

Map 7.1 Noninstitutional sterilization petition rates by county per 10,000 occupants (in 1940 census) in North Carolina, 1934–44. Sterilization data is compiled from a database created by Johanna Schoen of sterilization petitions submitted by county, 1934–44 (note that data before 1937 are less complete). I am very grateful to Schoen for sharing this information with me. Population data is from the 1940 U.S. *Census of Population*, vol. 1: *Number of Inhabitants*, 773. Map by Matt Simon.

mental defects. Almost without exception, Benson's case summaries mentioned the families' poverty. In fact, he proposed that people on public assistance or in institutions were natural candidates for sterilization. Since the public already bore the cost of their maintenance, he wrote, "the public in turn has a right to demand some protectionary measures against the possibilities of an increase in the future." Welborn's statewide study, likewise, found that in 13 percent of noninstitutional sterilization cases, the main "defect" was being a "pauper."[58]

Yet something set targets of sterilization apart from the average welfare recipient. In the cases Benson chronicled, families came to social workers' attention not only because of poverty but also because of criminal activity, alcohol use, and sex delinquency. Welborn, too, observed that just under half of people sterilized had been in court for at least one offense prior to the sterilization. Social workers were likely to interpret "deviant" behavior, in particular sexual behavior outside acceptable norms, as evidence that a person was feebleminded.[59] Eugenics Board forms asked for a medical and social history, including results of mental exams, a list of the person's children, and prompts about the patient's "social and economic status in their community" (see figure 7.1). Petitioners were specifically asked to describe "abnormal or anti-social behavior." Such behavior was clearly gendered; in Welborn's analysis, a quarter of the women sterilized had at least one illegitimate child, while none of the men sterilized had illegitimate children recorded as part of their petition.[60]

The application of the sterilization law thus reflected a common feature of eugenics programs: although programs were based on hereditarian logic, environmental factors loomed large in practice. The Eugenics Board petition asked for a family history of "defects," but petitioners did not have to show that the patient's condition was hereditary, as a strictly hereditarian eugenic approach would require. Instead, the law also allowed for sterilization when it was "believed to be for the public good" or for the "mental, moral, or physical improvement" of the patient. Brown even opened his introductory pamphlet on the Eugenics Board with a quote from a national eugenics publication that argued for the importance of environmental causes: "We do not know precisely to what extent mental defects and psychopathic conditions are inherited. But we do know that on the whole, feeble-minded and insane persons who are permitted to propagate their kind, raise families in a most unfavorable home environment." A study commissioned by the governor two years later echoed similar logic, arguing that "we find more reasons for sterilization [from an environmental viewpoint] than appear from the standpoint of eugenics. . . . Mentally handicapped parents are a liability."[61]

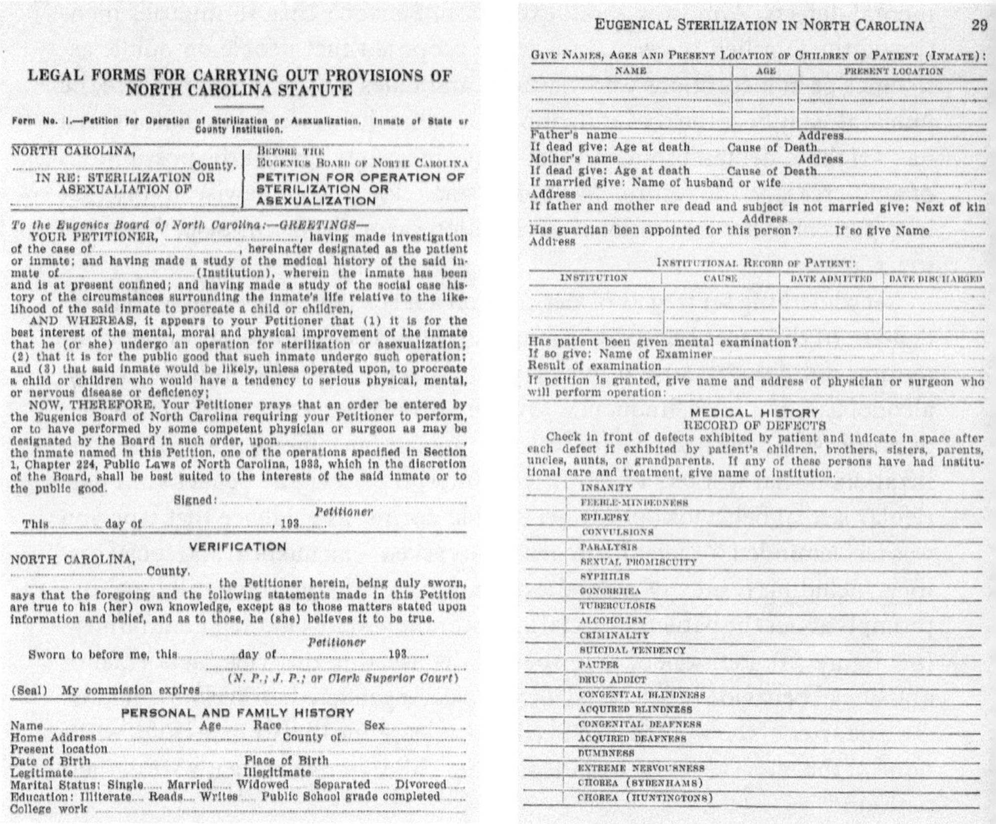

LEGAL FORMS FOR CARRYING OUT PROVISIONS OF NORTH CAROLINA STATUTE

Form No. 1.—Petition for Operation of Sterilization or Asexualization. Inmate of State or County Institution.

NORTH CAROLINA, ... County. IN RE: STERILIZATION OR ASEXUALIATION OF	BEFORE THE EUGENICS BOARD OF NORTH CAROLINA **PETITION FOR OPERATION OF STERILIZATION OR ASEXUALIZATION**

To the Eugenics Board of North Carolina:—GREETINGS—

YOUR PETITIONER, ..., having made investigation of the case of ...., hereinafter designated as the patient or inmate; and having made a study of the medical history of the said inmate of .... (Institution), wherein the inmate has been and is at present confined; and having made a study of the social case history of the circumstances surrounding the inmate's life relative to the likelihood of the said inmate to procreate a child or children,

AND WHEREAS, it appears to your Petitioner that (1) it is for the best interest of the mental, moral and physical improvement of the inmate that he (or she) undergo an operation for sterilization or asexualization; (2) that it is for the public good that such inmate undergo such operation; and (3) that said inmate would be likely, unless operated upon, to procreate a child or children who would have a tendency to serious physical, mental, or nervous disease or deficiency;

NOW, THEREFORE, Your Petitioner prays that an order be entered by the Eugenics Board of North Carolina requiring your Petitioner to perform, or to have performed by some competent physician or surgeon as may be designated by the Board in such order, upon ...., the inmate named in this Petition, one of the operations specified in Section 1, Chapter 224, Public Laws of North Carolina, 1933, which in the discretion of the Board, shall be best suited to the interests of the said inmate or to the public good.

Signed: ....
Petitioner

This .... day of ...., 193......

VERIFICATION

NORTH CAROLINA,
.... County.

........................, the Petitioner herein, being duly sworn, says that the foregoing and the following statements made in this Petition are true to his (her) own knowledge, except as to those matters stated upon information and belief, and as to those, he (she) believes it to be true.

....
Petitioner

Sworn to before me, this .... day of .... 193......

....
(N. P.; J. P.; or Clerk Superior Court)

(Seal) My commission expires ....

PERSONAL AND FAMILY HISTORY

Name .... Age ...... Race .... Sex ....
Home Address .... County of ....
Present location ....
Date of Birth .... Place of Birth ....
Legitimate .... Illegitimate ....
Marital Status: Single ...... Married ...... Widowed ...... Separated ...... Divorced ......
Education: Illiterate ...... Reads ...... Writes ...... Public School grade completed ......
College work ....

EUGENICAL STERILIZATION IN NORTH CAROLINA 29

GIVE NAMES, AGES AND PRESENT LOCATION OF CHILDREN OF PATIENT (INMATE):

NAME	AGE	PRESENT LOCATION

Father's name .... Address ....
If dead give: Age at death .... Cause of Death ....
Mother's name .... Address ....
If dead give: Age at death .... Cause of Death ....
If married give: Name of husband or wife ....
Address ....
If father and mother are dead and subject is not married give: Next of kin .... Address ....
Has guardian been appointed for this person? .... If so give Name ....
Address ....

INSTITUTIONAL RECORD OF PATIENT:

INSTITUTION	CAUSE	DATE ADMITTED	DATE DISCHARGED

Has patient been given mental examination? ....
If so give: Name of Examiner ....
Result of examination ....

If petition is granted, give name and address of physician or surgeon who will perform operation: ....

MEDICAL HISTORY
RECORD OF DEFECTS

Check in front of defects exhibited by patient and indicate in space after each defect if exhibited by patient's children, brothers, sisters, parents, uncles, aunts, or grandparents. If any of these persons have had institutional care and treatment, give name of institution.

	INSANITY	
	FEEBLE-MINDEDNESS	
	EPILEPSY	
	CONVULSIONS	
	PARALYSIS	
	SEXUAL PROMISCUITY	
	SYPHILIS	
	GONORRHEA	
	TUBERCULOSIS	
	ALCOHOLISM	
	CRIMINALITY	
	SUICIDAL TENDENCY	
	PAUPER	
	DRUG ADDICT	
	CONGENITAL BLINDNESS	
	ACQUIRED BLINDNESS	
	CONGENITAL DEAFNESS	
	ACQUIRED DEAFNESS	
	DUMBNESS	
	EXTREME NERVOUSNESS	
	CHOREA (SYDENHAMS)	
	CHOREA (HUNTINGTONS)	

Figure 7.1 Excerpt of blank forms for officials to nominate people to the Eugenics Board for sterilization under the 1933 law. Brown, *Eugenical Sterilization in North Carolina* (1935), 28–29, North Carolina Collection, Louis Round Wilson Special Collections Library, University of North Carolina at Chapel Hill.

The importance of social or environmental factors is clear in a comparison of sterilization victims to recipients of public assistance. Both sterilization targets and recipients of Mothers' Aid or ADC were more likely to be women than men. But social workers were inclined to think of sterilization in only some of these cases. According to Benson, people nominated for sterilization in Orange County were "quite undesirable," exhibited "degenerate traits," associated with "riff-raff," and were unwilling to support themselves. These were people the state welfare board would have categorized as incapable of benefiting from relief, "whose personal maladjustments have little direct relationship to economic distress."[62] Moreover, as one contemporary study noted, the financial considerations of local welfare departments made them particularly likely to notice "the dependent mother of one or more children and the promiscuous feeble-minded girl." Women's ability to bear children, the sexual double standard, and their economic insecurity made them more of a target for sterilizations outside of institutions, making up almost 90 percent of operations.[63]

In counties with low sterilization rates, the usual barrier to sterilization was cost. Each operation cost around thirty dollars. In 1938 an average ADC family with four members received sixteen dollars a month, and it cost a county an average of seventeen dollars per month to maintain one person in a county home.[64] The cost of a sterilization operation was thus roughly equivalent to the cost of two to eight months of public assistance for one person. Each superintendent, state officials believed, knew of "many cases where a few dollars for sterilization (either on mental or physical grounds) would constitute an excellent preventive measure. Failure to provide funds for this purpose will tremendously increase our public burden in the future." Moya Woodside, who wrote a book-length study of sterilization in North Carolina in 1950, reported that the majority of county social workers were "in favor of sterilization."[65] To them, the cost of an operation was money well spent, since they believed each operation would prevent the perpetuation of mental defects that led to poverty and delinquency—a short-term cost but long-term savings. The sticking point was convincing other county officials. The state law mandated that counties had to assume the costs of the operation, but by 1936 no county board of commissioners had allocated recurring funds for sterilizations. Instead, county officials had to be convinced to pay for each operation separately.[66] Closely related constraints were the limited capacity of county workers to prepare the petition paperwork along with their other duties, the lack of mental testing availability in counties far from clinics at Chapel Hill and Caswell, and limited surgical facilities. Of course, not all social workers supported eugenic sterilization, and some raised ethical objections or simply did not nominate their clients for operations.[67]

Ongoing pushback from would-be targets of sterilization was another significant barrier. Benson described one white teenage girl from Orange County whom the Eugenics Board approved for sterilization because of her sex delinquency and her "apparent" feeblemindedness. Although her parents and brother gave their consent for the operation, Annie did not want to be sterilized. She claimed to be sick so that welfare officials would not take her to the hospital, then was "hateful." Lawrence's staff eventually "persuaded" her by unspecified means to go to the hospital, where they took away her street clothes, hoping she would not try to run away dressed only in her nightgown. She was sterilized. In another Orange County case, a family's resistance was more successful. This white family was a "constant problem to the welfare office," and Lawrence applied to sterilize both parents and their six children.

The Human Element in the Modern Welfare State 205

After most of the family was "induced" to visit Harry Crane's office for a mental exam, they grew suspicious. They moved "during the darkness of some night" to a neighboring county, where welfare officials were less interested in sterilizing them. But the family could not move back home: Benson reported that if they returned without having been sterilized, "Orange County is ready for them."[68]

At least two people in the early years of the Eugenics Board went as far as challenging the law, but with results that only strengthened the state's hand. One person appealed their case to the superior court in March 1934. In the face of this resistance, the Eugenics Board quietly backed off, thinking they could obtain the consent of the family later. Another appeal in February 1935 went to the superior court, which upheld the Eugenics Board's decision.[69] The state responded to these early challenges by further tightening the law with a 1935 amendment that specified the appeals process and provided a path for "consent" to the operation. The vast majority of families did sign consent forms, although doubtless such consent was compromised by power imbalances between welfare officials (on whom families relied for relief funds) or by families' illiteracy or lack of information about the procedures.[70]

Another group of people—or at least their relatives—sought out or welcomed sterilization operations. In one case Benson described, a brother and a sister were engaged in incestuous relations. Their parents saw sterilization as the only way to prevent another pregnancy. In other cases, women saw sterilization as desirable for themselves because it was one way to protect against unwanted pregnancies in the absence of other effective contraceptive methods. One woman had suffered severe depression and attempted suicide because of her fear of pregnancy, and sterilization seemed to her an excellent alternative. This pattern of elective sterilization was a constant in the later decades of the Eugenics Board, highlighting the lack of viable alternatives as well as many poor women's creativity in navigating their limited options.[71]

A "Racial Responsibility": Public Perceptions of Sterilization

Brown, Bost, and their colleagues in the state welfare office were often frustrated with the slow growth of the eugenic sterilization program. In addition to cost constraints and procedural difficulties, some people objected to sterilization on principle. Some people opposed it on religious grounds, particularly fundamentalist Christian beliefs. For these people, sterilization was morally troubling in part because it allowed sterilized people to have sex without the possibility of pregnancy and, they believed, would lead to promiscuity or venereal disease. Others raised nonreligious ethical objections; some people viewed sterilization as an unnecessary punishment or worried about its effects in "unsexing" men, perhaps conflating vasectomy with castration. In 1938, one small-town theater screened *Tomorrow's Child*, an antisterilization film that critiqued state-sponsored sterilization as government overreach. Billing the film as "a gripping drama of a beautiful girl caught in the meshes of the sterilization law," they invited preachers, doctors, and mayors to attend for free. A few critics with medical training saw sterilization laws as a good step but criticized them on scientific grounds. The degree of uncertainty in inherited qualities, they argued, meant that "to attempt to breed a certain type of individual is absurd, to say nothing of the difficulties arising as to who should be the judge of the standard we are to produce."[72]

Yet public opinion often favored sterilization for economic reasons. When the 1933 law first passed, the *News and Observer* highlighted its usefulness in limiting the size of feebleminded families who "now contribut[e] so largely to county and State expense." In 1934, the leaders of the Charlotte Junior League used their annual space in the newspaper to contemplate the future of welfare work as emergency relief funds dried up. Even when able-bodied people could return to work and take care of themselves, they said, governments would still spend increasing amounts on "indigent, diseased, mentally deficient beings," which would require raising taxes. The solution they proposed was "a more liberal application" of the sterilization law. Targeting families with "no hope of ever becoming self-sustaining again" would "do more to improve, if not solve, the social and economic condition of our state than anything else." Moreover, they argued, sterilization was humane because it prevented the birth of people who were "diseased at birth, with no hope or opportunity to ever enjoy life." Editorials in small-town papers sounded similar notes, calling for sterilizing the "indigent class" or "all those who persistently and permanently remain on the relief or unemployment rolls." They acknowledged that some people were not at fault for needing charity, but argued others were "too lazy" to help themselves. Some editorials pointed to more active sterilization efforts in Germany as a rational economic response.[73]

Official support for sterilization as part of "mental hygiene" efforts was also increasing. In 1935, the governor appointed a commission to study "the care of the insane and mental defectives." Chaired by Frederic M. Hanes, a professor of neurology at Duke's School of Medicine, the commission also included a Duke professor of psychiatry, a Baptist minister, a newspaper editor, and a lawyer. After eighteen months of work funded by the Rockefeller Foundation, the commission released a 377-page report. They focused largely on the extent of these problems among white people, while also claiming that the intelligence of Black people was generally lower and the incidence of insanity just as high. By conservative estimates, they said, there were 27,734 mentally defective white children in the state who needed institutionalization, sterilization, or special classes in schools. Among their sixteen recommendations was continuing sterilization "on the same basis but on a larger scale," including "milder borderline cases." All mentally defective people, they argued, were always near the possibility of "social failure." The commission also recommended supporting UNC's training programs with an emphasis on "the mental hygiene principles that pervade all social work." They echoed Board of Charities and Public Welfare opinions that "extreme need of money" often indicated a person was "psychopathic" or had "underlying maladjustments in the realm of physical and mental health, family relationships, [or] past training and experience."[74]

Like policymakers in the previous two decades, the commission was concerned with the capacity of state institutions. As the commission composed their report, new cottages were being built at Caswell to bring the capacity to over eight hundred beds. This construction was the result of a $900,000 commitment to increasing the size of state institutions for the insane and feebleminded, the combination of a state bond issue and Public Works Administration funds. Yet Caswell's waiting list was over eight hundred names long, and the commission calculated that by conservative estimates there were 16,700 "socially maladjusted mental defectives" in the state, of whom 10 percent should be institutionalized. They called for adding a second training school for mentally defective children, perhaps including space for Black children.[75]

The commission's work built public sentiment to increase provisions for mental diseases and led to some concrete changes for North Carolina. Newspapers published its recommendations, and some pointed out that North Carolina's lack of provisions for the insane and feebleminded was out of step with recent progress it had made in other areas. Perhaps thanks to the report, in 1937, a new law criminalized both aiding Caswell inmates in escaping and engaging in "prostitution" with any inmate. The report generated interest in passing additional sterilization requirements, including a failed 1937 bill that would have required women to be sterilized before marriage if either partner was an "idiot, imbecile, or of unsound mind." The commission's work also led to discussions with the governor about consolidating mental hospitals and other mental hygiene services into a unified "state psychiatric service." This idea came to fruition with a 1943 law creating a unified state Hospitals Board of Control.[76]

White reformers, who had been so influential in building support for eugenics in the 1910s and 1920s, were still interested onlookers. Members of the Conference for Social Service continued to discuss the need for eugenics programs. In 1932 they elected as president Ella Waddill, who had been superintendent of public welfare in Vance County for ten years. The state welfare office sent a special invitation to the state's social workers to attend the 1932 Conference gathering.[77] There, Waddill spent much of her hourlong speech discussing the need for stronger eugenics programs, arguing that "we have been *so busy* trying to provide care for those [children] already born, that I fear we have not stressed enough the importance of working for a *better born child*, or a *better average child*." Waddill warned against the "constant stream of physically and mentally unfit" and was adamant that "people of unsound mind have no right to bring their kind into the world" or "further contaminate the race." The "only way to attack this problem," she argued, "is through a study of *Eugenics*," including marriage laws and greater use of sterilization. Among those who should be sterilized, she argued, were "chronic criminals" and "chronic paupers." Waddill spoke with the authority of a veteran, acknowledging the huge time demands for social workers who tried to "adjust" feebleminded families to their communities. Still, she was hopeful that "our sense of social responsibility is becoming a sense of *racial* responsibility ... which renders possible what we call the regeneration of the race."[78] In other meetings during the decade, Conference members covered a range of related topics. They were early supporters of birth control as part of mental hygiene efforts, supporting federal funding for birth control in 1934; three years later, North Carolina became the first state to sponsor distribution of contraceptives. The Conference endorsed training teachers about mental hygiene and offering college courses on it. They also supported more stringent physical exams before marriage, aiming at syphilis and its related effects on mental health.[79]

But the Conference lost some of its political influence during the 1930s. In the first part of the decade, it was still a meeting ground for key reformers: John Bradway, the architect of the 1933 sterilization law; Alexander McAlister and the Conference founders; Ella Waddill and county social workers; Annie Kizer Bost and state officials; Grace Robson, head of Samarcand Manor; and Harry Crane and UNC faculty—all routinely crossed paths on Conference committees and Board meetings.[80] In 1934, however, the Conference claimed just over 140 members, a notable decline from the many hundreds who had regularly attended annual meetings in the past. By 1940, membership rebounded but the composition of the group changed, with 85 percent of paying members being professional social workers. The Conference struggled to maintain the interest of the lay reformers who had been the organization's foundation, were more likely to make financial contributions, and served as vital gateways to the rest of North Carolina's white elite.

Other organizations stepped in as advocates for eugenics programs. First was a resurrected Mental Hygiene Society. The original society, founded in 1913, had petered out. In 1936, a group of enthusiasts, many with links to the Conference for Social Service, organized a new society. Ernest Groves, the

UNC professor who supervised J. McLean Benson's study of Orange County sterilizations, was the president, succeeded by Crane and Bradway. The Eugenics Board's R. Eugene Brown was also an officer.[81] The state society oversaw the growth of local mental societies, starting with existing mental hygiene clinics in Charlotte and Durham. By 1952, there were half a dozen functioning mental hygiene clinics and as many as twenty local mental hygiene societies.[82]

Another powerful advocacy group was the Human Betterment League of North Carolina, founded in 1947 to promote sterilization after concerns about mental deficiency once again surged during wartime. The organization reflected the long-standing pro-eugenics partnerships between public and private, academics and practitioners, medical doctors and social workers: George H. Lawrence, the former Orange County welfare superintendent and UNC social work professor, was its first president. Early financial support came from geneticist Clarence Gamble and textile magnate James Hanes, the brother of Lucy Hodgins Hanes Chatham, who had been frustrated by Mary Brewer's appearance at her door in the early 1930s. Other charter members included four UNC faculty and staff members (one then director of UNC's Institute for Research in Social Science and another the director of the university's news bureau); C. Nash Herndon, a geneticist who taught at Wake Forest's Bowman Gray School of Medicine; and Helen Hunter, the president of the state Mental Hygiene Society. For the next four decades, the Human Betterment League stridently promoted sterilization, family planning, and genetic counseling through a publicity onslaught built on principles of eugenics.[83]

Buoyed by public support, state welfare leaders expanded sterilization programs. Annie Kizer Bost's successor in 1944 was Ellen Winston, another strong advocate of eugenic sterilization. A high school teacher in the Raleigh area, Winston had become interested in sociology, thanks in part to Howard Odum's extension courses, and she went on to earn a PhD in sociology. Her first published article investigated rates of mental illness and its relationship to modern civilization. As early as 1934, she was involved in the Conference for Social Service's mental hygiene committee. She worked for FERA and the WPA in Washington during the New Deal, then returned to North Carolina, where she taught, wrote, and was active in multiple white women's clubs. After taking office in 1944, Winston pushed to further professionalize the public welfare staff and expand welfare services to both white and Black recipients.[84]

Thanks in part to Winston's advocacy, the number of sterilizations grew in new directions. Social workers' active use of the sterilization law resulted in a notable increase in the number of noninstitutional sterilizations. Before 1950, noninstitutional sterilizations constituted 40 percent of sterilizations, but between 1950 and 1966, they were over 70 percent of sterilizations.[85] Winston also mounted a campaign to expand the programs as part of the fight against poverty. The Eugenics Board's justification shifted further away from hereditary theories and toward "culture of poverty" rhetoric that posited the transmission of undesirable traits through socialization. At the same time, the extension of welfare benefits to African Americans, fears about Black women's fertility, and concern about rising welfare costs led to a "significant shift in the racial composition" of the program. Whereas African Americans had been sterilized at lower rates than white people in the early years of the program, by the mid-1950s, they were sterilized at higher rates, with Black women targeted in particular. From 1957 onward, the majority of people sterilized were African Americans.[86]

We usually think of the New Deal as a radical modernization of the South. In some ways it was: it ushered in mechanized agriculture, which later forced a massive shift in the region's political economy. The New Deal left a lasting mark on the South's infrastructure, paving the way (sometimes literally) for postwar suburban expansion. FDR's appeal to a broad coalition, and the backlash among some conservative Democrats to New Deal policies, was the beginning of the demise of the Solid South. The New Deal created major new channels of federal funding, linked to regulations that enshrined at least the principle of equality into many citizens' interactions with state and federal governments.

At the same time, people who administered New Deal programs everywhere had to deal with local circumstances. In many cases the success of federal programs was predicated on administrators' ability and willingness to tolerate existing structures, many of which were far from equitable. The implementation of federal relief and Social Security programs in North Carolina was a case in point. In the realm of social welfare, the net effect of the New Deal was not to reshape the purpose of welfare, but rather to drastically expand the resources available to welfare officials—whose social vision, including a desire to eliminate mental defects among white people—remained unchanged.[87]

At least one historian has seen the persistence of North Carolina's county-based welfare programs during the New Deal as part of its "backwardness," its stubborn resistance to modernization.[88] Local politicians could indeed be obstinate in their refusal to raise taxes or adequately fund welfare services. Some historians have condemned state welfare officials, too, for their reluctance to cede power over welfare programs to new agencies, as officials in Washington would have preferred.[89]

But viewing North Carolina's politics from the perspective of frustrated Washington New Dealers or characterizing the New Deal as a radical departure from a retrograde past obscures important historical patterns. First, North Carolina's decision in 1935 to shift Social Security programs to the established framework of the Board of Charities and Public Welfare allowed welfare officials' personal relationships and intimate knowledge of local practices to smooth the transition. In this sense, North Carolina's dedication to localism had benefits as well as drawbacks. Second, the professional acumen of the welfare board's staff and their influence on new social workers after federal funds arrived meant that workers administering federal programs were trained with the priorities of the North Carolina's existing welfare program in mind. Those priorities included sterilization and teaching social workers to divide their clients into "normal" and "abnormal," a modern reinterpretation of the old dichotomy of worthy and unworthy poor. When the New Deal expanded public welfare, it also cemented eugenics practices as an integral part of the state's social work model.

In practice, North Carolina's welfare workers in the 1930s and early 1940s provided different kinds of social safety nets for what they saw as different kinds of people, using casework techniques to determine who was eligible. White, "self-respecting," and usually self-supporting people fallen on hard times received old-age pensions, ADC or other public assistance, or work relief jobs. For the "unfit"—chronic paupers or criminals, mentally defective people, the insane—social workers tended to use a different set of options: institutionalization, sterilization, or denial of benefits as a cudgel-like tool to push poor people to curb undesirable behaviors. Black people, even if not deemed "defective," were often denied the benefits accorded to the "fit" as a result of both policy and practice during Jim Crow.[90]

Even in the midst of the Depression, then, as families across the country were struggling to make ends meet, North Carolina county officials sometimes considered chronic poverty or "undesirable" social behavior grounds for sterilization. Their training predisposed them to make this decision. In their coursework, the social problems of poverty, delinquency, and feeble-mindedness were linked in numerous ways, and instructors posited that all these conditions were hereditary. Their mandate included both caring for clients and stretching welfare budgets as far as possible—and as long as government programs fell short of addressing the fundamental inequities of the Southern political economy, poverty persisted. Pulled in two different directions, they sometimes offered solutions for poverty and mental disease driven more by financial constraints than their clients' wishes. In addition, one of the basic principles of casework was regular and repeated contact with clients in order to reshape their behavior. Caseworkers who had average loads of twenty to thirty cases at a time were stretched thin, especially with limited travel budgets and many miles to cover between their rural clients. For particularly intransigent cases, where repeated visits produced few improvements, social workers may have seen sterilization as the most expedient solution for the long-term prevention of social problems.

Focusing on the training that social workers received reminds us of a persistent strain of American thought: the assumption that poverty is pathological or a result of immorality. During the Depression (when, after all, many people suffered from poverty and mental distress), the state labeled some poor, uneducated people as "feebleminded" and treated them as incapable or unworthy of raising children. Even as New Dealers challenged the stigmatization of poverty and celebrated the right of every person to live above certain minimum standards, many Americans believed some people were an undue burden on the rest, products of an abnormal type of poverty that would continue regardless of economic cycles. By the end of the 1930s, many North Carolinians with power to enact their ideas believed that dealing with this "indigent class" required both eugenic segregation and sterilization.

Epilogue

The human impact of North Carolina's embrace of eugenics ideology goes beyond the devastating effects for people who were sterilized. In the decades leading up to and during active eugenic sterilization programs, state and local officials embraced policies and practices that blamed chronically poor people for their own problems. By publicizing the supposed benefits of institutional segregation and the work of the Eugenics Board in sterilizing "abnormal" people, state officials built public acceptance of their work to make poor but "normal" families self-supporting. They did so for complex reasons: misplaced faith in their own ability to diagnose social problems, reliance on contemporary ideas about heredity that reinforced existing race and class prejudice, and a political environment that forced welfare workers to justify every penny spent on public assistance. As a result, reformers and welfare officials established in the public's mind the idea that "unfitness" was reason enough to deny a person the benefit of a social safety net, as well as to deny the possibility of having children.

Of course, the lack of a guarantee of public assistance was a national phenomenon, not unique to North Carolina. The inadequacy of the social safety net in the United States even after the New Deal was the result not of a single state's decisions but rather the product of widespread reluctance to invest in the common weal.[1] In North Carolina's history, however, we see quite clearly how eugenics helped carry that reluctance forward into the welfare state established during the New Deal years. Eugenics ideology, as purveyed by its believers in North Carolina, posited that some people simply were not fit to be part of society: they did not deserve assistance in hard times because, for them *and* for their offspring, hard times would never end. They were not elderly people who had already produced value for society, nor hard workers who needed temporary help or food, nor mothers whose labor in raising future citizens was worth supporting. Instead, they were people beyond help—chronic paupers, feebleminded people, people "unfit" to be parents. The very belief that such groups of people existed led naturally to the routine scrutiny of everyone receiving public assistance.

This pairing of full citizenship rights with fitness aligned with the assumptions of a white patriarchal society. Most white reformers, officials, and policymakers at the turn of the century accepted the natural superiority of men, white people, and middle-class or elite people. The eugenics policies they espoused, in turn, reinforced these assumptions. Their successes in rationalizing and normalizing biased policies embedded hierarchies of race, class, and gender into the modern state a century ago.[2] Even as modern society has rejected these reformers' most sordid views, many of our present ideas about welfare recipients and women's bodies reflect the legacy of eugenics. The state itself linked eligibility for public assistance to rigid moral standards for women's sexual behavior and for decades targeted poor women in an effort to "preserve" the "white race." We should not be surprised, then, at the continued appeal of sexist or white supremacist ideologies. The underlying logic of modern white supremacy—that not all Americans belong here or deserve full citizenship rights—owes an intellectual debt to the hundreds of white social reformers, welfare officials, legislators, and other advocates who embraced eugenics programs in the name of preserving the white race.

The close linkage of welfare and eugenics was not inevitable. On an institutional level, there were several moments when oversight of eugenic segregation or sterilization might have become the purview of medical doctors or public health officials. Many of these officials held similar views about eugenics and the need to target "unfit" white people. But social workers had unusual access to poor people's lives, making the housing of eugenics programs in welfare agencies particularly powerful. At the same time, from an intellectual perspective, welfare officials had other models for social work that were more equitable and less biased. Leftist social workers at the time were exploring ways to address the deeper structural issues responsible for endemic poverty, including exploitative labor systems and racial hierarchies. But North Carolina's politics and economy made those models unlikely to gain traction, as welfare officials faced pushback to their spending, particularly spending on Black recipients. Greater state and local support for public assistance would have required higher tax rates, which would have lowered profits in the state's industrial and agricultural sectors. More generous "outdoor relief" programs were unpopular until the Great Depression made them a near-necessity. Even then, business leaders pushed hard to keep payments for relief jobs low in order to maintain a cheap labor pool. These economic and political realities shaped the bounds of possibility for reformers and social workers, and they added appeal to arguments that eugenics programs could ultimately reduce costs for taxpayers. North Carolina's welfare officials and social workers chose to emphasize mental defects—individual failings, rather than societal ones—as they interacted with poor people.[3]

North Carolina's sterilization program lasted for four decades. It expanded after World War II, even as most states shuttered their programs. (For those interested, historian Johanna Schoen's *Choice and Coercion* is an excellent account of the state's sterilization program under the Eugenics Board.) Finally, thanks to the efforts of women's and civil rights activists, the program ended in 1977 when the legislature disbanded the Eugenics Commission (the successor to the Eugenics Board). The program then faded from public view for thirty years. Beginning in 2002, however, public attention to the state's history of eugenics grew, sparked by a series about the sterilization program in the *Winston-Salem Journal* that drew on Schoen's research. That year, Governor Mike Easley issued a formal apology for the state's sterilization program. A small group of survivors and their allies began to call for the state to provide financial remuneration in recognition of their suffering and inability to have children. The fight for compensation took a decade, but in 2013 the legislature created a system for victims to submit their claims. In late 2014 North Carolina became the first state to compensate people who were sterilized as part of its eugenics program, paying each eligible person at least $20,000. Because the sterilization program reached its peak in the 1950s and 1960s, and because many of the people sterilized were teenagers, officials estimated that as many as three thousand sterilization survivors might still be alive.[4]

As North Carolina has tried to come to terms with its eugenic past, the rhetoric surrounding sterilization survivors indicates, in some ways, how little things have actually changed. News coverage of the push for compensation legislation routinely focused on sterilization victims as mostly "poor minorities." While that statement is true for the program's most active years in the 1950s and 1960s, it is not true for the program's earlier years. It also misses larger points about the impact of eugenics on welfare programs.

The first point is about the striking gender dynamics of the sterilization program. Over the program's duration, approximately 84 percent of those sterilized were women, with a gradually increasing percentage over time. From the beginning of discussions about eugenics and feeblemindedness, reformers focused on women and girls. North Carolina's welfare and medical experts, like national eugenics experts, often argued that "high-grade" feebleminded girls were the most dangerous because they looked normal. Experts believed that these girls or women had an unusually high sex drive. White women's expressions of sexuality out of wedlock, which threatened ideas about white female purity, made them candidates for sterilization. In addition, because gendered roles assigned caregiving labor to women, their behavior was more likely to draw the attention of social workers evaluating a home. Proponents of eugenics often viewed parenting and housekeeping practices as evidence of someone's mental status, so women were more likely to be targeted as feebleminded or as unfit parents, as in the case of Mary Brewer. Despite these striking and consistent patterns, during the five years when the legislative fight for compensation was at its height, few news articles or opinion pieces focused on gender.[5]

Second, a focus on only the later years of North Carolina's sterilization program obscures the ways that strategies for maintaining racial and gender hierarchies evolved over time. For pro-eugenics reformers in the early twentieth century, rationales for targeting white women were always linked to racial ideologies and shaped by white fears of miscegenation. White women who were "oversexed" or challenged the racial order, especially those who bore children, threatened the racialized foundation of Southern society. In the mid-1950s, the state's sterilization programs began to focus on Black women. The turn was a response to the extension of welfare benefits to African Americans as Jim Crow was dismantled, the subsequent vilification of poor Black women as undeserving of public support, fears about Black women's fertility, and rising welfare costs. The shift in the racial demographics of sterilization targets was thus a product of the continuation of earlier white supremacist ideology, even as external conditions and the subjects in question shifted.[6]

The question, then, is why public discussions of North Carolina's eugenic past have neglected such obvious features. One answer may lie in the fact that many Americans share the assumptions about women's reproductive and social roles that framed eugenic segregation and sterilization a century ago. To many people, it makes sense that the programs targeted women, because women bear children. Yet sterilization programs could easily have targeted men as equally responsible for the genetic makeup or rearing of their offspring. Other people today might assume that targeting someone because of their race or gender was merely another mistake of the past that has since been corrected.

The tenor of recent public discussion has also been shaped by the political coalition that formed to pass the compensation bill, one last testament to the complicated politics of eugenic policies. The first champion of a compensation bill was Larry Womble, a Democrat, who received only a lukewarm reception from his party for the first several years. Democratic Governor Beverly Perdue later appointed a task force to study compensation, but it was not until Republicans gained control of both houses that compensation began to look like a real possibility. Thom Tillis, the speaker of the House after Republicans swept to victory in 2010 (and later a US senator), became the bill's new champion. A Catholic and opponent of abortion, Tillis was motivated by religious principles to support compensation for people who were forcibly sterilized. He and other conservative supporters of compensation framed the eugenic sterilization program as "big government run amok." The John Locke

Foundation, a Raleigh think tank, issued a 2011 report and subsequent editorials arguing that compensation would help "ensure that . . . such gross violations of natural, inalienable rights never happen again." The support of Tillis and other conservatives allowed a bipartisan victory, but their anti–big government and "pro-family" stance did not set up an easy alliance with reproductive rights activists. In this atmosphere, even the most liberal Democrats in this political coalition were unlikely to alienate their conservative allies by starting a discussion about the gender dynamics of sterilization.[7]

Apology or compensation efforts in other states have followed similar patterns. In Georgia, as Paul Lombardo has noted, the legislature passed a resolution apologizing for the state's eugenics programs only when a Republican senator joined the campaign. His version of the resolution highlighted links between eugenics and "Darwinian evolutionary theory" and claimed that eugenics legislation was adopted "despite 'religious objections'"—a claim of questionable historical accuracy. The resolution also expressed hope that Georgia citizens would be educated about eugenics in order to "foster a respect for the fundamental dignity of human life and the God given rights recognized by our Founding Fathers." In Virginia, the second state to agree to compensate sterilization victims, a similar coalition emerged between political liberals and religious conservatives, shepherded by Mark Bold, a Liberty University–trained lawyer who founded the Christian Law Institute, which defined itself as a "think tank . . . dedicated to advancing biblical principles through ideas and action." The rhetoric of Bold and his Republican ally emphasized compensation as an opportunity for "healing and forgiveness."[8]

The politics of these compensation debates have thus rendered unlikely any discussion of sterilization survivors as women with reproductive rights. As a result, we have not reckoned with the sex discrimination built into eugenic sterilization. By ignoring the assumptions that led to this sex discrimination, we may reduce women to their biological role in reproduction. The public has lost an opportunity to challenge long-standing but overly simplistic links between women, childbearing, and child-rearing. Finally, news that fails to untangle the importance of sex discrimination in these programs also fails to acknowledge the struggle against forced sterilization as a struggle for reproductive choice. From the perspective of reproductive rights activists, framing sterilization abuse as a nongendered question of sanctity of life rather than a women's issue undermines the movement for women's right to self-determination and control of their bodies.

I wrote this book because I want all people with a stake in the future of North Carolina to understand this complicated past—and because the issues of power and poverty at the heart of the history of eugenics are unlikely to disappear anytime soon. In fact, as public knowledge of eugenics programs has grown in the past two decades, politicians on both the left and right have tried to invoke aspects of the history to score political points. For example, when North Carolina's legislature passed a (pre–*Dobbs v. Jackson*) bill to ban abortions based on race, gender, or Down syndrome, one proponent called such procedures "eugenics in its worst form." Another legislator quickly pointed out that an abortion obtained by choice would be very different from forcible sterilization. The invocation of eugenics is often newsworthy; it is a concept with a fraught past, and many people have an immediate emotional response to hearing the term. My hope is that readers of this book will be better able to recognize modern forms of eugenics when they do appear, and to bring their historical understanding to bear on related ethical questions emerging from new technologies such as gene-editing.[9]

The widespread nature of eugenics ideology and programs is, in fact, important. Only by understanding how pervasive eugenics beliefs were for white elites and policymakers in the first half of the twentieth century can we see the effects of eugenics on the institutions they built and trace the elements of them that remain. We can also learn from the history of eugenics by remembering that dangerous ideologies can hold popular appeal: pro-eugenics reformers focused on fiscal necessity, efficiency, and thinly veiled threats of racial catastrophe. Eugenics ideology today might look different, but it is not yet a relic of the past. The history of eugenics, with its emphasis on racialized fitness and restrictive definitions of citizenship, has left an indelible mark on our contemporary institutions.

Acknowledgments

After working on a project for nearly two decades, writing acknowledgments is nearly as hard as writing the book itself. My list of people to whom I am grateful is longer than this space permits. Still, I am delighted to acknowledge the ways I have benefited from the support of many people, a few of whom I name here.

Above all, I am grateful to the many students, friends, colleagues, and even strangers who have expressed interest in this topic. I have talked to many people who did not know the history of eugenics in our state and nation, and who were interested to learn more. Conversations like these always renewed my sense of purpose and drove me to share my research with a broader audience. I would not have written this book without their encouragement.

I have been lucky to be part of many supportive academic communities that have made me a better scholar. Early in my academic career, Ira Bashkow and Lori Schuyler helped me to see myself as an intellectual peer. An amazing group of historians connected to UNC have been professional and personal lifelines for many years: Friederike Bruehoefener, Nora Doyle, Shannon Eaves, Rob Ferguson, Brad Proctor, Jonathan Hancock, Rachel Hynson, Kim Kutz Elliott, Sarah McNamara, Elizabeth Lundeen, Katy Smith, Jessie Wilkerson, David Williard, and many others. I am also fortunate to be a faculty member in a multidisciplinary department where I constantly learn from my colleagues. I particularly appreciate the support from Cassandra Davis, Dan Gitterman, Steve Hemelt, Will Goldsmith, Rebecca Kreitzer, Doug MacKay, Elizabeth Sasser, and Tricia Sullivan. Beyond my department, I am grateful for the friendship and intellectual conversations I have shared with Mara Evans, Jackie Kruszewski, Bob Pleasants, and Caela O'Connell.

I am grateful for the institutional support I received to write this book. The Institute for the Arts and Humanities at UNC–Chapel Hill provided an incredible semester of research and writing leave through its Faculty Fellowship Program, along with a vibrant peer cohort. In addition, the IAH provided an Arts and Humanities Publication Support Grant. I also received funding for research at the Virginia Historical Society from the Mellon Research Fellowship. No less important were the small army of librarians and archivists who helped find sources or produce scans of images (including at the last minute!) at each of the collections I used, which are listed in the bibliography. There are too many people to name, but I am especially grateful to the staff at North Carolina Collection and Southern Historical Collection, both at UNC's Louis Round Wilson Special Collections Library. For superb assistance with a whole range of research tasks, I thank Kaitlyn Davis and Andy Hill (whose work was funded by the Duncan MacRae Jr. Public Policy Mentored Research Assistant Grant), as well as the stellar Aaron Pattillo-Lunt. Thank you also to Matt Simon for putting his love of maps in service to this book.

Many people have offered their thoughts on some piece of this project. I am thankful to all of them for their time and generosity in sharing ideas and feedback, and I have done my best to incorporate as many suggestions as I could. Thanks to the two anonymous readers for the press, whose careful feedback helped me sharpen key concepts. For valuable commentary at conferences or workshops, I thank Gwendoline Alphonso, Tony Harkins, and Steven Noll. I am also grateful to Fitz Brundage, Laura Edwards, Rob Ferguson, Will Goldsmith, Jacquelyn Hall, Tina Irvine, Bob Korstad, Joan Krause, Elizabeth Krome, Jim Leloudis, Viji Sathy, Johanna Schoen, Ben Waterhouse, and Jessie Wilkerson for reading all or part of the manuscript (sometimes multiple times!). Tina and Jessie are the world's best writing partners, and together they have made this book immeasurably better than I could have made it on my own.

Finally, in a book about families, I will end by thanking my own amazing family. I grew up with the most supportive parents and sibling anyone could ask for. They all have modeled for me the importance of integrity and the value of seeking the truth. I thank them for pushing me to be my best while always making me feel that I'm already the best. My husband has been my anchor and foremost ally in my best and worst moments. He and the rest of my family (and many friends) have made this book possible through their own contributions of time, meals, laundry-folding, and encouraging words. Finally, during the process of writing this book, I had two children. Their very existence changed my perspective on this topic and underscored my reasons for writing this book. Their energy, curiosity, and kindness are a constant source of joy, and they give me hope for a better future.

Notes

Abbreviations in the Notes

Bickett Papers	Papers of Governor Thomas Walter Bickett, State Archives of North Carolina, Raleigh, NC
BCPW	Board of Charities and Public Welfare
BCPW Report	*Biennial Reports of the North Carolina Board of Charities and Public Welfare*, 1917–38.
BPC Report	*Annual Reports of the North Carolina Board of Public Charities*, 1899–1916.
BPW Records	Board of Public Welfare Records, Social Services Record Group, State Archives of North Carolina, Raleigh, NC
Bradway Papers	John S. Bradway Papers, David M. Rubenstein Rare Book and Manuscript Library, Duke University, Durham, NC
Branson Papers	E. C. Branson Papers, Collection #2610, Southern Historical Collection, Wilson Library, University of North Carolina at Chapel Hill, Chapel Hill, NC
Brewer v. Valk Records	*Brewer v. Valk* Records, NC Supreme Court Records, 33S-363, North Carolina State Archives, Raleigh, NC
Caswell Biennial Report	*Biennial Reports of the North Carolina School for the Feeble-Minded*, 1911–14 and *Biennial Reports of the Caswell Training School for Mental Defectives*, 1915–34.
Caswell Records	Unprocessed records, Caswell Center, Kinston, NC
Coon Papers	Charles L. Coon Papers, 1775–1831, Collection #177, Southern Historical Collection, Wilson Library, University of North Carolina at Chapel Hill, Chapel Hill, NC
Corr. with Associations	Commissioner's Office: Correspondence with Associations and Committees, 1918–58, Board of Public Welfare Records, Social Services Record Group, State Archives of North Carolina, Raleigh, NC
Corr. with State Agencies	Commissioner's Office: Correspondence with State Agencies, Boards, and Commissions, 1917–58, Board of Public Welfare Records, Social Services Record Group, State Archives of North Carolina, Raleigh, NC
CSS Papers	North Carolina Conference for Social Service Records, Org. 100, State Archives of North Carolina, Raleigh, NC
Davenport Papers	Charles B. Davenport Papers, Mss.B.D27, American Philosophical Society Library, Philadelphia, PA
Denson Papers	Denson Family Papers, PC #1230, State Archives of North Carolina, Raleigh, NC

ECU Hyatt Papers	Sybil Hyatt Papers, Manuscript Collection #778, East Carolina University Special Collections, Greenville, NC
ERO Records	Eugenics Record Office Records, Mss.Ms.Coll.77, American Philosophical Society Library, Philadelphia, PA
FWC Records	North Carolina Federation of Women's Clubs Records, North Carolina Federation of Women's Clubs Headquarters, Raleigh, NC
FWC Yearbook	*North Carolina Federation of Women's Club Yearbooks*
General Corr. of the Board	Commissioner's Office: General Correspondence of the Board, 1891–1922, Board of Public Welfare Records, Social Services Record Group, State Archives of North Carolina, Raleigh, NC
House Journal	*Journal of the House of Representatives of the General Assembly of North Carolina*
Kinston-Lenoir Hyatt Papers	Sybil Hyatt Papers, Kinston-Lenoir Public Library, Kinston, NC
LSRM Records	Laura Spelman Rockefeller Memorial Records, Rockefeller Center Archive, Sleepy Hollow, NY
McAlister Papers	Alexander W. McAlister Papers, Collection #4318, Southern Historical Collection, Wilson Library, University of North Carolina at Chapel Hill, Chapel Hill, NC
Mental Hygiene Society Records	North Carolina Mental Health Association (NC Mental Hygiene Society, 1913–55) Records, Org. 117, State Archives of North Carolina, Raleigh, NC
Miller Papers	Papers of Dean Justin Miller, 1929–34, Deans Papers, School of Law Records, 1914–2010s, David M. Rubenstein Rare Book and Manuscript Library, Duke University, Durham, NC
NC Public Laws	*Public Laws and Resolutions of the State of North Carolina Passed by the General Assembly*
Poteat Papers	William Louis Poteat Papers, 1856–1938, MS 91, Z. Smith Reynolds Library Special Collections and Archives, Wake Forest University, Winston-Salem, NC
RF Records	Rockefeller Foundation Records, Rockefeller Center Archive, Sleepy Hollow, NY
Scales Papers	Alfred Moore Scales Papers, Collection #4037, Southern Historical Collection, Wilson Library, University of North Carolina at Chapel Hill, Chapel Hill, NC
Senate Journal	*Journal of the Senate of the General Assembly of North Carolina*
Session Records	Session Records, North Carolina Senate and House of Representatives, 1919, 1923, 1925, 1929, 1933, State Archives of North Carolina, Raleigh, NC
State Board Corr.	Commissioner's Office: State Board Correspondence, 1897–1947, Board of Public Welfare Records, Social Services Record Group, State Archives of North Carolina, Raleigh, NC

Transactions	*Transactions of the Medical Society of the State of North Carolina*
UNC Trustee Minutes	Board of Trustees of the University of North Carolina Records, Series 1: Minutes, Collection #40001, University Archives, Wilson Library, University of North Carolina at Chapel Hill, Chapel Hill, NC
Unprocessed BPW records	Unprocessed Board of Charities and Public Welfare papers, MARS ID 97.101, Old Records Center, State Archives of North Carolina, Raleigh, NC
WCR Records	Woman's Club of Raleigh Records, State Archives of North Carolina, Raleigh, NC

Introduction

1. "Inaugural Address of T. W. Bickett, Governor of North Carolina," *North Carolina Public Documents, Session 1917*, 3–19.

2. Accurate totals of sterilizations performed are difficult to find. Largent estimates that North Carolina ranks seventh in per capita sterilizations but records only 5,993 sterilizations for North Carolina, while Schoen was able to find documentation of only 5,704 sterilizations performed. Other reports indicate that either 7,600 or over 8,000 people were sterilized. Unfortunately, North Carolina has restricted access to records of the Eugenics Board (under NC General Statute 132-1.23) as well as records that pertain to recipients of public assistance, with no sunset provision for older records (NC General Statute 108A-80). These restrictions have limited researchers' ability to reconstruct the nuances of social workers' and state officials' decisions. For estimates of sterilization totals, see Lombardo, *Three Generations, No Imbeciles*, 293–94; Largent, *Breeding Contempt*, 77–80; Schoen, *Choice and Coercion*, 82; Johanna Schoen, email message to author, July 21, 2025.

3. On the program's later years generally, see Schoen, *Choice and Coercion*. On racial bias against Black people, 1958–68, see Price, Darity, and Sharpe, "Did North Carolina Economically Breed-Out Blacks?"

4. The foundational scholarship on eugenics focused on leaders of national eugenics organizations. More recently, scholars have been interested in eugenics programs at the state level and in the multifaceted cultural manifestations of eugenics. On the importance of state studies, see Ladd-Taylor, *Fixing the Poor*, 9.

5. I aim for an approach similar to what Canaday calls a "social history of the state," seeing "the state through its practices"; Canaday, *Straight State*, 5. On the importance of mid-level actors and "bureaucratic and mundane" eugenic strategies, see also Ladd-Taylor, *Fixing the Poor*, 16, 224. For a similar phenomenon among professional psychiatrists, see Dowbiggin, *Keeping American Sane*; and for analysis of a similarly intertwined group of academics, private actors, and government officials that shows shared public and private culpability for redlining, see Winling and Michley, "Roots of Redlining."

6. Some of the best scholarship on eugenics and welfare explores the links between those two fields. Although she focuses on a later period of North Carolina history, Schoen (*Choice and Coercion*) describes the links between sterilization programs and welfare and public health programs. Ladd-Taylor's *Fixing the Poor* argues that Minnesota's child welfare

and sterilization programs were linked both administratively and ideologically, and that eugenic strategies were part of broader efforts to "fix the poor."

7. Ring, *Problem South*.

8. On whiteness as a salient identity for reformers, see Sallee, *Whiteness of Child Labor Reform*; Ring, *Problem South*; and Wray, *Not Quite White*.

9. Powell, *North Carolina Through Four Centuries*, 415–18; Rabinowitz, *First New South*, 18, 23. For descriptions of farm life in North Carolina beginning around 1900, see Jones, *Mama Learned Us to Work*. On income, see Sylla, "Long-Term Trends," 851.

10. For debates about the essence of the Progressive movement, see Hofstadter, *Age of Reform*; Filene, "Obituary for 'The Progressive Movement'"; Rodgers, "In Search of Progressivism"; Link and McCormick, *Progressivism*; Gilmore, *Who Were the Progressives?*; and McGerr, *A Fierce Discontent*. On "positive statism" as the core belief of Progressives, see Gendzel, "What Progressives Had in Common."

11. No single state, of course, represents a regional or national movement, but because North Carolina's reformers were so deeply embedded in larger networks and conversations, the state is a valuable entry point into Southern approaches to Progressivism. North Carolina's reformers discussed their state's approaches with others in the state or region, helping to define the modern welfare state not just in their state but also for outside observers. On the Progressive movement in the South, see Grantham, *Southern Progressivism*; Link, *Paradox of Southern Progressivism*; Ring, *Problem South*; Kirby, *Darkness at the Dawning*. On liberalism, reform, and modernity in the Jim Crow South, see Johnson, *Reforming Jim Crow*, esp. 19–42; Gilmore, *Gender and Jim Crow*; Haley, *No Mercy Here*; McGerr, *Fierce Discontent*, 182–220; Singal, *War Within*, 46; Higham, *Strangers in the Land*, 131–93; and Stein, "Nature Is the Author."

12. Phenotype was not a reliable indicator of race, particularly as people began moving around the South more and their backstory was unknown. As Brundage writes, there was no "easy or consistent definition of whiteness. Only in the abstract did white southerners agree on a definition of whiteness. In practice they changed their minds many times about how and on what grounds to draw the line between the races." Brundage, "Introduction," 7. On the making of racial categories in legal, political, academic, and cultural realms see Pascoe, *What Comes Naturally*; Ritterhouse, *Growing Up Jim Crow*; Hale, *Making Whiteness*; Schultz, *Rural Face of White Supremacy*; Wray, *Not Quite White*; and Jacobson, *Whiteness of a Different Color*. On Lumbee efforts to claim their identity in the context of racial segregation, see Lowery, *Lumbee Indians*; on Indians and the Jim Crow South generally, see Perdue, "Southern Indians and Jim Crow."

13. In the last three decades, scholarship on various aspects of the American eugenics movement has exploded. For key texts on eugenics and related fields, see Kevles, *In the Name of Eugenics*; Stern, *Eugenic Nation*; Kline, *Building a Better Race*; Lombardo, ed., *Century of Eugenics*; Paul, *Controlling Human Heredity*; Larson, *Sex, Race, and Science*; Ladd-Taylor, *Fixing the Poor*; Trent, *Inventing the Feeble Mind*; Schoen, *Choice and Coercion*; Dorr, *Segregation's Science*; Noll, *Feeble-Minded in Our Midst*. For global perspectives, see Bashford and Levine, eds., *Oxford Handbook of the History of Eugenics*.

14. For examples, see the Individual Analysis Cards in the files of the Eugenics Record Office, such as "Crane, H. W.—Pedigree of Harry Wolven Crane taken by K. M. Cowdery, 1915," Series VI, card file, ERO Records.

15. On terminology, see Trent, *Inventing the Feeble Mind*, xix–xx; Noll, *Feeble-Minded in Our Midst*, 1–4. On feeblemindedness as a term that signified "tainted whiteness," see Stubblefield, "Beyond the Pale."

16. On the appeal of eugenics to white and Black middle-class and elite people, see Currell and Cogdell, eds., *Popular Eugenics*; Lovett, "Fitter Families"; Selden, *Inheriting Shame*; Pernick, *Black Stork*; Dorey, *Better Baby Contests*; Kevles, *In the Name of Eugenics*, esp. 57–84; Lombardo, "From Better Babies to the Bunglers"; Dorr and Logan, "Quality, Not Mere Quantity, Counts"; Mitchell, *Righteous Propagation*. On social and political questions surrounding eugenics as science, see Paul, *Politics of Heredity*, esp. 117–32; Selden, *Inheriting Shame*.

17. The lack of federal eugenics policies was related to the general weakness of the US federal government in the early twentieth century, a contrast to industrialized European nations, where powerful centralized governments enabled the creation of strong social safety nets but also made possible coordinated, nationwide eugenics programs. For analyses of the relationship between welfare and eugenics in Scandinavian countries, see Broberg and Roll-Hansen, eds., *Eugenics and the Welfare State*.

18. On sterilization laws, see Reilly, *Surgical Solution*, 45; Stern, *Eugenic Nation*, 2. On Virginia, see Dorr, *Segregation's Science*, esp. 141–43; and Smith, *Managing White Supremacy*, esp. 76–106. On Vermont, see Gallagher, *Breeding Better Vermonters*, 42–70. On California, see Kline, *Building a Better Race*, 32–60. On the racial ideologies of eugenicists, see Turda, "Race, Science, and Eugenics," and on racial dynamics of eugenics in the South, see Lindquist Dorr, "Arm in Arm"; Schoen, *Choice and Coercion*; Larson, *Sex, Race, and Science*; Noll, *Feeble-Minded in Our Midst*, 1, 39, 89–103.

19. On a parallel process in public health, using the ideology of white supremacy as justification, see Stein, "Nature Is the Author." On the "untidy" process of creating Jim Crow, see Brundage, "Introduction," 5; Smith, *Managing White Supremacy*; Johnson, *Reforming Jim Crow*; Ritterhouse, *Growing Up Jim Crow*; Hale, *Making Whiteness*; Hanchett, *Sorting Out*.

20. Julian M. Baker, "Dr. Baker Addresses Welfare Conference," *Public Welfare Progress* 9, nos. 10–11 (October–November 1928): 1–2. On ideas about an "Anglo-Saxon" race and ways reformers deployed the term to defend poor whites and "resurrect myths about an old 'classless' South to combat New South class strife," see Sallee, *Whiteness of Child Labor Reform*, 4, 92–113. See also Wray, *Not Quite White*; Smith, *Managing White Supremacy*. On gendered constructions of Black inferiority, deviance, and disease, as well as Black resistance to these constructions, see Hunter, *To 'Joy My Freedom*; Haley, *No Mercy Here*; Roberts, *Killing the Black Body*; Feimster, *Southern Horrors*; Gilmore, *Gender and Jim Crow*; Cahn, *Sexual Reckonings*; Hickey, *Hope and Danger*; Bederman, *Manliness and Civilization*.

21. On the category of "fitness" and its relationship to categories of feeblemindedness and disability, see Carlson, *The Unfit*; Trent, *Inventing the Feeble Mind*; Rose, *No Right to Be Idle*.

22. On the history of the modern state, particularly the formation of the welfare state, see Tani, *States of Dependency*; Michelmore, *Tax and Spend*; Piven and Cloward, *Regulating the Poor*, 407–80; Trattner, *From Poor Law to Welfare State*; Green, *Business of Relief*; Kotch, *Lethal State*.

23. Cott, "Marriage and Women's Citizenship," 1441, quoted in Canaday, *Straight State*, 8. I draw here on Margot Canaday's helpful framing and historiography; see Canaday, *Straight State*, 7–10.

24. In keeping with the insights of scholars such as Julian Zelizer, Edward Berkowitz, and Paul Pierson, I do not assume linear or causal connections between the outcomes of a policy and policymakers' original intent. Rather, I aim to examine the influence of early decisions to establish eugenics policies on the subsequent range of possibilities and to analyze long-term structural causes that enable seemingly sudden policy changes.

25. C. Banks McNairy, "Eugenics" (reprint of address before Onslow County Medical Society), *Greensboro Daily News*, February 6, 1916; G. G. Dickson, "Lydia Spruill and Sally Bryson Are Pronounced Imbeciles After Examination by Expert Authority," *Greensboro Daily News*, January 26, 1919.

26. Eligibility for welfare benefits, in fact, is a critical piece of citizenship. British sociologist T. H. Marshall identified "social citizenship," the ability to access all social benefits the state grants, as a phase of citizenship that most often follows the establishment of equality under the law and voting rights. Marshall, *Citizenship and Social Class*; see also Katz, *Price of Citizenship*.

27. An important strain of scholarship looks at the roles of race, class, and gender in the creation of the welfare state and how the state reinforced those identities. For example, see Skocpol, *Protecting Soldiers and Mothers*; Gordon, *Pitied but Not Entitled*; Mettler, "Stratification of Social Citizenship"; Mink, *Wages of Motherhood*; Fraser and Gordon, "A Genealogy of Dependency." On the American welfare state generally, see Evans, Rueschemeyer, and Skocpol, eds., *Bringing the State Back In*; Ruswick, *Almost Worthy*; Alphonso, "From Need to Hope"; Trattner, *From Poor Law to Welfare State*. On the balance between federal and state governments, see Tani, *States of Dependency*.

28. Annie Kizer Bost, "State Citizenship," in McMahon, ed., *Studies in Citizenship*, 11; *Biennial Report of the North Carolina Board of Charities and Public Welfare* (hereafter *BCPW Report*), 1928–30, 15; William Allen Blair to Daisy Denson, October 6, 1904, Records of the State Board of Public Welfare (State Archives of North Carolina, Raleigh; hereafter, BPW Records), State Board Correspondence, 1897–1947 (hereafter State Board Corr.), Box 1, Folder: Correspondence of W. A. Blair, Chairman of the Board, 1903–4.

29. Benson, "Sterilization," 89. On the categorization of people with disabilities as "unproductive citizens," see Rose, *No Right to Be Idle*, 3.

30. On changes in North Carolina, see Ready, *Tar Heel State*, 301–41; Link, *North Carolina*, 317–91. On the importance of administrative infrastructure and knowledge creation, see Pearson, *Birth Certificate*; Pascoe, *What Comes Naturally*, esp. 131–59; Scott, *Seeing Like a State*; Wiebe, *Search for Order*, 293–301.

31. "Prime Objects of N.C. Public Welfare Board," *Public Welfare Progress* 4, no. 1 (May 1923): 1.

32. "State Adopts Usable Law for Sterilization of Defectives," *Public Welfare Progress* 10, no. 3 (March 1929): 1.

33. "Eugenics and Social Work," *Public Welfare Progress* 11, no. 4 (April 1924): 6; "State Adopts Usable Law for Sterilization of Defectives," *Public Welfare Progress* 10, no. 3 (March 1929): 1.

34. Schoen, *Choice and Coercion*, 105–11.

35. Sixty-three percent of those sterilized received some welfare benefit, and between 1950 and 1966, noninstitutional residents constituted over 70 percent of sterilizations. Schoen, *Choice and Coercion*, 89–90, 95, 100.

Chapter 1

1. *BPC Report, 1905*, 15.

2. On the New South, its political economy, racial politics, and tensions between tradition and modernization, see Woodward, *Origins of the New South*; Boles and Johnson, eds., *Origins of the New South*; Ayers, *Promise of the New South*; Kuhn, *Contesting the New South Order*; Hunter, *To 'Joy My Freedom*. On industry in North Carolina, see Ready, *Tar Heel State*, 277; Ayers, *Promise of the New South*, 105–10.

3. "Denson, Daisy," in Hill Directory Company, *Raleigh City Directory*, 1905, 144; "Margett M. Denson," 1910 US Census, Wake County, North Carolina, population schedule, Raleigh City, Ward 2, roll T624_1136, page 13B, enumeration district 118, dwelling 245, family 245; Powell, *North Carolina Through Four Centuries*, 415, 440–41; National Park Service, "Raleigh: A Capital City—Early History," archived June 8, 2023, https://web.archive.org/web/20230608081413/https://www.nps.gov/nr/travel/raleigh/earlyhistory.htm. On urban populations, see table 13, "Population of the 100 Largest Urban Places: 1900," in Gibson, "Population of the 100 Largest Cities"; and table 8, "Population of Incorporated Cities, Towns, Villages, and Boroughs in 1900, with Population for 1800," US Census Bureau, 1900 Census of the Population, vol. 1: Population, Part 1, 466–67; Ready, *Tar Heel State*, 281.

4. J. D. Lewis, "North Carolina Railroads—Pittsboro Railroad," 2018, https://www.carolana.com/NC/Transportation/railroads/nc_rrs_pittsboro.html; Ingram, *Dixie Highway*; Hall et al., *Like a Family*, 24–33, 39, 56, 114; Ayers, *Promise of the New South*, 113–14; Gilmore, *Gender and Jim Crow*, 23.

5. North Carolina had fewer tenant farmers than other Southern states. Rabinowitz, *First New South*, 18, 23; Powell, *North Carolina Through Four Centuries*, 415–18. For descriptions of farm life in North Carolina beginning around 1900, see Jones, *Mama Learned Us to Work*.

6. Most scholars of Progressivism have focused on reformers in cities in the Northeast and Midwest as the model for their analysis, viewing Southern Progressivism as a deviation rather than reorienting their views of Progressivism to encompass Southern efforts. I build on scholarship that uncovers numerous intellectual links between the South and other regions, acknowledges the variety of reform efforts in the South, and explores the "paradox" of Southern Progressivism, in which humanitarian concerns stood alongside racial segregation, industrialists' desires, and other antidemocratic tendencies. See Grantham, *Southern Progressivism*; Link, *Paradox of Southern Progressivism*; Hall, "O. Delight Smith's Progressive Era"; Szymanski, "Beyond Parochialism"; Green, "Gendering the City, Gendering the Welfare State"; Ring, *Problem South*; Matthews, *Capturing the South*; Link, *Frank Porter Graham*.

7. On income, see Sylla, "Long-Term Trends," 851. On racial segregation in textile mills and other industries, see Matthews, *Capturing the South*; Ayers, *Promise of the New South*, 114; and Hall et al., *Like a Family*, 66–67. On poverty, see Hall et al., *Like a Family*; Jones, *Mama Learned Us to Work*; and Green, ed., *Before the New Deal*.

8. Hall et al., *Like a Family*, 150–51; Ettling, *Germ of Laziness*.

9. Green, *Before the New Deal*, x–xii, xvii; Ready, *Tar Heel State*, 256; North Carolina Constitution of 1868, Article XI, Section 7. For the history of North Carolina's welfare bureaucracy, see Aydlett, "The North Carolina State Board of Public Welfare"; Dobelstein, "Public Welfare in the American System"; Saxon, *Social Services in North Carolina*; and Brown, *Public Poor Relief in North Carolina*.

10. NC Public Laws 1868–69, chapter 170; Aydlett, "The North Carolina State Board of Public Welfare," 7–9.

11. *BPC Report, 1901*, 181–82; *BPC Report, 1902*, 40–41, 43–44, 67. For an example of inmate labor, see *BPC Report, 1902*, 57; on expenditures for the poor, see *BPC Report, 1902*, 43.

12. *BPC Report, 1903*, 140; *BPC Report, 1902*, 44–45.

13. Hall et al., *Like a Family*, 131–39.

14. On state board powers, see *BPC Report, 1907*, 19–20. Even after the state provided funds for the state board to travel on inspection trips until 1909, it was impossible for one staff member alone to inspect each institution. Aydlett, "The North Carolina State Board of Public Welfare," 12, 15.

15. Denson to James C. Matchitt (Sec., Board of State Visitors, St. Paul, MN), November 11, 1912, BPW Records, Commissioner's Office: General Correspondence of the Board, 1891–1922 (hereafter General Corr. of the Board), Box 3 (1910–13), Folder: July–December 1912.

16. From 1872 to 1887, the share of state revenues spent on welfare ranged from 6.3 to 7.8 percent, and from 1892 to 1907 welfare made up 11.9 to 15.2 percent of state spending. Sylla, "Long-Term Trends," 823–26, 830, 836, 839–41, 850–51; see also Link, *Paradox of Southern Progressivism*.

17. *BPC Report, 1912*, 12; "Resignation of Miss Denson: First Woman to Hold an Executive Position in North Carolina," *News and Observer* (Raleigh, NC), July 14, 1921; and Mrs. Al Fairbrother, "Miss Daisy Denson," *Everything Weekly* (Greensboro, NC), January 24, 1914.

18. For Denson family biographical details, see Claudius Ashborn Denson's gravestone at St. Bartholomew's Episcopal Church, Pittsboro, North Carolina; "Thomas Cowan," 1860 US Census Slave Schedules, Brunswick County, North Carolina, Town Creek District, 173; "Claudius B. Denson," 1880 US Census, Chatham County, North Carolina, population schedule, Center Twp., page 9, enumeration district 26, dwelling 75, family 76; R. Beverly Raney, "Denson, Claudius Baker," in Powell, ed., *Dictionary of North Carolina Biography*; Wilkerson-Freeman, "Women and the Transformation of American Politics," 120; and Fairbrother, "Miss Daisy Denson."

19. Battle, *Early History of Raleigh*, 5, 106–27, 131–33.

20. Fairbrother, "Miss Daisy Denson"; Hood, *To the Glory of God*, 49–50; Daisy Denson to Dr. W. L. Poteat, December 2, 1912, BPW Records, General Corr. of the Board, Box 3, Folder: July–December 1912. The Order of King's Daughters was a nondenominational Christian organization whose members were often from elite families. Sims, *Power of Femininity*, 45–46.

21. White and Hopkins, *Social Gospel*, xviii; Rosen, *Preaching Eugenics*, 15–16. For the central tenets of the social gospel and variants of more radical and conservative social Christianity, see Handy, *Social Gospel in America*, 5–6, 10–11. On the social gospel and its adherents in the South, see Harvey, "Religion in the American South"; and Hall, *William Louis Poteat*. On Southern women and religious justification, see Sims, *Power of Femininity*;

Higginbotham, *Righteous Discontent*; Turner, *Women, Culture, and Community*; Hall, *Revolt Against Chivalry*; and McDowell, *Social Gospel in the South*.

22. On Claude's political connection, including serving as an officer of the North Carolina Confederate Veterans' Association, see Battle, *Early History of Raleigh*; Raney, "Denson, Claudius Baker." On Denson's appointment, see Claude Denson to Daisy Denson, November 1, 1897, Denson Papers, Box 1, Folder: Correspondence, 1850–1944; Diary of the Secretary, 1898–1904, 38–39, BPW Records; Raney, "Denson, Claudius Baker"; Report of the Assistant Secretary, January 1 to July, 1903, in *BPC Report, 1903–5*, 156–61; "Resignation of Miss Denson," *News and Observer* (Raleigh, NC), July 14, 1921.

23. McKee to Denson, February 24, 1904, BPW Records, General Corr. of the Board, Box 1 (1891–1905), Folder: January–July 1904; Wilkerson-Freeman, "Women and the Transformation of American Politics," 130–31, 162n36; "Quarterly Report, January to April, 1904," and "Quarterly Report, July 1 to October 1, 1904," printed with *BPC Report, 1904*, 306, 313.

24. *BPC Report, 1912*, 9; Thomas S. Morgan, "Blair, William Allen," in Powell, ed., *Dictionary of North Carolina Biography*.

25. William Blair to Daisy Denson, October 1, 1913, BPW Records, State Board Corr., Box 1, Folder: Correspondence, W. A. Blair, 1913. On female officeholders, see Wilkerson-Freeman, "Women and the Transformation of American Politics," 126.

26. On the shift from benevolent reform to supposedly rational, gender-neutral, and professional casework, see Kunzel, *Fallen Women, Problem Girls*; Walkowitz, *Working with Class*; Ruswick, *Almost Worthy*.

27. *BPC Report, 1908*, 27; *Proceedings of the National Conference of Charities and Correction*, 1903–15. For examples of Denson sharing recommendations, see *BPC Report, 1907*, 22–23; *BPC Report, 1908*, 6, 26; *BPC Report, 1909*, 19; *BPC Report, 1910*, 9.

28. Blair to Denson, May 24, 1905, BPW Records, State Board Corr., Box 1, Folder: Correspondence, W. A. Blair, 1905; Denson to Carl Kelsey, May 4, 1905, BPW Records, General Corr. of the Board, Box 1 (1891–1905), Folder: January–July 1905; *BPC Report, 1905*, 15; Denson to Secretary, Chicago School of Civics and Philanthropy, April 8, 1910, BPW Records, General Corr. of the Board, Box 2, Folder: January–July 191; Denson to Mr. M. E. Robinson, May 3, 1916, BPW Records, General Corr. of the Board, Box 4, Folder: January–July 1916.

29. 1903 report to NCCC, reprinted in *BPC Report, 1903*, 160; and BPC Quarterly Report, July–October 1903, printed in *BPC Report, 1903*, 162–63.

30. Denson to James C. Matchitt, November 11, 1912, BPW Records, General Corr. of the Board, Box 3, 1910–13, Folder: July–December 1912.

31. *North Carolina Federation of Women's Clubs Yearbook, 1915–16* (hereafter *FWC Yearbook*), 56, FWC Records. Many clubwomen's campaigns fell under the rubric of "public housekeeping," which capitalized on women's distinct responsibility for overseeing the well-being of women and children. Scholars have labeled clubwomen's approach as "maternalism." For the most comprehensive account of North Carolina clubwomen's reform activities on all fronts, see Sims, *Power of Femininity*, esp. chapter 3; and Gilmore, *Gender and Jim Crow*. For similar analysis of South Carolina, see Johnson, *Southern Ladies, New Women*, esp. chapter 5.

32. Sims notes that Black women had their own parallel branches of the WCTU and the King's Daughters. The WCTU was the site of early attempts at racial cooperation in the 1880s and early 1890s, but the racist politics of the late 1890s killed these efforts. Gilmore

argues that Black women's efforts to collaborate with white women in the 1910s bore some fruit, reshaping Southern white Progressivism in the process, but the debate over woman suffrage strained these interracial efforts. Sims, *Power of Femininity*, 24, 40–46, 114–15, 119–20; Gilmore, *Gender and Jim Crow*, esp. chapters 6–8. On the differences between Black and white women's welfare activism, see also Gordon, "Black and White Visions of Welfare."

33. Cotten, *History of the North Carolina Federation*, 53, 57; *FWC Yearbook, 1912–13*, 34; for departments, see *FWC Yearbooks* for various years.

34. Scrapbook 3, Cotten Collection, and coverage of Stiles's speech in *News and Observer*, May 7, 1909, cited in Martha K. Shaw, "The Development of the North Carolina Federation of Women's Clubs: As Reflected in Its Activities from 1902 Until 1915," November 28, 1962, copy in FWC Records, Folder: 2708-2, History of Some Things Accomplished by the Federation; Cotten, *History of the North Carolina Federation of Women's Clubs*, 59; "North Carolina Federation of Women's Clubs Now in Session," *Greensboro Daily News*, May 7, 1913. Other national speakers included Howard L. Baldensperger of the National Committee on Prisons and Prison Labor and Dr. Rachelle S. Yarros, a pioneer in birth control and sex education. On Baldensperger's address, see "State Federation at Durham," *Winston-Salem Journal*, May 4, 1917; on Yarros, see 1919 convention minutes, FWC Records, Convention Minutes (bound volume), 83; P. S. Ward, "Rachelle Slobodinsky Yarros," in Trattner, ed., *Biographical Dictionary of Social Welfare in America*, 813–16.

35. *FWC Yearbook, 1911–12*, 48–50.

36. Raleigh Woman's Club *Yearbook*, 1904–5, 17–18, Denson Papers, Box 2, Folder: Yearbooks; Mrs. Isaac M Taylor (S. E. Taylor) to Denson, December 16, 1913, BPW Records, General Corr. of the Board, Box 3, Folder: August–December 1913; Daisy Denson to Mrs. B. A. Hocutt, September 30, 1912, BPW Records, General Corr. of the Board, Box 3, Folder: July–December 1912.

37. Daisy Denson to Mrs. B. A. Hocutt, September 30, 1912, BPW Records, General Corr. of the Board, Box 3, Folder: July–December 1912. For other examples of Denson's educational efforts, see Denson to Mrs. T. R. Garner, August 31, 1916, BPW Records, General Corr. of the Board, Box 4, Folder: August–December 1916; Denson to Miss W. A. White, March 21, 1917, BPW Records, General Corr. of the Board, Box 4, Folder: 1917; Denson to Mrs. Thomas, November 25, 1912, BPW Records, General Corr. of the Board, Box 3, Folder: July–December 1912.

38. Charles Duffy to C. B. Denson, March 1, 1894, BPW Records, State Board Corr., Box 2, Folder: Correspondence of Dr. Charles Duffy, Chairman of Board, 1897–1908; *BPC Report, 1899–1900*; Denson to Miss Clara I. Cox, June 25, 1912, BPW Records, General Corr. of the Board, Box 2, Folder: January–June 1912; *BPC Report, 1909*, 48–54; *FWC Yearbook, 1912–13*, 40–41; *FWC Yearbook, 1914–15*, 45; *FWC Yearbook, 1916–17*, 59.

39. Shaw, "The Development of the North Carolina Federation of Women's Clubs." In 1915, the FWC had 121 member clubs, with about 4,000 members; see "The Part of Club Women in Social Service," *Social Service Quarterly* 3, no. 2 (July–September 1915): 37. On the limitations of women's independent power and the ways their authority derived from agreements with men about social work priorities, see Sims, *Power of Femininity*, 3–4, 82–83, 109–27.

40. Cotten, *History of the North Carolina Federation of Women's Clubs*, 57; *FWC Yearbook, 1912–13*, 34.

41. Sims, *Power of Femininity*, 82–83. See also Johnson, *Southern Ladies, New Women*, esp. 130–32, 152–54.

42. Gilmore, *Gender and Jim Crow*, 36.

43. Sims, *Power of Femininity*, 58, 66–67, 83–84; Gilmore, *Gender and Jim Crow*, esp. 147–75; Higginbotham, *Righteous Discontent*; Gordon, "Black and White Visions of Welfare"; Johnson, "The Colors of Social Welfare"; Johnson, *Southern Ladies, New Women*, 4.

44. Sims, *Power of Femininity*; Gilmore, *Gender and Jim Crow*.

45. Quarterly Report, April to July 1904, printed in *BPC Report, 1904*, 310; Report of the Secretary, July 1 to October 1, 1903, printed in *BPC Report, 1903–5*, 165; Daisy Denson to Mr. L. B. Myers, August 27, 1912, BPW Records, General Corr. of the Board, Box 3, Folder: July–December 1912.

46. Denson was ill and did not attend the initial gathering of the SSC, but soon afterward she became the state's corresponding secretary. See Shivers, "The Social Welfare Movement in the South," 51–62; Kirby, *Darkness at the Dawning*, 51; "N.C. Conference for Social Service," *Public Welfare Progress* 3, no. 1 (1923); Secretary's Diaries and Reports, May 1912, BPW Records; Denson to J. E. McCulloch, May 9, 1912, BPW Records, General Corr. of the Board, Box 2, Folder: January–June 1912.

47. *BPC Report, 1912*, 23; Denson to Dr. W. S. Rankin, October 16, 1912, BPW Records, General Corr. of the Board, Box 3, Folder: July–December 1912. On the history of the Conference, see Ella Waddill's "President's Report," 1932, CSS Papers, Accession 2, Box 1, Folder: Historical—President's Report—1932—Mrs. W. B. Waddill; Gulledge, *North Carolina Conference for Social Service*, esp. 12–13.

48. "Social Workers Meet Here Feb 11," *News and Observer*, February 2, 1913; "Senator Owen to Speak Here," *News and Observer*, January 15, 1913; "For Co-Ordinated Social Service," *News and Observer*, February 2, 1913.

49. "Four Hundred in Social Service First Congress," *News and Observer*, February 13, 1913; "The Success of the Social Service Conference," *News and Observer*, February 14, 1913; "Day's News Events from State Capitol," *Greensboro Daily News*, February 11, 1913; "Social Service Congress Makes Good Beginning," *News and Observer*, February 12, 1913. For sympathetic coverage, see "Social Service Conference," *Raleigh State Journal*, February 14, 1913. Reprinted articles ran in urban newspapers including the *Wilmington Dispatch*, *High Point Enterprise*, *Winston-Salem Journal*, Asheville *Citizen-Times*, Asheville *Gazette News*, and *Greensboro Daily News*, as well as more rural papers such as the *Salisbury Evening Post*, *Lincoln County News*, *Taylorsville Mountain Scout*, and *Wadesboro Messenger*.

50. 1913 conference program, CSS papers, Acc. 2, Box 1, Folder: Historical Material—Dr. Poe; "Social Service Congress Makes Good Beginning."

51. Poteat address at CSS, February 11, 1913, "The Correlation of Social Forces," reprinted in *Raleigh State Journal*, March 21, 1913.

52. "Social Workers Meet Here Feb 11"; "Social Service Congress Makes Good Beginning"; Poteat, "The Correlation of Social Forces."

53. Draft of circular letter, "You Are Asked to Join," n.d. [1922 or 1923], CSS Papers, Acc. 2, Box 1, Folder: Historical Material—Dr. Poe; "Social Service Congress Makes Good Beginning."

54. "A Plea for the Forgotten Child," address by J. Y. Joyner at CSS, February 12, 1913, reprinted in *Raleigh State Journal*, March 14, 1913. On the organization of the Anglo-Saxon Clubs of America around similar principles, see Dorr, *Segregation's Science*, 137–66.

55. Gilbert T. Stephenson, "We Must Lift the Negro Up or He Will Drag Us Down," *Social Service Quarterly* 1, no. 1 (May–June 1913): 17–18; "Resolutions Adopted by the State Conference," *Social Service Quarterly* 1, no. 1 (May–June 1913): 29; "Resolutions Adopted at Second Annual Session North Carolina Conference for Social Service," *Social Service Quarterly* 2, no. 1 (April–June 1914): 6. On the ubiquity of racist beliefs among Progressive white Southerners and the instability of relations between Black and white Southerners even after disfranchisement and segregation, see Ayers, *Promise of the New South*, 426–37; Ritterhouse, *Growing Up Jim Crow*; and Herbin-Triant, *Threatening Property*. On the importance of Anglo-Saxon identity, see Johnson, *Southern Ladies, New Women*, 69–70; Dorr, *Segregation's Science*.

56. Charles Aycock Poe, "Clarence Hamilton Poe," in Powell, ed., *Dictionary of North Carolina Biography*; Kirby, *Darkness at the Dawning*, 130, 134–35; Herbin-Triant, "Southern Segregation South Africa–Style," 182–84, 188; Clarence Poe, "What We Need for the Improvement of Country Life," *Social Service Quarterly* 1, no. 1 (May–June 1913): 20; and "Resolutions Adopted by the State Conference," *Social Service Quarterly* 1, no. 1 (May–June 1913): 20; Clarence Poe, "Negroes Should Buy Land in Communities to Themselves," *Social Service Quarterly* 1, no. 2 (July–September 1913): 37. On Poe and the racism of the Country Life movement, see Kirby, "Clarence Poe's Vision"; Crow, "An Apartheid for the South"; Baker, "Race and Romantic Agrarianism"; Bowers, *Country Life Movement*.

57. "The Story of the NC CSS," 1926 program for Conference for Social Service, Alexander W. McAlister Papers, Collection #4318, Southern Historical Collection, Wilson Library (hereafter McAlister Papers), Folder 291: Conference for Social Service, other materials; Gulledge, *The North Carolina Conference for Social Service*, 15; Margaret Clark Neal, *North Carolina Conference for Social Service: The Record of Twenty-Five Years, 1912–37* (typed manuscript, North Carolina Collection, Wilson Library, University of North Carolina at Chapel Hill), 10; W. T. Bost, "Raleigh Postoffice Fight Is Interesting; Social Service Program," *Greensboro Daily News*, January 25, 1915; "Program of the Fourth Annual Session," *Social Service Quarterly* 4, no. 1 (January–March 1916): 3–7; "State Conference on Social Service Has First Session," *News and Observer*, January 22, 1917.

58. "Social Service Congress Makes Good Beginning"; "Four Hundred in Social Service First Congress," *News and Observer*, February 13, 1913. Progressive reformers tended to frame their political opponents in militaristic terms of "forces" making "great and lasting conquests," as well as hinting at conspiracy, as with Owen's call to "overthrow the plutocracy." "For Co-Ordinated Social Service," *News and Observer*, February 2, 1913.

59. Powell, *North Carolina Through Four Centuries*, 433–34; "The North Carolina Conference for Social Service," undated pamphlet [ca. 1933], BPW Records, Subject Files: NC CSS, Folder: n.d., 1913–33, NC Conference for Social Service.

60. Denson to Eugene T. Lies, April 27, 1914, BPW Records, General Corr. of the Board, Box 4, 1914–17, Folder: January–July 1914; Gilmore, *Gender and Jim Crow*, 66–67; Downs, "University Men," 270; Neal, *North Carolina Conference for Social Service*, 5; CSS Program, March 28–30, 1922, in BPW Records, Subject Files: NC CSS, Folder: n.d., 1913–33, NC Conference for Social Service.

61. These statements are based on 1910 Census records for approximately 185 Conference members. Thank you to Kaitlyn Davis for her help in compiling this database.

62. "Board of Public Charities," *News and Observer,* February 12, 1913; "Who's Who in the North Carolina Conference for Social Service," *Social Service Quarterly* 1, no. 4 (January–March 1914): 106–11; *BPC Report, 1909,* 16–17; Denson to Mrs. E. W. Cole, June 14, 1912, BPW Records, General Corr. of the Board, Box 2, Folder: January–June 1912.

63. Sallie Southall Cotten, "Women and Social Service," *Social Service Quarterly* 1, no. 4 (January–March 1914): 101.

64. The only group more likely to be active were male clergy and rabbis. I base my calculations of "active" rates on a membership list published in early 1914 and on members who had selected a committee to join, and I used professional titles as well as Census records to divide members into groups. Percentage of each group that was active (with number of members in that group in parentheses): married women (110), 49 percent; unmarried women (64), 61 percent; clergy and rabbis (62), 68 percent; legislators or elected officials (16), 50 percent; doctors (76), 42 percent; professors (18), 33 percent; other men (380), 48 percent. "Who's Who in the North Carolina Conference for Social Service."

65. Mary Institute and St. Louis Country Day School, "Our History At-a-Glance"; Mrs. Gordon M. Finger, "Echoes from Clubdom," *Charlotte Observer,* January 23, 1916; "Rev. Dr. Thomas W. Lingle," *Charlotte Daily Observer,* June 17, 1911; "Dr. Lingle the Man," *Charlotte Daily Observer,* August 15, 1908; "Of a Religious Turn," *Charlotte Daily Observer,* July 17, 1897; Lingle, *Memories of Davidson College,* 95–96; "Five Quiet Weddings; Lingle-Souther," *St. Louis Republic,* July 3, 1901; "Bought by the Linden," *Charlotte Daily Observer,* September 1, 1898.

66. Lingle, *Memories of Davidson College,* 95–96; "The Fund Is Complete," *Charlotte Daily Observer,* June 2, 1908; *FWC Yearbook, 1912–13;* "Rev. Dr. Thomas W. Lingle"; "County and Suburbs," *Charlotte Daily Observer,* September 20, 1911. One article indicates that Clara and the children spent almost a year and a half in Europe on this trip: "County and Suburbs," *Charlotte Daily Observer,* October 7, 1911.

67. Sims, *Power of Femininity,* 167–68; Flynt, *Southern Religion and Christian Diversity,* 102; Mrs. T. W. Lingle, "Woman's Share in Social Service Through the Club Movement," *Social Service Quarterly* 3, no. 2 (July–September 1915): 58–61.

68. Weathers, *A Century to Celebrate,* 25; Lingle to Poe, May 29, 1915, CSS Papers, Acc. 2, Box 1, Folder: Historical Material—Dr. Poe; *FWC Yearbook, 1916–17,* 68. Likewise, before the 1917 Conference gathering Lingle encouraged all the state's clubwomen to attend: Lingle to clubwomen (circular letter), January 5, 1917, BPW Records, General Corr. of the Board, Box 4, 1914–17, Folder: 1917.

69. Cotten, "Women and Social Service," 101.

70. "Editorial," *Social Service Quarterly* 3, no. 3 (October–December 1915): 68; "Mrs. T. W. Lingle," photograph and caption, *Social Service Quarterly* 4, no. 1 (January–March 1916): 13.

71. Lingle to clubwomen (circular letter), January 5, 1917, BPW Records, General Corr. of the Board, Box 4, 1914–17, Folder: 1917. The committee on the "negro problem" was also the Conference's smallest, with only eight members. The committee on industrial conditions and child labor had only two women among its seventeen members—surprising, given scholars' usual understanding that child labor was a particular concern of women. "Who's Who in the North Carolina Conference for Social Service."

72. There were no women on the first conference program. See also conference programs for 1914, 1916, and 1917 in Neal, *North Carolina Conference for Social Service,* 10,

20–24, 29. On Ella P. Waddill's presidency, see McAlister Papers, Folder 282: Conference for Social Service, other materials. On the integration of women's groups into the conference and the alignment of their goals, see Sims, *Power of Femininity*, 115–16. For a different interpretation that argues that the Conference was "a clear recognition of women's political influence, see Wilkerson-Freeman, "Women and the Transformation of American Politics," 176–77.

73. E. C. Lindeman, "Social Progress in NC," *NC Community Progress* 3, no. 16 (May 20, 1922), copy in CSS Papers, Acc. 2, Box 1, Folder: Historical Material—Dr. Poe.

Chapter 2

1. On invitations, see, for example, "School for Feeble-Minded," *Hickory Times-Mercury*, May 1, 1912; "We Acknowledge," Elizabeth City *Advance*, May 3, 1912. For descriptions of the campus and buildings, see *BPC Report, 1911*, 33; *Biennial Report of the North Carolina School for the Feeble Minded* (hereafter *Caswell Biennial Report*), *1911–12*, 7–8; Minutes, Executive Committee, February 2, 1912, Caswell Records, Executive Committee Reports of the Trustees of the North Carolina School for the Feebleminded, 1911–32 (bound volume; hereafter Caswell Executive Committee Reports), 18; Executive Committee Report to Trustees, in Minutes, Trustees, December 6–7, 1912, Caswell Records, Caswell Executive Committee Reports, 34–46.

2. "Formal Laying of Cornerstone," *News and Observer*, May 7, 1912; "Cornerstone Has Been Laid," *Greensboro Daily News*, May 8, 1912; Brown and Genheimer, *Haven on the Neuse*, 31; Charles O. Laughinghouse, "The Problem of the Feeble-Minded," *Bulletin of the North Carolina State Board of Health* 27, no. 5 (August 1912): 177–83; Minutes of Trustees, May 6, 1912, Caswell Records, Executive Committee Reports, 27–28; and Exec. Committee Report to Trustees, in Minutes, Trustees, December 6–7, 1912, Caswell Records, Executive Committee Reports, 34–46. See also Noll, *Feeble-Minded in Our Midst*, 22.

3. Edward Larson has traced similar patterns in the Deep South, arguing that physicians and state medical associations were key players in making the case for eugenic segregation between 1910 and 1920, but noting that "a broader coalition of forces was required to embed [these concepts] into public policy." Larson's analysis, however, gives little attention to social welfare professionals. See Larson, *Sex, Race, and Science*, 62. For the appeal of eugenics to white Progressives in the South, see also Noll, *Feeble-Minded in Our Midst*, 4–5, 11–15.

4. *BPC Report, 1912*, 10.

5. Similar patterns played out in many other states across the country, as well as internationally. For the US eugenics movement, see Lombardo, ed., *Century of Eugenics in America*; for an overview of the eugenics movement from an international perspective, see Bashford and Levine, eds., *Oxford Handbook of the History of Eugenics*.

6. On shifting and imprecise definitions and categories of feeblemindedness, see Trent, *Inventing the Feeble Mind*, esp. 65–73, 129–77; Zenderland, *Measuring Minds*, esp. 74–84; Rose, *No Right to Be Idle*, 15–19; Noll, *Feeble-Minded in Our Midst*, 29–32; Haller, *Eugenics*, 45–46.

7. Helen MacMurchy, "The Relation of Feeble-Mindedness to Other Social Problems," *Proceedings of the National Conference of Charities and Corrections* 43 (May 1916): 229–325; Trent, *Inventing the Feeble Mind*, 137–38. Goddard's *Feeble-Mindedness* (1914) also argued that feeblemindedness was a recessive, single-gene trait and that many "normal-minded"

people were actually carriers. On Goddard and *The Kallikak Family*, see Trent, *Inventing the Feeble Mind*, 152–61; Zenderland, *Measuring Minds*; Zenderland, "Parable of the Kallikak Family"; and Paul, *Politics of Heredity*, 119–22.

8. Virginia and Texas were among the states with a private institution only. Tennessee and West Virginia housed some of feebleminded people at other institutions but did not have a dedicated public institution. Department of Commerce, Bureau of the Census, "Table 1, Feeble-Minded in Institutions, 1910: Summary by Individual Institutions," *Insane and Feeble-Minded in Institutions, 1910: General Tables* (Bulletin 119) (Government Printing Office, 1914), 80–83.

9. Trent, *Inventing the Feeble Mind*, 9, 95; Rose, *No Right to Be Idle*, chapters 1–2.

10. On eugenicists' focus on mental defects, see Kevles, *In the Name of Eugenics*, 76–84, 92. Ironically, Trent notes, these calls to restrict the growth of the feebleminded came after institutional populations more than doubled from 1890 to 1904. See Trent, *Inventing the Feeble Mind*, 160, 181; Haller, *Eugenics*, 129. On the shift in the late nineteenth century from a model of social reintegration to one of permanent custodial care linked to changes in the economy and in charity policies, see Rose, *No Right to Be Idle*, 49–50. On the colony model and "total institutionalization," see Trent, *Inventing the Feeble Mind*, 9, 95, 138; and Rose, *No Right to Be Idle*, 14–90. On the emergence of the category of "moron," see Trent, *Inventing the Feeble Mind*, 155–60; Paul, *Controlling Human Heredity*, 50–71; and Gould, *Mismeasure of Man*, 188–201. For the perceived threat of feeblemindedness in the South, see Noll, *Feeble-Minded in Our Midst*, esp. 2–6, 12–14, 19–20.

11. Paul V. Anderson, "Mental Hygiene in the Young," *Transactions of the Medical Society of the State of North Carolina* (hereafter *Transactions*) 57 (1910): 449–58; "Resolution of Thanks to Greensboro," *Transactions* 62 (1915): 339; J. T. J. Battle, "The Artificial Life a Cause of the Increase of Degenerative Diseases," *Transactions* 63 (1916): 147; Cyrus Thompson, "Public Sentiment in the State and in the Individual," *Transactions* 57 (1910): 127–52; C. Banks McNairy, "Heredity's Relation to Feeble-Mindedness," *Transactions* 62 (1915): 324; Ira Hardy, "Feeble-Mindedness from a Medical Standpoint," *Transactions* 59 (1912): 271, 282; and F. R. Harris, "Eugenics and Conservation," *Transactions* 59 (1912): 462–71. Haller points out that the Progressive reformers most likely to be drawn to hereditarian ideas were physicians, social workers, and others who had the most contact with people who became wards of the state. Haller, *Eugenics*, 77. On interest in eugenics from mental health officials and local physicians, see Larson, *Sex, Race, and Science*, 40–62; Dorr, *Segregation's Science*, 112–18. On psychiatry and eugenics, see Dowbiggin, *Keeping America Sane*. On common understandings of heritability of mental defects in the 1910s and 1920s, see Paul, *Politics of Heredity*, 117–32. On the relative weight given to environment and heredity at different historical moments—not a linear path—see Cooke, "The Limits of Heredity"; Paul, *Politics of Heredity*, 81–93, Paul, *Controlling Human Heredity*, 40–49; Stern, *Eugenic Nation*, 14–16, 54–55.

12. H. D. Stewart, in discussion of Charles O. Laughinghouse, "One of the State's Immediate Needs," *Transactions* 57 (1910): 103; and Thompson, "Public Sentiment in the State and in the Individual," 145. For scriptural passages see Exodus 20:5, Exodus 34:7, Numbers 14:18, and Deuteronomy 5:9. See also W. J. McAnally, "Hope and Menace of Heredity," *Transactions* 62 (1915): 317–19. On race suicide, see Oliver Hicks, "National Recognition of the Medical Profession," *Transactions* 53 (1906): 642–45; F. R. Harris, "Eugenics and Conservation" and discussion, *Transactions* 59 (1912): 233–34, 462–66. For comments on African

Americans' sterility from gonorrhea, see L. B. McBrayer, "The Role of Infection in Relation to Diseases of the Uterus and Adnexae," and discussion of this paper, *Transactions* 57 (1910): 61, 303–4; on other extensions of eugenics, see H. D Stewart, "Traits and Taints," *Transactions* 58 (1911): 178–91. For analysis of medical scientists' views of disease among African Americans in this period, see Stein, "Nature Is the Author."

13. "Resolutions Adopted: In Regard to Outside Insane," *Transactions* 47 (1900): 208; Charles O. Laughinghouse, "Annual Oration: A Few Hints in Medico-Social Ethics," *Transactions* 44 (1897): 39. One doctor advocated marriage restrictions even for tubercular patients; see Charles Roberson, "The Reduction of Infant Mortality," *Transactions* 58 (1911): 549–56.

14. P. L. Murphy, "President Murphy's Address," *Transactions* 44 (1897): 15–23; A. K. Tayloe, "A Protest Against Indiscriminate Surgical Operations upon the Female Organs of Generation," *Transactions* 51 (1904): 433–42; George K. Collier, "Epilepsy, Its Treatment," *Transactions* 54 (1907): 136–48; Stewart, "Traits and Taints"; Charles J. O'Hagan, "Address at Conjoint Meeting with State Board of Health," *Transactions* 47 (1900): 189–93; C. S. Grayson, "Tuberculin Therapy," *Transactions* 55 (1908): 446. For a similar critique of public health efforts as enabling the survival of "many physically and mentally deficient individuals," see William M. Jones, "President's Address," *Transactions of the Health Officers' Association* (1915): 5–10. On arguments that sterilization could make inmates more manageable (at least by controlling their sexual behavior), see Trent, *Inventing the Feeble Mind*, 185–88.

15. Patrick L. Murphy, "Care of the Insane and Treatment and Prognosis of Insanity," *Transactions* 42 (1895): 61–73; *BPC Report, 1904*, 196–98. For another early call for an institution for all feebleminded, see G. T. Sikes, "Law vs. Justice," *Transactions* 44 (1897): 224–29.

16. *BPC Report, 1899–1900*, 67–69.

17. *BPC Report, 1903*, 10–11, 152–55; *BPC Report, 1912*, 10–11; Daisy Denson to Charles L. Coon, January 2, 1911, BPW Records, General Corr. of the Board, Box 3 (1910–13), Folder: January–July 1911; *BPC report, 1899–1900*, 67–69. For discussion of prevention instead of care alone, see also *BPC Report, 1916*, 7.

18. *BPC Report, 1903*, 10–11, 141–46; *BPC Report, 1908*, 5–6. Denson continued to study eugenics throughout the 1910s, including joining the national committee on insane and mental defectives of a new organization, the American Association of Officials of Charity and Correction, in 1912. Her 1912 report was the first in which she talked about eugenic segregation as aiming for the "ultimate decrease" of the feebleminded. Her reports in the 1910s contain frequent mentions of eugenics, and to correspondents she quoted Charles Davenport and recommended eugenics experts as speakers. See *BPC Report, 1912*, 11; Denson to Robert W. Hebberd (President, AAOCC), August 27, 1912, BPW Records, General Corr. of the Board, Box 3, Folder: July–December 1912; Denson to Mrs. T. R. Garner, August 31, 1916, BPW Records, General Corr. of the Board, Box 4, Folder: August–December 1916; and Denson to McAlister, December 22, 1915, BPW Records, General Corr. of the Board, Box 4, Folder: August–December 1915. The NCCC discussed sterilization at multiple meetings, including 1906, 1907, 1909, and 1910. See *Proceedings* from 1906 (280, 468), 1907 (10), 1909 (420), 1910 (37).

19. Trent describes how the cottage or colony plan, the dominant model by 1890, facilitated the classification of types of feebleminded people. Despite officials' rhetoric, such

distinctions were often in service of institutional needs rather than inmates' treatment. Trent, *Inventing the Feeble Mind*, 83–88.

20. Women's clubs continued to support the school, including by raising funds to build an additional cottage. Clubwomen were also important lobbyists in establishing other state institutions, building on their maternalist role in caring for children and other members of society who needed special care and protection. Cotten, *History of the North Carolina Federation of Women's Clubs*, 41–42; *FWC Yearbook, 1912–13*, 30; Sims, *Power of Femininity*; Pascoe, *Relations of Rescue*; Zipf, *Bad Girls at Samarcand*.

21. In 1905, a bill to create four reformatories segregated by race and gender died in committee in the House. "Addenda," *BPC Reports 1903–5*, 331–32. On Jackson and on clubwomen's role in establishing and maintaining reformatories, see Sims, *Power of Femininity*, 119–26. On Samarcand, see Zipf, *Bad Girls at Samarcand*.

22. HB 339, *Journal of the House of Representatives of the General Assembly of North Carolina* (hereafter *House Journal*), Session 1905, 149, 178; Denson's report to NCCC, July 1905, printed in *BPC Report, 1905*, 165; Denson's report to NCCC, June 1907, printed in *BCP Report, 1907*, 132–35; reports from Goodwin and Ray in *BPC Report, 1907*, 28–31, which depart from their recent practice of calling for an institution for the feebleminded; *BPC Report, 1907*, 6–7; *BPC Report, 1909*, 7–8; and Denson's report to NCCC, June 1909, printed in *BPC Report, 1909*, 202–3.

23. "Rites Dr. Hardy to Be from Church at 2 p.m. Tuesday" [no source; probably *Kinston Free Press*], [November] 22, 1948, clipping in Sybil Hyatt Papers, Kinston-Lenoir Public Library (hereafter Kinston-Lenoir Hyatt Papers), Personal Files, Obituary Clippings.

24. Brown and Genheimer, *Haven on the Neuse*, 26; Noll, *Feeble-Minded in Our Midst*, 21; and "Hardy, Ira," 1910 US Census, Beaufort County, North Carolina, population schedule, Washington Twp., [page illegible], enumeration district 16, dwelling 58, family 61; Ira M. Hardy, "What It Costs," December 8, 1910, copy in Caswell Records; Trent, *Inventing the Feeble Mind*, 155–57; and Zenderland, *Measuring Minds*, 61–62, 65–68.

25. Hardy, "What It Costs," 2.

26. "Medicoes Gathering for Annual Meeting," *Kinston Free Press*, December 6, 1910; "Seaboard Convention Drawing to a Close," *Kinston Free Press*, December 8, 1910; "Seaboard Medical Convention Closes," *Kinston Free Press*, December 9, 1910.

27. On Hardy's participation, see *Transactions* 57 (1910): 7, 507. For papers on related topics at the 1910 session, see Thompson, "Public Sentiment in the State and in the Individual"; and Paul V. Anderson, "Mental Hygiene in the Young," *Transactions* 57 (1910): 449–58.

28. Hardy, "What It Costs," 3–8. On similar rhetoric (appealing to pity but also playing on fears) by the head of Minnesota's institution, see Ladd-Taylor, *Fixing the Poor*, 35–36.

29. "What It Costs," *Kinston Free Press*, December 10, 1910; "A Neglected Obligation," *Charlotte Observer*, December 14, 1910; "The State's Duty to Feeble-Minded," *News and Observer*, December 11, 1910; "For the Feeble-Minded," *News and Observer*, February 1, 1911.

30. "Paralysis and Death," *News and Observer*, December 21, 1910; "For the Feeble-Minded." Bills were introduced in both the House and Senate on January 31, 1911, with the Senate bill ultimately passing. The sponsor of the Senate bill, Dr. R. V. Cartwright, first had a private discussion with Hardy. The sponsor of the House bill was W. A. Thompson, who represented Hardy's home county of Beaufort. On Cartwright's conversation with Hardy,

see Brown and Genheimer, *Haven on the Neuse*, 27. For the two bills, see *House Journal*, 1911, 208–10; *Journal of the Senate of the General Assembly of North Carolina* (hereafter *Senate Journal*), 1911, 148–49, 517, 664.

31. Finding Aid, Coon Papers; circular letter, Charles Coon to educators, December 25, 1910; Coon to Denson, December 31, 1910; and replies, all in Coon Papers, Folder 30: November–December 1910; Denson to Coon, January 6, 1911; Coon to Denson, January 7, 1911; Coon to Kesler, January 9, 1911, all in Coon Papers, Folder 31: January 1911; Daisy Denson to Charles Coon, February 1, 1911, in Coon Papers, Folder 32: February 1911. For examples of correspondence with other states, see Coon to Henry Goddard, January 6, 1911; Elsie M. Seguin to Coon, January 9, 1911; Elsie Gordon to Coon, January 10, 1911; A. W. Wilmarth to Coon, January 11, 1911; J. W. Wilbur to Coon, January 11, 1911; and Coon to Walter Fernald, January 11, 1911, all in Coon Papers, Folder 31: January 1911.

32. There is no evidence in correspondence that Denson was aware of Hardy's bill before it was introduced or knew of Hardy at all. The *News and Observer* had covered his speech favorably but did not discuss his plans for a bill beforehand. In fact, Denson seems to have worked with *News and Observer* editor Josephus Daniels to spur public interest in *her* version of the bill, and she discovered only on the day that her bill was introduced that Hardy's had been introduced the day before. See "For the Feeble-Minded"; and Denson, entries for February 1911, Diary of the Secretary, BPW Records, Assistant Commissioner's Office: Minutes of the State Board of Social Services, Reel 1 (S.98.1–S. 98.3).

33. Denson, entries for February 6–15, and February 25, 1911, Diary of the Secretary, BPW Records, Assistant Commissioner's Office: Minutes of the State Board of Social Services, Reel 1 (S.98.1–S. 98.3); "Feeble Minded Are Provided For," *News and Observer*, February 26, 1911.

34. Cost had been the objection of the nine senators who voted against the bill, who asked whether the state could afford a new institution; see "Editorial Briefs," *Washington Progress*, March 2, 1911. One alternative suggested was to house the school at one of the existing mental hospitals; see "Bills Pour In," *Greensboro Daily News*, February 26, 1911.

35. "Feeble Minded Are Provided For"; "Bills Pour In"; "School for Feeble Minded Passes," *News and Observer*, March 4, 1911; *House Journal*, 1911, 963, 1002, 1050; *BPC Report, 1911*, 10.

36. Virginia's Lynchburg State Colony opened in 1910 as an institution for epileptics, but it did not admit feebleminded people until 1914. For a list of Southern institutions and the year they first admitted patients, see Noll, *Feeble-Minded in Our Midst*, 12.

37. Minutes, Board of Trustees, April 6, 1911, Caswell Records, Caswell Executive Committee Reports; *Caswell Biennial Report, 1911–12*, 9–17. On tours of institutions, see Noll, *Feeble-Minded in Our Midst*, 22–23.

38. "Report of Committee of Visitation," *Caswell Biennial Report, 1911–12*, 9–17.

39. On North Carolina's consultations with experts, see Minutes, Executive Committee, September 13, 1911, Caswell Records, Caswell Executive Committee Reports; Denson to W. B. Streeter, September 6, 1911, BPW Records, General Corr. of the Board, Box 3, Folder: August–December 1911. Many Southern states had similar relationships with the Russell Sage Foundation. Hart was a strong advocate of permanent segregation for feebleminded women, and he pushed for institutions in several Southern states. North Carolina was actually unusual in starting its institution "on its own initiative." See Noll, *Feeble-Minded in Our Midst*, 14–21. On national eugenics organizations' interest in the South, see Larson, *Sex, Race, and Science*, 56–62; and Haller, *Eugenics*, 125–28.

40. NC Public Laws 1911, chapter 87, section 1.

41. Noll, *Feeble-Minded in Our Midst*, 93.

42. Other Southern states had similar arrangements. The only exceptions before 1940 were Virginia, which had a colony for Black feebleminded at a hospital for the Black insane, and Kentucky and Louisiana, which had segregated space at a single institution for the feebleminded. See Noll, *Feeble-Minded in Our Midst*, 89–103. On calls for a separate school in North Carolina, see Noll, *Feeble-Minded in Our Midst*, 95–96; and *Caswell Biennial Report, 1917–18*, 36–37.

43. "Dr. Hardy the Inspiration," *News and Observer*, March 28, 1911; Minutes, Trustees, June 8, 1911, and June 26, 1911, Caswell Records, Caswell Executive Committee Reports.

44. Institutional heads thought urbanization was a cause of feeblemindedness, and they also recognized the importance of agricultural production to the institutions' financial sustainability. See Noll, *Feeble-Minded in Our Midst*, 25–26; Trent, *Inventing the Feeble Mind*, 97–87. Hastings Hart, however, thought Caswell was too isolated. See Noll, *Feeble-Minded in Our Midst*, 108, quoting Hart to Beasley, January 24, 1919, BPW Records, State Commissioner's Office files, Box 29, Folder: Russell Sage Foundation.

45. The crowd included the mayor, "judges, merchants, bankers, physicians, the editor of the Daily Free Press, and ladies in the finest carriages." "Committee of Seventeen," *Kinston Free Press*, May 17, 1911; Brown and Genheimer, *Haven on the Neuse*, 30.

46. Executive Committee Report to Trustees, in Minutes, Board of Trustees, December 6–7, 1912; and Minutes, Trustees, June 26, 1911, both in Caswell Records, Caswell Executive Committee Reports; Brown and Genheimer, *Haven on the Neuse*, 31; "Masonic Ceremonies—Cornerstone Placed," *Kinston Free Press*, May 6, 1912; "Report of School for the Feeble-Minded," *BPC Report, 1911*, 33.

47. On landscaping, see Executive Committee Report to Trustees, Minutes, Board of Trustees, December 6–7, 1912, Caswell Records, Caswell Executive Committee Reports; and Brown and Genheimer, *Haven on the Neuse*, 31.

48. On Caswell and other institutions as part of a nascent support system for people with disabilities, see Castles, "Little 'Tardies.'"

49. A. A. Kent, "The Profession and the State," *Transactions* 59 (1912): 38–39. On Kent and other trustees, who included members of the Seaboard Medical Society and legislators who had advocated establishing the school, see Brown and Genheimer, *Haven on the Neuse*, 27–28; and *Caswell Biennial Report, 1911–12*, 3.

50. Ira Hardy, "The Feeble-Minded from a Medical Standpoint," *Transactions* 59 (1912): 292.

51. Bix, "Experiences and Voices of Eugenics Field-Workers," 629, 632.

52. Most fieldworkers did work in the Northeast, the Midwest, and California. See card file of fieldworkers, ERO Records, Series VII, Box 2. For quote about Davenport, see "Field Worker Makes an Interesting Report," *Kinston Free Press*, December 9, 1912. For Davenport's views of the South, see "Notes on Meeting of Eugenics Field Workers and the Eugenics Research Association Held on June 23d 1916 at Cold Spring Harbor," Davenport Papers, Series II, Subseries B, Box 116, Folder: ERO Field Workers' Conference, 1916.

53. Noll does not address this topic directly, but he stresses Southern reformers' acute awareness of national, professional standards of care. Noll, *Feeble-Minded in Our Midst*, 25.

54. Telegram from Hardy to Davenport, n.d. [1913], Davenport Papers, Series II, Subseries B, Box 116, Folder: ERO Field Workers' Conference, Correspondence, 1913.

55. Hyatt was either the third or fourth fieldworker stationed in the South. Fieldworkers from the class of 1911 were from Louisiana and Kentucky, and by 1913 another member of the class of 1911 was also in Kentucky. See "Eugenics Class 1910" and "Eugenics Class 1911," both in Davenport Papers, Series II, Subseries B, Folder: ERO Summer Class.

56. On Hyatt's family and history, see "Henry Otis Hyatt, MD," typescript of entry for Cyclopedia of Eminent and Representative Men of the Carolinas of the Nineteenth Century, 1892, Kinston-Lenoir Hyatt Papers, Henry Otis Hyatt Files, Personal Files. On Hyatt's education and graduation in 1895, see Sybil Hyatt, "North Carolina Hiatts—Hyatts," ECU Hyatt Papers, Box 3, Folder D: Hyatt, Sybil, and Hyatt Family. On keeping house, see "Hyatt, Sybil," 1900 US Census, Lenoir County, North Carolina, population schedule, Kinston Town, Ward 1, page 5, enumeration district 44, dwelling 95, family 107. On work as a bookkeeper, see letter from Royall and Borden, February 21, 1907, ECU Hyatt Papers, Box 3, folder e: Hyatt, Sybil—Testimonials. On Hyatt's teaching, see "Historical Note," Finding Aid to Delia Hyatt Papers (PC.1529), State Archives of North Carolina, Raleigh; and letters from Dr. W. E. Headen, July 9, 1909, and Zeb V. Judd, April 25, 1910, both in Kinston-Lenoir Hyatt Papers, Personal Files, Letters of Reference for Sybil Hyatt.

57. Anderson attended UNC and Maryland, graduating in 1910. "Historical Note," Finding Aid to Delia Hyatt Papers (PC.1529), State Archives of North Carolina, Raleigh. On Columbia, see Registration Book, Columbia University, Kinston-Lenoir Hyatt Papers, Personal Papers, Sybil Hyatt's Education Documents.

58. Finding Aid to Delia Hyatt Papers (PC.1529), State Archives of North Carolina, Raleigh; Daughters of the American Revolution Applications, Kinston-Lenoir Hyatt Papers, Personal Files; Mr. Jesse M. Hiatt to Hyatt, December 1907, ECU Hyatt Papers, Box 3, Folder B: Delia Hyatt; Stephen Hyatt Jr. to Sybil Hyatt, February 28, 1904, and April 10, 1904, ECU Hyatt Papers, Box 3, Folder D: Hyatt, Sybil, and Hyatt Family.

59. Amy Sue Bix notes that Davenport particularly sought out and gave scholarships to people with previous experience in psychology, zoology, and anthropology. Bix, "Experiences and Voices of Eugenics Field-Workers," 625, 633, 637–38, 642; on 1912 class, see *Eugenical News* 2, no. 6 (June 1917): 44–45; for example of pedigree card, see "Crane, H. W.—Pedigree of Harry Wolven Crane Taken by K. M. Cowdery, 1915," ERO Records, Series VI: Fitter Family Contests, card file.

60. In the 1910s, dozens of ERO-trained fieldworkers did research and submitted reports on twenty-eight locations, some focusing on specific topics such as Huntington's chorea or insanity. Hyatt's work was funded by the Carnegie Institute in Washington, thanks to Dr. Hardy's mediating efforts. Bix, "Experiences and Voices of Eugenics Field-Workers," 629; "Training Class Statistics," *Eugenical News* 2, no. 6 (June 1917): 44; Minutes, Board of Trustees, December 7, 1912, Caswell Records, Caswell Executive Committee Reports; Brown and Genheimer, *Haven on the Neuse*, 32; card file of fieldworkers, ERO Records, Series VII, Box 2.

61. *Caswell Biennial Report, 1911–12*, 44–45. On ERO fieldworkers playing similarly complicated roles in Minnesota, see Ladd-Taylor, *Fixing the Poor*, 37–41.

62. Handwritten notes on meeting in Brooklyn, June 24, 1915, ERO Papers, Series VII: Field Worker Files, Folder: Meeting of the Field Workers, June 23, 1915; Handwritten notes, Kinston-Lenoir Hyatt Papers, Personal Files, SH's Eugenics Field Work; Bix, "Experiences and Voices of Eugenics Field-Workers," 641.

63. Minutes, Board of Trustees, December 7, 1912, Caswell Records, Caswell Executive Committee Reports; "Field Worker Makes an Interesting Report"; "Feeble-Minded: Report of Field Worker for North Carolina Institution," *Charlotte Observer*, December 14, 1912. Hyatt's report was also reprinted as part of the school's report for 1911–12; see *Caswell Biennial Report, 1911–12*, 44–45.

64. On Hyatt and Hardy's attendance at the ABA, see untitled clipping, n.d. [1913], no source [*Kinston Free Press*?], in Kinston-Lenoir Hyatt Papers, Personal Files, Articles About Sybil Hyatt. For Ward's article and commentary, see editorial comment, *Carolina and the Southern Cross* 1, no. 8 (October 1913): 10; Robert DeC. Ward, "The Call of Today—Eugenic Immigration," *Carolina and the Southern Cross* 1, no. 8 (October 1913): 11–13. For examples of subsequent articles on immigration, see editorial comment, *Carolina and the Southern Cross* 1, no. 10 (January 1914): 10–11; Peter Clark MacFarlane, "Japan in California," *Carolina and the Southern Cross* 1, no. 10 (January 1914): 13; editorial comment, *Carolina and the Southern Cross* 1, no. 11 (February 1914): 9; Edward Alsworth Ross, "American and Immigrant Blood," *Carolina and the Southern Cross* 1, no. 11 (February 1914): 11; "Menace of Immigration," *Carolina and the Southern Cross* 1, no. 12 (March 1914): 11–12. For Hyatt's views about the plant, see "Predicts Deplorable State," *Kinston Daily Free Press*, January 29, 1914.

65. Bix argues that the 1913 conference provides evidence that fieldworkers critiqued some aspects of ERO methodology, both scientifically and ethically. Hyatt may have been aware of such critiques, but she did not join the conversations about methods at the 1913 gathering. Hardy and trustee Charles O'Hagan Laughinghouse were also invited but did not attend. Hyatt attended another ERO fieldworkers' conference in July 1916. On the 1913 conference and attendance, see Bix, "Experiences and Voices of Eugenics Field-Workers," 625, 658; Transcript of the ERO Eugenics Conference, June 20–21, 1913, Davenport Papers, File: "ERO Field-Workers' Conference 1913," Folder 3: Proceedings; "Child Rescued from Vicious Bull Dog [Kinston news]," *Greensboro Daily News*, June 18, 1913; Charles Davenport to Alexander Graham Bell, February 21, 1913, Davenport Papers, File: "ERO Field Workers' Conference 1913," Folder 1: Correspondence; Registration Book, Columbia University, Kinston-Lenoir Hyatt Papers, Personal Papers, Sybil Hyatt's Education Documents. On Hyatt's attendance in 1916, see "Eugenics Conference," *Eugenical News* 1, no. 7 (July 1916): 49.

66. *Eugenical News* also contained summaries of the latest eugenics research or legal changes in various states. Hyatt at first tried to find a job with established genealogical researchers, but she failed. For a while she also worked for the federal government's income tax division. This pattern of brief employment with the ERO but a continuing interest in related fields was typical of ERO fieldworkers, although most worked in fields more directly connected to biology. On ERO fieldworkers, see Bix, "Experiences and Voices of Eugenics Field-Workers," 636, 652–53. On Hyatt's subsequent career, see "Eugenics Field Workers," *Eugenical News* 1, no. 2 (February 1916): 9; and *Eugenical News* 1, no. 11 (November 1916): 81. On Hyatt's views of eugenics and genealogical work as linked, see "Monument to the Palatines," *New Bern Journal*, January 11, 1914.

67. On public attention to Hyatt's work, see "Communications and Resolutions," *Transactions* 60 (1913): 273; Brown and Genheimer, *Haven on the Neuse*, 32. On applications, see Report of the North Carolina School for the Feeble Minded, Ending November 30, 1913, in Caswell Records, Caswell Executive Committee Reports; and Report of North Carolina School for the Feeble Minded, in *BPC Report, 1913*, 32.

68. Although funding struggles were common, Noll describes North Carolina's public political battles over Caswell as an exception to the pattern that most Southern superintendents of institutions for the feebleminded "ran their institutions as virtual private fiefdoms" with little interference from outside. Noll, *Feeble-Minded in Our Midst*, 52–60.

69. On funds, see "School for Feeble Minded Passes," *News and Observer*, March 4, 1911; and NC Public Laws 1913, Extra Session, chapter 64; on committee to investigate, see NC Public Laws 1913, chapter 121. Although Hardy was charged with mismanagement, his real failure may have been the bad judgment to hire and pay staff before the school was open. On McNairy's resignation, see "Dr. C. B. M'Nairy Is Hardy's Successor," *Charlotte Observer*, February 19, 1914; "New Regime at Kinston," *Charlotte Observer*, February 20, 1914. On the difficulties of superintendents across the nation between 1890 and 1920, as they faced "pressures to admit more and different types of inmates" and administered increasingly large and complex institutions, see Trent, *Inventing the Feeble Mind*, 93–127.

70. For McNairy's appointment, see *Caswell Biennial Report, 1913-14*, 5; on the school's renaming, see "Report of Superintendent, December 16, 1914," *Caswell Biennial Report, 1913-14*, 17–18; and NC Public Laws 1915, chapter 266, section 2. On McNairy, see "Funeral at Lenoir for Dr. C. B. M'Nairy," *Greensboro Daily News*, October 31, 1928.

71. Brown and Genheimer also mention a young woman, presumably a Caswell employee, who spent a year studying the techniques used at Vineland. Brown and Genheimer, *Haven on the Neuse*, 36.

72. On Southern institutions, see Noll, *Feeble-Minded in Our Midst*, 12. Virginia opened an institution for epileptics in 1910, and in 1914 the state legislature approved a colony for feebleminded women there; see Noll, *Feeble-Minded in Our Midst*, 24–25; see also Lombardo, *Three Generations, No Imbeciles*, 15. On the perception that feebleminded women needed special protection, see Noll, *Feeble-Minded in Our Midst*, 40–42, 112–16; and Noll, "A Far Greater Menace." For an example of McNairy's concern, see *Caswell Biennial Report, 1915-16*, 14.

73. In 1915, after the legislature failed to appropriate money for Caswell, McNairy traveled to Raleigh to plead for money in person. In 1917, the trustees asked for $258,000 to increase capacity but got only $75,000. This situation of drastically inadequate funding and long waiting lists was common in the South. On funding, See Brown and Genheimer, *Haven on the Neuse*, 44–47, 51; "Caswell Schools Asks for $258,000," *News and Observer*, January 14, 1917; "Caswell School Is Given $75,000," *News and Observer*, March 21, 1917; Noll, *Feeble-Minded in Our Midst*, 48–51. On waiting lists, see *Caswell Biennial Report, 1913-14*, 14–15.

74. "Report of Superintendent, December 16, 1914," *Caswell Biennial Report, 1913-14*, 14–15.

75. Nearly every institution for the feebleminded faced similar questions, particularly in the South, where the other options for institutional care were more limited than in the North and Midwest and funding complicated the realization of schools' dual functions of protecting feebleminded people from society and protecting society from them. Noll notes that superintendents were reluctant to take low-grade idiots because they were untrainable and were reluctant to take high-grade morons because of their deviant behavior. He also notes they wanted to admit children so that they could "train" them. See Noll, *Feeble-Minded in Our Midst*, 44, 47–48, 108–12. North Carolina officials' emphasis on older moron women, more in keeping with principles of eugenic segregation, seems unusual in this regard.

76. Brown and Genheimer, *Haven on the Neuse*, 47. The school's original charter said it should admit all feebleminded persons over six years of age "capable of being benefitted by school instruction." See "An Act to Establish the North Carolina School for the Feeble-Minded," NC Public Laws 1911, chapter 87.

77. *BPC Report, 1913*, 10; *BPC Report, 1912*, 11; Daisy Denson to Dr. Hubert Work, January 26, 1912, BPW Records, General Corr. of the Board, Box 3, Folder: January–June 1912. On the initial plans that included adult women, see Minutes, Caswell Board of Trustees, September 30, 1913, Caswell Records, Caswell Executive Committee Reports. On a law in late 1913 that limited admission to youth under twenty-one, see NC Public Laws 1913, chapter 64; and *BPC Report, 1913*, 10. On the debates leading to the 1915 change in admission policy, see "Report of Superintendent, December 16, 1914," *Caswell Biennial Report, 1913–14*, 17–18; and NC Public Laws 1915, chapter 266, section 2.

78. After another change to the institution's charter in 1919 and more years of urging from Caswell and welfare officials, the legislature lifted the age restriction in 1923. See NC Public Laws 1923, chapter 34. On disputes about the nature of patients admitted, see Noll, *Feeble-Minded in Our Midst*, 56–60. In institutions nationwide, male inmates were younger and there for shorter periods, partly because of concerns about women's sexuality. On institutionalization by gender and age, see Noll, *Feeble-Minded in Our Midst*, 42, 113, 132–33; and Trent, *Inventing the Feeble Mind*, 97.

79. See *Caswell Biennial Report, 1915–16*, 13; and Mary Schwarberg, "Some Impressions from Study of Feeble-Minded in Our State," *Greensboro Daily Record*, March 14, 1920.

80. As Noll notes, families' financial problems worsened during the Great Depression, resulting in an increased burden on institutions. Noll, *Feeble-Minded in Our Midst*, 134–35. On typical education at institutional schools and links with the emerging special education movement, see Trent, *Inventing the Feeble Mind*, 105–8, 142–51. For examples of family petitions from 1925 to 1936, see Noll, *Feeble-Minded in Our Midst*, 50–52. On a parent's concern, see Noll, *Feeble-Minded in Our Midst*, 58. On familial reactions and power struggles at other institutions, see Trent, *Inventing the Feeble Mind*, 111–14; Ladd-Taylor, *Fixing the Poor*, 39–41; and Chamberlain, "Challenging Custodialism."

81. "Schools Appeal for State Funding," *Charlotte Observer*, February 5, 1919. On other institutions' funding context, see Noll, *Feeble-Minded in Our Midst*, esp. 47–64; Trent, *Inventing the Feeble Mind*, 85–86, 103. On staff and their (lack of) training, see C. Banks McNairy, "Some Phases of Construction, Organization and Administration of an Institution for the Feebleminded in the South," *Journal of Psycho-Asthenics* 29 (1924): 271–75; Brown and Genheimer, *Haven on the Neuse*, 40; Noll, *Feeble-Minded in Our Midst*, 139–53; and Trent, *Inventing the Feeble Mind*, 120–25.

82. Mrs. J. F. Parrott, "A Visit to Caswell Training School," *Social Service Quarterly* 5, no. 1 (January–March 1917): 24–27; Brown and Genheimer, *Haven on the Neuse*, 38–40. At institutions nationwide, such a need for labor, particularly in caring for other inmates, was part of superintendents' desire for "higher-grade" cases. On inmate labor at institutions nationwide, particularly inmates caring for other inmates, see Trent, *Inventing the Feeble Mind*, 77–78, 83–84, 101–5, 108; Noll, *Feeble-Minded in Our Midst*, 148–50; and Rose, *No Right to Be Idle*, esp. 78–88. Caswell's trustees acknowledged the value of inmates' labor as one of their reasons for admitting boys. Minutes, Board of Trustees, September 30, 1913, Caswell Records, Caswell Executive Committee Reports.

83. Parrott, "A Visit to Caswell Training School."

84. Brown and Genheimer, *Haven on the Neuse*, 42–43. This kind of public relations campaign was typical. See Noll, *Feeble-Minded in Our Midst*, 25. On Caswell as a model institution, see Noll, *Feeble-Minded in Our Midst*, 107.

85. For example, see Susan Iden, "Federation Chooses Department Heads," *Greensboro Daily News*, May 8, 1915; C. Banks McNairy, "Cause and Prevention of Feeble-Mindedness," speech at Tri-State Medical Association, reprinted in *Charlotte Medical Journal*, 71, no. 6 (June 1915): 314–18; C. Banks McNairy, "Eugenics," address at Onslow County Medical Society, reprinted in *Greensboro Daily News*, February 6, 1916; and *Caswell Biennial Report, 1915–16*, 9, 15.

86. The first Conference gathering included a discussion of eugenics, and one of its standing committees was dedicated to it. See 1913 Program, CSS Papers, Acc. 2, Box 1, Folder: Historical Material—Dr. Poe, North Carolina Conference for Social Service Records; Dr. L. B. McBrayer, "The Problem of Feeble-Mindedness and Eugenics—Six Recommendations," *Social Service Quarterly* 1, no. 1 (May–June 1913): 16–17. On CSS membership, see "Who's Who in the North Carolina Conference for Social Service," *Social Service Quarterly* 1, no. 4 (January–March 1914): 106–11; *Caswell Biennial Report, 1911–12*, 3.

87. For examples of discussions of eugenics at Conference meetings, see L. B. McBrayer, "Importance of Giving More Attention to Eugenics," *Social Service Quarterly* 1, no. 1 (May–June 1913): 6–8; L. B. McBrayer, "The Problem of Feeble-Mindedness and Eugenics—Six Recommendations," *Social Service Quarterly* 1, no. 1 (May–June 1913): 16–17; L. B. McBrayer, "Mental Hygiene, Feeble-Mindedness, Insanity, and Eugenics," *Social Service Quarterly* 2, no. 1 (April–June 1914): 15–17; C. B. McNairy, "Feeble-Mindedness," *Social Service Quarterly* 3, no. 1 (April–June 1915): 17–18; and H. W. Chase, "Heredity as Related to Mental Deficiency," *Social Service Quarterly* 5, no. 1 (January–March 1917): 42–45. One expert who visited the conference was Alexander Johnson, who worked with the Committee on Provision for the Feebleminded, founded in 1914. See Haller, *Eugenics*, 125–28; "A Visitor's Estimate of the Recent Conference," *Social Service Quarterly* 5, no. 1 (January–March 1917): 10.

88. On the mental hygiene movement, which focused on prevention and drew lessons from public health, see Zenderland, *Measuring Minds*, 224–25. North Carolina was the seventh state, and the first in the South, to organize a mental hygiene society, with movement founder Clifford Beers in attendance. See Lewellys F. Barker, "The First Ten Years of the National Committee for Mental Hygiene, with Some Comments on Its Future," *Mental Hygiene* 2, no. 4 (October 1918): 564; "The Mental Hygiene Exhibit," *News and Observer*, November 28, 1913; "Hygiene Exhibit Is Open Today," *News and Observer*, November 30, 1913. "Expert" members of the North Carolina Mental Hygiene Association included Daisy Denson, William Louis Poteat, Charles Laughinghouse, and Albert Anderson (head of the Raleigh mental hospital). Of 106 charter members, most were in related professions, but twenty were laypeople. See Minutes of the Organization Meeting of the North Carolina State Society for Mental Hygiene, Mental Hygiene Society Records, Box 1, Folder: Minutes of the Mental Hygiene Society, 1913–15; Speas, *Voluntary Mental Health Movement*.

89. Only about a quarter of the Conference members were female, but women constituted almost half of the members of the committee on feeblemindedness and eugenics. "Who's Who in the North Carolina Conference for Social Service." On women's membership in eugenics organizations, see Kevles, *In the Name of Eugenics*, 64; and Larson, "'In the Finest,

Most Womanly Way.'" For examples of clubwomen studying eugenics, see Denson to Lucille Ellington Hocutt, September 30, 1912, BPW Records, General Corr. of the Board, Box 3, Folder: July–December 1912; Denson to Mrs. T. R. Garner, August 31, 1916, BPW Records, General Corr. of the Board, Box 4, Folder: August–December, 1916; L. B. McBrayer, "Report of Committee Chairman, Mental Hygiene, Feeble-Mindedness, Insanity, and Eugenics," *Social Service Quarterly* 2, no. 1 (April–June 1914): 16; Mary Schwarberg, "The Care of the Feeble-Minded," *Social Service Quarterly* 3, no. 3 (October–December 1915): 75–76.

90. "Dr. Lewis Burgin McBrayer; A Big Man and His Big Work," *Charlotte Observer*, September 27, 1914; Benjamin Ransom McBride, "McBrayer, Louis Burgin," in Powell, ed., *Dictionary of North Carolina Biography*; *Transactions* 62 (1915); Neal, *North Carolina Conference for Social Service*.

91. Gatewood, *Preachers, Pedagogues, and Politicians*, 60; Hall, *William Louis Poteat*, 36–37. See Hall for analysis of how Poteat's ideas on eugenics developed.

92. L. B. McBrayer, "Importance of Giving More Attention to Eugenics," 6–8; H. W. Chase, "Heredity as Related to Mental Deficiency," *Social Service Quarterly* 5, no. 1 (January–March 1917): 42–46. On the interaction between livestock breeding and "human racecraft," see Rosenberg, "No Scrubs." See also Lovett, *Conceiving the Future*, esp. 132–62.

93. As the social gospel was the religious analog of the Progressive movement, eugenics appealed to both Progressives and social gospelers. Some religious leaders embraced eugenics as congruent with both modern science and biblical ideas of heredity; see Rosen, *Preaching Eugenics*, esp. 184. On the South, I diverge from Larson, who argues that religion in tandem with strong family ties made the South tight-knit and more impenetrable; see Larson, *Sex, Race, and Science*, 15, 167. I argue that Protestant religion actually paved the way for acceptance of eugenics because of the influence of the social gospel in the South, as it did elsewhere.

94. *BPC Report, 1912*, 10–11; *BPC Report, 1916*, 7; McBrayer, "Importance of Giving More Attention to Eugenics," 7. Note that McBrayer sidestepped the question of evolution, asserting that natural selection was compatible with divine creation because human selection took place only after the creation of the human species.

95. On common views of racial difference and their intersections with eugenics in the United States and Britain, see Kevles, *In the Name of Eugenics*, 46–47, 73–76; Paul, *Controlling Human Heredity*, 106–14; Jacobson, *Whiteness of a Different Color*.

96. For examples of discussion of feebleminded people as a distinct race, see Hasting Hart, quoted in Roland F. Beasley, "Save the Feeble-Minded Girl," *BCPW Bulletin* 1, no. 2 (April–June 1918): 15; and Martin W. Barr, "Defective Children: Their Needs and Their Rights," *International Journal of Ethics* 8 (July 1898): 487–88, quoted in Trent, *Inventing the Feeble Mind*, 139–40. For an analysis of how one scientist linked idiocy to contemporary anthropological formulations of ethnicity and degeneracy, see Wright, "Mongols in Our Midst." On immigration, "race suicide," and "race degeneration," see Baynton, *Defectives in the Land*; Paul, *Controlling Human Heredity*, 97–114; Lovett, *Conceiving the Future*, 78–108; Ring, *Problem South*, 90–92; Haller, *Eugenics*, 144–59. For analysis of how the discourse of civilization linked male power and white supremacy at the turn of the century, see Bederman, *Manliness and Civilization*.

97. This doctor argued that better public health conditions were inhibiting natural conditions of the "survival of the fittest." See William M. Jones, "President's Address,"

Transactions of the North Carolina Health Officers' Association, 1915, 5-10. For another example, see F. R. Harris, "Eugenics and Conservation," *Transactions* 59 (1912): 462-71.

98. E. L. Daughtridge, "Three Things Needed for Our Rural Development," *Social Service Quarterly* 2, no. 3 (October-December 1914): 91; Clarence Poe, "What We Need for the Improvement of Country Life," *Social Service Quarterly* 1, no. 1 (May-June 1913): 18-19; and Bion Butler, "The Immigration Question," *Social Service Quarterly* 2, no. 2 (July-September 1914): 65-68. Butler presented a bill in 1917 that aimed to recruit this type of settler from other parts of the country; see "Plan to Get People Outside of State to Settle in NC," *News and Observer*, January 22, 1917.

99. Poteat used some version of this language repeatedly. For a few examples, see Poteat, "The New Fates and the Web of Destiny," April 3, 1914, Poteat Papers, Box 9, Folder 969; Poteat, "The Wealth of North Carolina," October 20, 1916, Poteat Papers, Box 12, Folder 1245; Poteat, "The Population and Its Prospects," 1924, handwritten notes, Poteat Papers, Box 9, Folder 1008. See also Thompson, "Public Sentiment in the State and in the Individual," 143.

100. Daisy Denson to S. D. Love, March 27, 1911, BPW Records, General Corr. of the Board, Box 3, Folder: January-July 1911. In arguing that even poor white people had potential and were influenced more by environment than heredity, North Carolina's Progressive reformers were pushing back against national narratives of white Southern degeneracy. For a discussion of white Northerners' views of the South and poor white people as threatening the linkage of American identity and whiteness, see Ring, *Problem South*, esp. 90-92, 135-74. On the importance of "Anglo-Saxon" heritage to the American eugenics movement, see Paul, *Controlling Human Heredity*, 102-4. For similar views about Anglo-Saxons and a similar fascination with genealogy among Virginia's pro-eugenic elites, see Dorr, *Segregation's Science*, 10-11, 13, 49-50, 87-88.

101. On the contributions of medical and social science to legitimizing Jim Crow by framing African Americans as a biological threat, see Stein, "Nature Is the Author." For an example of a UDC article alerting "mothers of the south" to the need to protect their daughters from sexual advances of Chinese men, see [Editorial Comment], *Carolina and the Southern Cross* 1, no. 8 (October 1913): 10. On reformers' concerns about feeblemindedness, delinquency, sexuality, and the "girl problem," see Noll, "A Far Greater Menace"; Cahn, *Sexual Reckonings*; Brice, "Undermining Progress"; Kline, *Building a Better Race*, 15-20; 40-48; Polansky, "I Certainly Hope"; and Holloway, *Sexuality, Politics, and Social Control*.

102. Daisy Denson to Charles L. Coon, January 2, 1911, BPW Records, General Corr. of the Board, Box 3, Folder: January-July 1911.

103. L. B. McBrayer, "President's Address," *Transactions of the North Carolina Health Officers' Association, Second Annual Meeting* (1912): 649-56. In this speech, McBrayer paired eugenics with preventive medicine and public health measures as keys to North Carolina's "race betterment." William Louis Poteat, "The Conservation of the Resources of North Carolina," address at Conservation Dinner, Greensboro, September 7, 1916, reprinted in *Bulletin of Wake Forest College*, in Poteat Papers, Box 7, Folder 832; Poteat, "Notes of Address at Reunion and Picnic on Lawn of Dr. Oscar Haywood, Montgomery Co., Aug. 17, 1912," Poteat Papers, Box 12, Folder 1245; "Governor Delivers His Annual Message," *News and Observer*, January 5, 1917; discussion following F. R. Harris's paper on "Eugenics and Conservation," *Transactions* 59 (1912): 233-35. On the high white birth rate, see "Governor Delivers His Annual Message." For similar language of children as a crop in Kansas, see Lovett, "'Fitter Families for Future Firesides.'"

104. See Kline, *Building a Better Race*; Ladd-Taylor, *Fixing the Poor*, 48–52; Larson, "In the Finest, Most Womanly Way."

105. For examples of white clubwomen hearing about eugenics, see Mrs. Gordon M. Finger, "Echoes from Clubdom," *Charlotte Observer*, January 23, 1916, 20; "Would Put a Crime in Some Tricks of Cupid, the Sly Wag," *Kinston Free Press*, January 22, 1917; Schwarberg, "The Care of the Feeble-Minded."

106. "Better Babies Contest," *Greensboro Patriot*, August 14, 1913; "Western North Carolina Day Will Mark Close of Annual Fair," *Asheville Citizen*, October 10, 1913; "Better Babies Health Contest," *Greensboro Patriot*, October 16, 1913; "Better Babies Contest at the Coming Fair, *Greensboro Patriot*, September 7, 1914; "More Concerning Better Babies," *Greensboro Patriot*, September 14, 1914; "Interest Lively in Baby Contest," *News and Observer*, October 10, 1915. For a description of North Carolina's contests from 1913 until 1922, see Brabble, "Save the Babies," 25–38. On race in contests, see Dorey, *Better Baby Contests*, 80–81, 142–45. On the intersection of public health and eugenics in infant health campaigns, see Ladd-Taylor, "Saving Babies and Sterilizing Mothers"; and Stern, "Making Better Babies," 750. On fitter family contests, which merged concerns for health and hygiene with a more explicitly eugenic focus on heredity, see Lovett, "'Fitter Families for Future Firesides."

107. Poteat, "The Conservation of the Resources of North Carolina." For another condemnation of the reluctance to talk openly about sex, see Kate Burr Johnson, "Welfare of Women and Children in Wartime," *BCPW Bulletin* 1, no 3 (July–September 1918): 12.

108. For comments about eugenics as "faddish," see discussion of Paul V. Anderson's paper, "Fallacies Concerning Insanity," *Transactions* 60 (1913): 76–85. For examples of comments about possible controversy or overreaching "fanatics," see discussion of H. D. Stewart, "Traits and Taints," 189–91; and J. F. McKay, "Have Alcoholics a Place in Medical Therapeutics?" *Transactions* 62 (1915): 108.

109. For examples, see discussion of Paul V. Anderson's "Dementia Praecox with Special Reference to the Pre-Dementia Stage," *Transactions* 59 (1912): 253–54; M. L. Kesler's comments in "Four Hundred in Social Service First Congress," *News and Observer*, February 13, 1913; Mrs. LeRoy Farinholt's comments in "Additional Social and Personal Notes, *Asheville Gazette-News*, February 4, 1914, 9; "Lady Hystery and Her New Utopia Called the Land of Eugenics," *Charlotte Evening News*, August 16, 1913. On how criticism of eugenics did not necessarily mean rejecting it, see Paul, *Controlling Human Heredity*, 11, 17.

110. See Lombardo, *Century of Eugenics*, 7.

111. John Hay Williams's comment on J. A. Hodges, "The Conservation of Nerve and Mental Health," *Transactions* 60 (1913): 55. For one example of questions about heritability of mental defect, see H. W. Chase, "Heredity as Related to Mental Deficiency." For a debate about cousin marriage, see "Four Hundred in Social Service First Congress."

112. "Report of Committee Chairman, Mental Hygiene, Feeble-Mindedness, Insanity, and Eugenics," *Social Service Quarterly* 2, no. 1 (April–June 1914): 15.

113. Parrott, "A Visit to Caswell Training School"; "Parrot, Mattie," 1920 US Census, Lenoir County, North Carolina, population schedule, Kinston Township, Kinston, Ward 1, page 8, enumeration district 58, dwelling 148, family 150.

114. Parrott, "A Visit to Caswell Training School."

115. Inaugural address of T. W. Bickett, January 11, 1917, *Public Documents, Session 1917*, 19.

Chapter 3

1. "Lydia Spruill Again Is at Large, Kinston Hears," *Charlotte Observer*, January 14, 1920.
2. On the Progressive movement in the 1910s, see Link, *Paradox of Southern Progressivism*, esp. 124–238; and Grantham, *Southern Progressivism*, esp. 351–85.
3. "Lydia Spruill Again Is at Large, Kinston Hears."
4. Wendy Kline writes about eugenics as an "appealing solution to the problem of moral disorder," evoking support from middle-class white people because it linked race and gender. Kline, *Building a Better Race*, 2.
5. Neal, *North Carolina Conference for Social Service*, 26.
6. "State Laws Regulating Marriage of the Unfit," *Journal of the American Institute of Criminal Law and Criminology* 4, no. 3 (1913): 423–25; Jessie Spaulding Smith, "Marriage, Sterilization and Commitment Laws Aimed at Decreasing Mental Deficiency," *Journal of Criminal Law and Criminology* 5 (1914): 364–65; Kuby, *Conjugal Misconduct*, 109–45, esp. 115. The push for uniform marriage laws was related to raising the age of consent, tracking venereal diseases, creating bureaus of vital statistics, and strengthening anti-miscegenation statutes. See Kuby, *Conjugal Misconduct*; Holloway, *Sexuality, Politics, and Social Control*; Canaday, Cott, and Self, eds., *Intimate States*; Pearson, *Birth Certificate*; Lindquist Dorr, "Arm in Arm." On the Commission on Uniform State Laws, which ultimately did not make specific recommendations about eugenic marriage laws, because of opponents' fears over "overexten[ding] the state's police power," see Kuby, *Conjugal Misconduct*, 133–36. On marriage laws in the United States and Britain and their relationship to other eugenic policies, see Kevles, *In the Name of Eugenics*, 92–93, 99–100; Kuby, *Conjugal Misconduct*, 109–45. On the influence of Protestant leaders, see Rosen, *Preaching Eugenics*, 53–67.
7. Dr. Albert Anderson, "For Our Insane—Recommendations of the Society for Mental Hygiene," *Social Service Quarterly* 3, no. 1 (April–June 1915): 25; H. D. Stewart, "Present Medical Conditions in North Carolina," *Transactions* 65 (1918): 95–96; John E. Ray, "Address at Fifty-Ninth Annual Meeting of the Medical Society of the State of North Carolina," *Transactions* 59 (1912): 61–66.
8. "Resolutions Adopted at the Different Sessions of the Charlotte Conference," *Social Service Quarterly* 4, no. 2 (April–June 1916): 52; "Resolutions," *Social Service Quarterly* 5, no. 1 (January–March 1917): 5; Neal, *North Carolina Conference for Social Service*, 26. See also McNairy's calls for marriage restrictions in Dr. C. B. McNairy, "Feeble-Mindedness," *Social Service Quarterly* 3, no. 1 (April–June 1915): 17–18.
9. Johnson's language is unclear. She was likely concerned about the effects of syphilis, as were many reformers during World War I, but she also discussed heredity. Kate Burr Johnson, "Welfare of Women and Children in Wartime," *BCPW Bulletin* 1, no. 3 (July–September 1918): 12; "Resolutions Adopted by the State Orphanage Association," *BCPW Bulletin* 1, no. 2 (April–June 1918): 4–5; "Amend the Marriage Law," *BCPW Bulletin* 1, no. 2 (April–June 1918): 3; Neal, *North Carolina Conference for Social Service*, 31, 36.
10. Clara (Mrs. T. W.) Lingle, "Club Women and the Social Service Conference," *Social Service Quarterly* 4, no. 2 (April–June 1916): 60–61.
11. Although the motion did not specifically refer to marriage restrictions, that was almost certainly its intent, given the similarity to the Conference's phrasing earlier that year. Council Minutes, October 24, 1917, FWC Records, "Convention Minutes, 1915–20, Council Minutes 1915–21, Bd. of Directors 1915–22" (bound volume), 114.

12. "Would Put a Crime in Some Tricks of Cupid, the Sly Wag," *Kinston Free Press*, January 22, 1917, 1; NC Public Laws 1917, chapter 135 (on cousins) and chapter 38 (on marriage licenses).

13. On the 1903 law, see North Carolina Code, Revisal of 1905, chapter 50, sections 2083, 2086, 3369; on the 1917 proposal (Senate Bill 762, House Bill 1496), see *Senate Journal, 1917*, 379–80; *House Journal, 1917*, 487, 595, 627; and "House Passes the Grier Ouster Law by 50 to 29 Vote," *Winston-Salem Journal*, February 24, 1917; "Jones Suffrage Bill Is Beaten in Senate After Lively Debate," *Greensboro Daily News*, February 28, 1917; and "Teaching Profession Is Created by Law," *Greensboro Daily News*, March 4, 1917. On policing boundaries, see Pascoe, *What Comes Naturally*.

14. Poteat, "Address at Runion and Picnic on Lawn of Dr. Oscar Haywood, Montgomery County," August 17, 1912, Poteat Papers, Box 12, Folder 1245; Kate Burr Johnson, "Welfare of Women and Children in Wartime," *BCPW Bulletin* 1, no 3 (July–September 1918): 12. For other comments by Poteat on marriage, see The Wealth of North Carolina (1916), Folder 1245; The Population and Its Prospects (1924), Folder 1008; Marriage and Divorce, CSS (1932), Folder 939; The Old Method for the New World, Folder 982; Poteat, "The Conservation of the Resources of North Carolina," address at Conservation Dinner, Greensboro, September 7, 1916, reprinted in *Bulletin of Wake Forest College*, Box 7, Folder 832, all in Poteat Papers; "Earnestly Wants to Serve State," *News and Observer*, January 14, 1917, 1. For another call for eugenics education, see F. R. Harris, "Eugenics and Conservation," *Transactions* 59 (1912): 467. Southern white traditions prohibited open discussions of sexuality, which complicated many Progressive-Era campaigns, such as fights against the sexual double standard and against venereal disease. On Southern attitudes about female sexuality, see Scott, *The Southern Lady*.

15. On Virginia, see Noll, *Feeble-Minded in Our Midst*, 67; Lombardo, *Three Generations, No Imbeciles*, 61; Dorr, *Segregation's Science*, 122. For a list of eugenic sterilization laws, see Engs, *Eugenics Movement*, 55. Reilly charts 1913 as an early peak in eugenic sterilization legislation activity, followed by a trough from 1918 to 1922. Reilly, *Surgical Solution*, 67–68, 84–88.

16. See *Proceedings of the Annual Conference of Charities and Correction, 1903*, 253–54; *1906*, 280, 468; *1907*, 10; *1909*, 420; and *1910*, 37. For some discussion of sterilization in a Southern context, see John H. De Witt, "Present Charitable Needs of the South," *Proceedings of the Annual Conference of Charities and Correction, 1914*, 427–34. For examples of discussion of sterilization at the Southern Sociological Congress, see William Francis Drewry, "Mental Defectives and the Insane," in McCulloch, ed., *The Call of the New South*, 153–68; and Carolyn Geisel, "Alcohol's Health Toll," in McCulloch, ed., *Democracy in Earnest*, 297–305.

17. Note, however, that Denson seems to have never advocated sterilization. Alexander Johnson later became field secretary for the Committee on Provision for the Feeble-Minded. On NCCC discussion, see "Report of the State of North Carolina to the National Conference of Charities and Correction, May, 1903," reprinted in *BPC Report, 1903*, 152–55; *Proceedings of the Annual Conference of Charities and Correction, 1903*, 247–48, 250. On Johnson, see Cox, "Alexander Johnson."

18. F. R. Harris, "Eugenics and Conservation," and discussion, *Transactions* 59 (1912): 230–41, 467–68; Mary Schwarberg, "The Care of the Feeble-Minded," *Social Service Quarterly* 3, no. 3 (October–December 1915): 75–76; Reilly, *Surgical Solution*, 29–32.

19. Susan Iden, "Federation Chooses Department Heads," *Greensboro Daily News*, May 8, 1915; C. Banks McNairy, "Cause and Prevention of Feeble-Mindedness," speech read before Tri-State Medical Association of the Carolinas and Virginia, February 17–18, 1915, reprinted in *Charlotte Medical Journal* 71, no. 6 (June 1915): 316–17; Dr. C. B. McNairy, "Feeble-Mindedness," *Social Service Quarterly* 3, no. 1 (April–June 1915): 17–18.

20. Registration Book, Columbia, 1913, ECU Hyatt Papers, Folder: Hyatt, Sybil—Testimonials; Dr. H. O. Hyatt, "Feeble Mindedness and Physiologic Psychology," *Transactions* 60 (1913): 109–19.

21. McNairy, "Cause and Prevention of Feeble-Mindedness." McNairy's first discussion of euthanasia predated the release of *The Black Stork*, which brought to the screen the question of whether to offer medical treatments that might save the life of a severely disabled baby. The film ran in movie theaters in various versions through the 1920s. See Pernick, *Black Stork*.

22. "Open Formula Is Strongly Favored by Social Workers," *News and Observer*, January 23, 1917.

23. The critic was Alexander Johnson, former head of the Indiana school for the feeble-minded and now field secretary of the National Committee on Provision for the Feeble-Minded. On Johnson, see Cox, "Alexander Johnson." On Johnson at the 1917 CSS gathering, see Neal, *North Carolina Conference for Social Service*, 27.

24. "Open Formula Is Strongly Favored by Social Workers."

25. "Social Service Sessions Close," *News and Observer*, January 25, 1917. Perhaps because of Baggett's support of sterilization measures, McNairy later pushed to have him hired as state commissioner of public welfare. See C. Banks McNairy to Kate Burr Johnson, March 25, 1921; and McNairy to Carey J. Hunter, March 23, 1921, both in Unprocessed BPW Records, Box 1, Folder 8: SBCPW, 1919–28.

26. "Resolutions of 1917 Conference," in Neal, *North Carolina Conference for Social Service*, 31.

27. By 1919–20, Caswell staff estimated the number conservatively at 5,000; see McNairy and Schwarberg, "Information Concerning the Caswell Training Center"; and Mary Schwarberg, "Some Impressions from Study of Feeble-Minded in Our State," *Greensboro Daily Record*, March 14, 1920.

28. For calls for space, see superintendents' reports and legislative recommendations in *BCPW Report, 1919–20*, 18; *BCPW Report, 1920–22*, 43–45; *BCPW Report, 1922–24*, 11–12, 150–51; *BCPW Report, 1924–26*, 103; *BCPW Report, 1926–28*, 9, 22–23; and *BCPW Report, 1928–30*, 14, 99.

29. In 1917, Caswell received an annual appropriation of $45,000 for maintenance, plus another $75,000 for permanent improvements. *Caswell Biennial Report, 1917–18*, 9–10; "The Defective Child," *BCPW Bulletin* 4, no. 4 (October–December 1921): 20; "Committee Visits Training School," *News and Observer*, February 4, 1917.

30. *BPC Report, 1905*, 21–23; *BPC Report, 1910*, 22; *BPC Report, 1911*, 30–31; Paul V. Anderson, "Mental Hygiene in the Young," *Transactions* 57 (1910): 450. On reformers' attempts during the Progressive Era to redefine innocent children (dependent and delinquent children, although not defective children) as the ultimate "deserving poor," see Ladd-Taylor, *Fixing the Poor*, esp. 24–56.

31. On the importance of white girls to the race, see Polansky, "I Certainly Hope"; and Cahn, *Sexual Reckonings*, esp. 43–67. On female teenage delinquency more generally and

the threat of feebleminded girls and women, see Cahn, *Sexual Reckonings*, esp. 160; Noll, "A Far Greater Menace"; Kline, *Building a Better Race*; and Holloway, *Sexuality, Politics, and Social Control*. On the reformatory movement as a response to class-based conflict over adolescent girls' sexuality, see Bickford, *Southern Mercy*; Odem, *Delinquent Daughters*; Perry, *Policing Sex in the Sunflower State*; and Zipf, *Bad Girls at Samarcand*.

32. On Black reformatories, see Cahn, *Sexual Reckonings*, 46, 68–97. On efforts to establish Efland and two reformatories for Black boys, see Sims, *Power of Femininity*, 122–26. On Black women's uplift and reform strategies, see Higginbotham, *Righteous Discontent*.

33. Denson to White, March 21, 1917, BPW Records, General Corr. of the Board, Box 4, Folder: 1917; Cotten, *History of the North Carolina Federation*, 83, 108–9; Dr. E. Delia Dixon Carroll, "What Can Our Women's Clubs Do in the State's Upbuilding," *Social Service Quarterly* 2, no. 4 (January–March 1915): 110–11; "The Part of the Club Women in Social Service," *Social Service Quarterly* 3, no. 3 (October–December 1915): 80–84; NC Public Laws 1917, chapter 255. Without help from the Conference, women's groups likely would have faced a more protracted struggle. On a similar need for women's organizations to cultivate powerful male allies in their education reform efforts, see Sims, *Power of Femininity*, 163. On McGeachy as the "father of the whole effort," see Mrs. J. R. Chamberlain, "Samarcand Manor," *BCPW Bulletin* 1, no. 3 (July–September 1918): 5–7; and Cotten, *History of the North Carolina Federation*, 109. Funding for Samarcand and Caswell were passed together; one person resisted funding Samarcand alone, wanting to consider it in the context of the other state institutions' needs. On passage in the House, see Nell Battle Lewis, "Samarcand Not Different from World of Humanity," *News and Observer*, November 20, 1926.

34. "Feeble Minded Men Too Many," *Charlotte Observer*, January 4, 1918; Kevles, "Testing the Army's Intelligence"; Zenderland, *Measuring Minds*, 288–89, 293–94, 302, 311–19; Gould, *Mismeasure of Man*, 222–63.

35. Susan Cahn also points to the creation of Samarcand in 1917 as a result of increased wartime concern about female "sex delinquents." Cahn, *Sexual Reckonings*, 46–47. On World War I fears, see Sims, *Power of Femininity*, 149. On federal antiprostitution efforts, see Bristow, *Making Men Moral*. On the links between prostitution and feeblemindedness, see Noll, "A Far Greater Menace," 42, 45–47. On women activists' efforts in Minnesota to "uncouple sex delinquency and feeblemindedness," painting sexually active young girls as innocent while they villainized feebleminded children, see Ladd-Taylor, *Fixing the Poor*, esp. 24–56.

36. For the Conference convention, March 5–6, 1918, see "State and National Efficiency," *BCPW Bulletin* 1, no. 3 (July–September 1918), 4–5; for Bickett's address to the Federation of Women's Clubs on May 30, 1918, see "Social Purity," in *Public Letters and Papers of Thomas Walter Bickett*, 170–72.

37. Bristow, *Making Men Moral*; Perry, *Policing Sex*; Cahn, *Sexual Reckonings*, 44–45, 324n8. For efforts in North Carolina, see Zipf, *Bad Girls at Samarcand*, 27–43.

38. R. F. Beasley, "Save the Feeble-Minded Girl," *BCPW Bulletin* 1, no. 2 (April–June 1918): 12–15; Mrs. J. R. Chamberlain, "Samarcand Manor," *BCPW Bulletin* 1, no. 3 (July–September 1918): 5–7; Mrs. K. M. D. Krause, "Work of the Girls' Protective Bureau at Camp Greene," *BCPW Bulletin* 1, no. 3 (July–September 1918): 7–9; Mrs. R. L. Justice, "Welfare of Women and Children," *BCPW Bulletin* 1, no. 3 (July–September 1918): 13–15.

39. Mrs. J. R. Chamberlain, "Samarcand Manor," *BCPW Bulletin* 1, no. 3 (July–September 1918): 6; Zipf, *Bad Girls at Samarcand*, 17; *BCPW Report, 1917–18*, 33–35. The

question of what to do with merely delinquent girls versus prostitutes was on reformers' minds from the beginning. McGeachy and the Conference discussed whether there should be two institutions to separate "wayward girls" and "fallen women," and McNaughton advocated creating an additional institution in 1921. See "Social Service Meeting Ends," *Charlotte Observer*, January 27, 1916; Zipf, *Bad Girls at Samarcand*, 46–47.

40. On escape attempts, see Noll, *Feeble-Minded in Our Midst*, 131; Zipf, *Bad Girls at Samarcand*, 57.

41. "Spruill, Lydia," 1910 US Census, Craven County, North Carolina, population schedule, Eighth Township, New Bern, Fourth Ward, page 9A, enumeration district [20], dwelling 176, family 187; "Public Pulse: Dr. Joyner in Re Lydia Spruill," *Greensboro Daily News*, July 27, 1918; Letter to the Editor from W. M. Bouterse, Adjutant, Salvation Army, Durham, in "Public Pulse: The Case of Lydia Spruill," *Greensboro Daily News*, July 9, 1918; "Greensboro Man Tells About Lida Spruill," *Greensboro Daily News*, July 6, 1918; *Greensboro Directory, 1915–16*, 448; Image 31 of Sanborn Fire Insurance Map from Greensboro, Guilford County, North Carolina, Sanborn Map Company, March 1919.

42. "Lydia Spruill Again Is at Large, Kinston Hears"; Letter to the Editor from W. M. Bouterse; "Public Pulse: Dr. Joyner in Re Lydia Spruill," *Greensboro Daily News*, July 27, 1918; "Action Unwarranted Declares Dr. M'Nairy," *Greensboro Daily News*, July 4, 1918; "Mrs. Townsend Wants Her Daughter in the School," *Greensboro Daily News*, July 17, 1918; "Beasley Files Report in Lida Spruill Case," *Charlotte Observer*, July 24, 1918.

43. "Action Unwarranted Declares Dr. M'Nairy"; "Lydia Spruill Case to Be Investigated Soon," *Greensboro Daily News*, July 9, 1918; "No Investigation of the Caswell School," *Greensboro Daily News*, July 16, 1918; "Beasley Files Report in Lida Spruill Case"; "Lydia Spruill Returns to School at Kinston," *Greensboro Daily News*, December 7, 1918; "Lydia Spruill Again Is at Large, Kinston Hears"; "Mrs. Townsend Wants Her Daughter in the School."

44. Letter to the Editor from W. M. Bouterse; "Action Unwarranted Declares Dr. M'Nairy." On the conflation of feeblemindedness and deviant sexuality in women, see Kline, *Building a Better Race*, esp. 32–60.

45. "Lydia Spruill Returns to School at Kinston"; Insurance Department Fire Investigation, no. 1908, January 10, 1919, Bickett's Papers, Box GP 380, Folder: Corr, January 1–31, 1919; "Spruill Girl Escapes from Training School," *Greensboro Daily News*, December 25, 1918; "Lydia Spruill Stirs Interest in Kinston," *Charlotte Observer*, July 26, 1920.

46. Little evidence at the time directly linked Spruill to the fires; the state investigation ultimately did not find her responsible. Still, people suspected her then and continued to suspect her for some time. The 1922 Board of Charities and Public Welfare report identified her as "Lyda [sic] Spruill, who set fire to the Caswell building," and newspaper reports later listed the series of Caswell fires as among Spruill's other "escapades." Spruill remained at Dix Hill through January 1920, when she once again escaped from state custody and sought refuge with her stepfather's family near Kinston. "Four Girls Started Caswell School Fire," *Greensboro Daily News*, January 9, 1919; *House Journal, 1919*, 20–21; Deputy Insurance Commissioner [initials R. M. C.] to Hon. James R. Young Insurance Commissioner, January 10, 1919, Bickett Papers, Box GP 380, Folder: Corr., January 1–31, 1919; *BCPW Report, 1920–22*, 101; "Lydia Spruill Again Is at Large, Kinston Hears"; "Lydia Spruill Stirs Interest in Kinston."

47. Some legislators proposed emergency orders to bring the displaced Caswell residents to Raleigh more permanently, but others feared the temporary change might become permanent. "Refuse to Allow M'Nairy to Quit," *News and Observer*, January 11, 1919; "Shepherd Authors New Building Bill," *News and Observer*, January 16, 1919; "Senate Pays Tribute Martin Stacy Dean of State University," *Winston-Salem Journal*, January 22, 1919; "The Capital Punishment Bill Is Amended but Not Finally Passed," *Greensboro Daily News*, January 24, 1919; "Are Not in Favor of Moving School," *News and Observer*, January 25, 1919; "Part of M'Nairy's Outfit Moves to Raleigh for Time," n.d. [January or February 1919], copy in Caswell Records, news clippings volume, 37; *Senate Journal, 1919*, 74, 590; "Transfer of Training School Improbable," *Winston-Salem Journal*, January 26, 1919; "Budget Bill Goes into the Hopper," *News and Observer*, January 14, 1919; "Alexander's Hand Is Seen in House," *News and Observer*, January 14, 1919; "Tells How Army Aviators Learn," *Charlotte Observer*, January 15, 1919; "Rotarians Join in Tax Protest; Caswell School Indorsed," *Charlotte Observer*, January 29, 1919; "Caswell Training School: A Charlotte Lawyer Makes Relation in Behalf of That Institution," *Charlotte Observer*, February 1, 1919.

48. Bickett's Private Secretary to W. W. Faison, January 11, 1919; John McCampbell to Col. Santford Martin, January 18, 1919, both in Bickett Papers, Box GP 380, Folder: Corr., January 1–31, 1919.

49. At stake was not only whether Spruill was feebleminded or not, but also whether she was insane and thus should be sent to a mental hospital rather than Caswell. "Nash County Man Will Battle Alexander for Presidency of Union; Miss Lydia in Custody," *Winston-Salem Journal*, December 11, 1918; "The Capital Punishment Bill Is Amended but Not Finally Passed"; "Are Not in Favor of Moving School"; G. G. Dickson, "Lydia Spruill and Sally Bryson Are Pronounced Imbeciles After Examination by Expert Authority," *Greensboro Daily News*, January 26, 1919. On Barr's early contributions to classification of the feebleminded, see Zenderland, *Measuring Minds*, 75, 83. On Barr's approach at Elwyn Training School in Pennsylvania and his belief in the linkage of feeblemindedness and criminality, as well as the necessity of institutionalizing "high-grade" feebleminded people, see Chamberlain, "Challenging Custodialism."

50. Dickson, "Lydia Spruill and Sally Bryson Are Pronounced Imbeciles."

51. On prior criticism of Caswell's management, see "Schools Appeal for State Funding," *Charlotte Observer*, February 5, 1919. For a contemporary example of the links between feeblemindedness and delinquency, see state welfare commissioner Roland Beasley's address quoting Goddard that "*a priori* there is a well-paved road for the feeble-minded person to either the almshouse or to the prison or to the brothel." Beasley, "Save the Feeble-Minded Girl," 13.

52. "Caswell Training School," *Charlotte Observer*, February 1, 1919; "Capital Punishment Bill Is Amended but Not Finally Passed"; Dickson, "Lydia Spruill and Sally Bryson Are Pronounced Imbeciles."

53. NC Public Laws 1919, chapters 224 and 295.

54. The subcommittee's report about their visit did not include Barr's recommendation to sterilize inmates. Rather, they focused on doubling Caswell's current capacity, providing some institutional home for feebleminded Black children, and creating an outreach bureau. "Are Not in Favor of Moving School"; "Speaker Sponsors Governor's Plan," *News and Observer*, February 2, 1919; Dickson, "Lydia Spruill and Sally Bryson Are Pronounced

Imbeciles"; McNairy, Supplemental Superintendent's Report, January 1919, in *Caswell Biennial Report, 1917–18*, 39–40.

55. "Speaker Sponsors Governor's Plan"; "A Good Man for Speaker," *News and Observer*, January 8, 1919; "Pyromania Spreads to Boys Caswell Training School," *Kinston Free Press*, January 29, 1919, copy in Caswell Records, news clippings volume, 34.

56. "Speaker Sponsors Governor's Plan." Roy Melton Brown, an employee of the Board of Charities and Public Welfare from 1921 to 1925, wrote in the 1950s in an unpublished history of welfare in North Carolina that "Apparently there was careful avoidance [in the 1919 law] of any specific mention directly or indirectly of sterilization." Brown's analysis appears to have been based only on the text of the law (which did indeed avoid mention of sterilization), but it is possible that his interpretation was also based on transmitted knowledge from his colleagues at the Board of Charities and Public Welfare. Roy Melton Brown, "The Growth of a State Program of Public Welfare," n.d. [ca. 1950], unpublished manuscript, North Carolina Collection (Wilson Library, University of North Carolina at Chapel Hill), chapter 17, 26.

57. One newspaper reported that Josephus Daniels and the Conference endorsed the sterilization bill, but the Conference's records do not include an explicit endorsement of the bill. "Brummitt Bill Passes in House," *News and Observer*, March 8, 1919; Harry Stich, Letter to Editor, "The Open Forum: Legislation Commended," *Charlotte Observer*, March 17, 1919; "Resolutions," 1919, in Neal, *North Carolina Conference for Social Service*, 41.

58. The lawmakers who were "aghast" may have been so because they associated sterilization with castration as a punishment for criminals. "Message of Governor T. W. Bickett to the General Assembly, 1919," *Public Documents, Session 1919*, 6–7; "Speaker Sponsors Governor's Plan"; *House Journal, 1919*, 117, 214, 329; T. W. Bickett, "Address by His Excellency, T. W. Bickett, Governor of North Carolina," April 15, 1919, reprinted in *Transactions* 66 (1919): 268–73; Press Release, Gov. T. W. Bickett, "An Inspiring Record," released for publication in morning papers of Thursday, March 13, 1919, copy in Bickett papers, Box GP 381, Folder 1: Corr, March 1–31, 1919. On similar interest group politics necessary to pass Indiana's sterilization bill in 1907, see Lantzer, "Indiana Way."

59. Of the fourteen members of the House Committee on Health, six were also members of the special joint committee on Caswell, so they were certainly familiar with the situation. The committee approved the bill on February 15, but nine days later, on February 24, legislators returned it to the committee. The *News and Observer*'s legislative coverage does not indicate why the bill was sent back to committee on February 24. *House Journal, 1919*, 22, 214, 329, 620; "Brummitt Bill Passes in House"; W. J. Martin, "Neal Child Bill Passes Senate—Bickett Sends Message," *Charlotte Observer*, March 8, 1919, 1; *Senate Journal, 1919*, 544. On the language of "mercy" in Southern reform efforts, see Bickford, *Southern Mercy*.

60. Of Republicans, ten were absent, eleven voted no, and six voted yes. Of Democrats, seventeen were absent, fourteen voted no, and sixty voted yes. *House Journal, 1919*, 649–50; "Brummitt Bill Passes in House."

61. W. J. Martin, "Neal Child Bill Passes Senate—Bickett Sends Message," *Charlotte Observer*, March 8, 1919; "Brummitt Bill Passes in House." Brown's comments about the bill being "made in Germany" are puzzling. In 1919, Germany had no sterilization program, nor was it fascist. There were some Germans calling for racial hygiene at the time, but certainly no more than in the United States. See Paul Weindling, "German Eugenics and

the Wider World: Beyond the Racial State," in Bashford and Levine, eds., *Oxford Handbook of the History of Eugenics*.

62. "Clash over Bill for Welcome of Soldiers," *Greensboro Daily News*, March 9, 1919; "State Holidays Remain the Same; Senate Inclined to Kill Brummitt Bill," *News and Observer*, March 9, 1919; "Expect to Finish Up Work Tonight," *News and Observer*, March 10, 1919; "Act for Purification Passed by the House but Senate Kill It," *Greensboro Daily News*, March 11, 1919; "State Highway Bill Meeting All Demands Is Finally Adopted," *Winston-Salem Journal*, March 11, 1919; W. J. Martin, "Number of Acts Ratified 1, 130," *Charlotte Observer*, March 12, 1919; "'Solicitous' for Chairman Warren," *News and Observer*, March 11, 1919; *Senate Journal*, 1919, 585, 603; *House Journal*, 1919, 692, 710–11; HB 356, SB 1388, Session Records, House and Senate Proceedings, North Carolina State Archives.

63. "257 NC Physicians at Pinehurst Sessions," *Winston-Salem Journal*, April 16, 1919; "President's Address at Ninth Annual Meeting of NC Health Officers' Association, Pinehurst, April 14, 1919," reprinted as J. R. M'Cracken, "What Is North Carolina Doing for Her Unfortunates," *Charlotte Observer*, May 25, 1919.

64. Zipf, *Bad Girls at Samarcand*, 36; NC Public Laws, 1919, chapter 97; HB 213, *House Journal 1919*, 65, 139.

65. HB 111, *House Journal, 1919*, 39, 248; SB 50 and HB 1202, *House Journal, 1919*, 470, 562; NC Public Laws 1921, chapter 129; "The General Assembly of 1921," *Greensboro Patriot*, March 14, 1921. Under the 1921 law, male marriage license applicants had to show no venereal disease, tuberculosis, or mental deficiency/insanity (idiot, imbecile, unsound mind); female applicants had to show no tuberculosis or unsound mind. See *Mental Hygiene* 5 (1921): 881.

66. *Mental Hygiene* 5 (1921): 881; *Mental Hygiene* 5 (1922): 651; Zipf, *Bad Girls at Samarcand*, 47. On federal funding, see also Cahn, "Spirited Youth or Fiends Incarnate," 212; Rafter, *Partial Justice*, 54. For excerpts of McDonald's report, see *BCPW Report, 1919–20*, 33–34.

67. "Lydia Spruill Again Is at Large, Kinston Hears"; "Lydia Spruill Stirs Interest in Kinston"; *BCPW Report, 1920–22*, 101. The best match I can find for Lydia in later census records is "Lydia Spruill," 1920 US Census, Norfolk, Virginia, population schedules, Norfolk City, Monroe Ward, page 11A, enumeration district 123, dwelling 159, family 225.

68. Scholars who do not mention the 1919 law include Reilly, *Surgical Solution*, 138; and Schoen, *Choice and Coercion*. Two scholars mention it in passing: Noll, *Feeble-Minded in Our Midst*, 66; and Hoke, "Politics of Fertility," 34n18. On one state official's belief that no sterilizations were performed under the 1919 law, see R. Eugene Brown to Ezra S. Gosney, February 14, 1938, University of Minnesota Social Welfare History Archives, Association for Voluntary Sterilization Records, Box 6, Folder 53.

69. Virginia passed a law in 1916 that allowed Albert Priddy, the head of the Lynchburg colony, to perform "moral, medical, and surgical treatment" on his patients as he saw necessary, and for a brief period Priddy interpreted the law as permission to sterilize his patients. Virginia passed a statewide law in 1924. In September 1919, Alabama passed a law allowing sterilization at one institution. On Virginia's 1916 law, the *Mallory* case, and laws across the country, see Lombardo, *Three Generations, No Imbeciles*, 19, 60–77, 293–94. On Alabama's law, see 1919 Alabama Acts chapter 704, section 10; Larson, *Sex, Race, and Science*, 84, 105–6; Larson and Nelson, "Involuntary Sexual Sterilization," 411n69. On laws across the country, see Laughlin, *Eugenical Sterilization*.

Chapter 4

1. Ironically, by 1924, this superintendent (Seaford) had become the juvenile court judge for Davie County. See *BCPW Report, 1922–24*, 96.

2. "Sample Court Trial for Culprit Juveniles," *Charlotte Observer*, July 17, 1922.

3. Biographical information on Crane is compiled from "Crane, H. W.—Pedigree of Harry Wolven Crane Taken by K. M. Cowdery, 1915," ERO Records, Series VI, card file; "Juvenile Court Cases," *BCPW Bulletin* 4, no. 4 (October–December 1921): 12; "Sample Court Trial for Culprit Juveniles."

4. Ladd-Taylor, *Fixing the Poor*, 24–25; Gordon, "Social Insurance," 28. On the social work profession's relationship with eugenics, see O'Brien, *Eugenics, Genetics, and Disability*.

5. Annie Kizer Bost, "State Citizenship," in McMahon, ed., *Studies in Citizenship*, 10–12. Bost was commissioner of public welfare from 1930 until 1944.

6. G. G. Dickson, "Lydia Spruill and Sally Bryson Are Pronounced Imbeciles After Examination by Expert Authority," *Greensboro Daily News*, January 26, 1919.

7. Scholars have noted that the South's traditions of minimal state power, racial and class hierarchies, and a slow-changing agricultural economy affected the goals and strategies of Southern Progressives. See Tindall, *Emergence of the New South*.

8. "Kate Burr Johnson," in Starr, ed., *Prominent Families of New Jersey*, 575; "Walton, T. G.," in 1860 US Census, Burke County, North Carolina, population schedule (free inhabitants), Morganton Post Office, page 147, dwelling 1071, family 1071; "Johnson, Kate B.," in 1910 US Census, Wake County, North Carolina, population schedule, Raleigh Township, Raleigh City, First Ward, page 13B, enumeration district 113, dwelling 220, family 236; "Johnson, Kate B.," in 1920 US Census, Wake County, North Carolina, population schedule, Raleigh Township, Raleigh City, page 27B, enumeration district 130, dwelling 431, family 727; *Hill's Directory Co. (Incorporated) Raleigh, NC City Directory [1921–22]* (Hill Directory Co., 1921), 313; Mollie C. Davis, "Kate Ancrum Burr Johnson," in Powell, ed., *Dictionary of North Carolina Biography*; Kate Burr Johnson to J. B. Buell, October 30, 1922, BPW Records, Commissioner's Office: Correspondence with Associations and Committees, 1918–58 (hereafter Corr. with Associations), Box 25, Folder: American Association of Social Workers, 1922–24. In 1923–24, the Johnsons lived on Cowper Drive; Kate moved by 1926. *Hill's Directory of Raleigh, 1923–24*, 392; *Hill's Directory of Raleigh, 1926*, 328; Hayes Barton National Register Nomination, available at https://files.nc.gov/ncdcr/nr/WA4070.pdf.

9. "Mrs. Kate Burr Johnson," *North Carolina Clubwoman* (April 1935): 7, copy in FWC Records, Presidential Files, Kate Burr Johnson (Mrs. Clarence A.); Weathers, *Century to Celebrate*, 26; Convention Minutes, June 2–4, 1919, in FWC Records, "Convention Minutes, 1915–20, Council Minutes 1915–21, Bd. of Directors 1915–22" (bound volume), 72; *FWC Yearbook, 1918–19*, 45; "Message from the President," *FWC Yearbook, 1918–19*, 18.

10. Johnson joined the Conference by 1914 and was elected vice president in 1918. "Who's Who in the North Carolina Conference for Social Service," *Social Service Quarterly* 1, no. 2 (January–March 1914): 107; "Message from the President," *FWC Yearbook, 1918–19*, 18; Neal, *North Carolina Conference for Social Service*, 37.

11. A. W. McAlister, "A State Board of Public Welfare—Scope, Duties, Equipment, and Support," *Social Service Quarterly* 4, no. 2 (April–June 1916): 42; A. W. McAlister to Roland F. Beasley, December 8, 1943, in McAlister Papers, Folder 31. See also Thomas S. Morgan, "Alexander Worth McAlister," in Powell, ed., *Dictionary of North Carolina Biography*.

12. "Resolutions Adopted at the Different Sessions of the Charlotte Conference," *Social Service Quarterly* 4, no. 2 (April–June 1916): 51; McAlister, "A State Board of Public Welfare," 42.

13. A. W. McAlister, "Is the Child Safe" (presidential address at 1916 conference), *Social Service Quarterly* 4, no. 2 (April–June 1916): 29. For McAlister, the child was "the center around which our social welfare undertakings have ranged themselves." McAlister, "A Four Years' Record and a Look Forward," address at CSS, March 25, 1920, McAlister Papers, Folder 305. On the centrality of children to Progressive welfare reforms, see Bullard, *Civilizing the Child*; Ladd-Taylor, *Fixing the Poor*.

14. On the transition from "scientific charity" to professional social work, see Trattner, *From Poor Law to Welfare State*, 236; Katz, *Price of Citizenship*; Katz, *In the Shadow of the Poorhouse*.

15. McAlister to Beasley, December 8, 1943, McAlister Papers, Folder 31; Leroy Halbert, "A Plan for Co-Ordinating State Welfare Work," *Survey* 28, no. 21 (August 24, 1912): 660–61; John E. Hansan, "Origins of the Nation's First Department of Public Welfare Established April 14, 1910," www.socialwelfarehistory.com/organizations/public-welfare-the-first-department-of-public-welfare/. For a comparison of the Missouri and North Carolina bills, see Krome-Lukens, "The Reform Imagination," 169–70.

16. For examples of lobbying efforts, see "Open Formula Is Strongly Favored by Social Workers," *News and Observer*, January 23, 1917; "State Welfare Bill Is Favored," *News and Observer*, January 25, 1917; and W. T. Bost, "Conference of Social Service Comes to End," *Greensboro Daily News*, January 25, 1917. On Bickett's support, see "Inauguration of Thomas W. Bickett as Governor Is Attended by Brilliant Ceremony," *Charlotte Observer*, January 12, 1917; and "Inaugural Address of T. W. Bickett, Governor of North Carolina," *Public Documents, Session 1917*, 3–19. On details of McAlister's campaign, and complicated negotiations with the Board of Public Charities, see Krome-Lukens, "The Reform Imagination," 136–75.

17. NC Public Laws, 1917, chapter. 170; NC Public Laws, 1919, chapter 46.

18. "A State Board of Public Welfare," *Social Service Quarterly* 4, no. 4 (October–December 1916): 108–12.

19. Halbert, "A Plan for Co-Ordinating State Welfare Work."

20. My approach here differs from that of John L. Saxon, who sees North Carolina's "county-administered and state-supervised" system as less desirable than the more common arrangement of state-funded and state-administered social service programs. As a modern arrangement, North Carolina's decentralized system certainly leaves something to be desired, but North Carolina's county-unit system made sense for the rural context in which it was created. See Saxon, *Social Services in North Carolina*, 5. On rural welfare generally, see Martinez-Brawley, ed., *Pioneer Efforts*.

21. *BCPW Report, 1919–20*, 6. On political and funding challenges during Beasley's two years as Commissioner, see Krome-Lukens, "Reform Imagination," 179–87.

22. Beasley to McAlister, June 7, 1918, BPW Records, State Board Corr., Box 2, Folder: 1916–18; Beasley to McAlister, April 27, 1920, BPW Records, Corr. of the Board, Box 39: Corr. with Board Members, 1920–21; Branson to Beasley, June 30, 1919, BPW Records, Corr. with State Agencies, Box 10, Folder 5: UNC (Chapel Hill): General Correspondence, 1917–22.

23. On the appeal of North Carolina's plan in the South, see "Public Welfare Officers Meet," *Winston-Salem Journal*, January 15, 1922.

24. "Federal Worker Comes to State," *Brevard News*, May 16, 1924.

25. NC Public Laws, 1917, chapter 170. For examples of North Carolina laws that structured Jim Crow, see William Sturkey, "The Laws in Context" and other materials in "On the Books," https://onthebooks.lib.unc.edu/laws/the-laws-in-context/.

26. *BCPW Report, 1919–20*, 19–20.

27. NC Public Laws, 1917, chapter 170.

28. Beasley also attended meetings of the National Prison Association in New Orleans and the National Conference for Social Work in Kansas City, Missouri. Minutes of the Board, October 8, 1917, BPW Records, Minutes of State Board of Charities and Public Welfare, 1889–1918, vol. 1; "The Enlarged Sphere of the Board of Charities and Public Welfare," *Social Service Quarterly* 5, nos. 2–4 (April–October 1917): 57–59; *BCPW Report, 1917–18*, 2, 8. On Beasley's political acumen, see Roy Melton Brown, "The Growth of a State Program of Public Welfare," n.d. [ca. 1950], unpublished manuscript, North Carolina Collection (Wilson Library, University of North Carolina at Chapel Hill).

29. Johnson to Beasley, July 10, 1919; and Johnson to Beasley, July 26, 1919, both in Unprocessed BPW Records, Box 1, Folder 4: Reports of the State Board, 1919–25.

30. McAlister in particular was adamant that the job required a man; see McAlister to Mrs. "Clara" A. Johnson, June 1, 1921, BPW Records, State Board Corr., Box 2, Folder: 1920–21. Applicants ranged from an Elon professor of sociology and economics to a land appraiser. They offered the job to three men, including Dr. J. Henry Highsmith, a state public education official. On applicants, see Carey J. Hunter to McAlister, March 21, 1921, BPW Records, State Board Corr., Box 2, Folder: 1920–21; and W. C. Hammond to Roland F. Beasley, March 22, 1921, in Unprocessed BPW Records, Box 1, Folder 8: SBCPW, 1919–28. On training requirements, see NC Public Laws 1917, chapter 170, section 3914g. On Beasley's background in newspapers, prison reform, and the Conference for Social Service, see R. F. Beasley, "Poverty and Charity," *Social Service Quarterly* 2, no. 1 (April–June 1914): 19–22; R. F. Beasley, "The Palace and the Hovel," *Social Service Quarterly* 1, no. 4 (January–March 1914): 94–95; and R. F. Beasley, "The Problem of Tenancy," *Social Service Quarterly* 3, no.1 (April–June 1915): 15–16.

31. Lingle to Johnson, July 10, 1921, BPW Records, State Board Corr., Box 2, Folder: 1920–21, emphasis in original; Minutes, Directors Meeting, June 7, 1921, in FWC Records, "Convention Minutes, 1915–20, Council Minutes 1915–21, Bd. of Directors 1915–22" (bound volume), 184–86. See also "Woman on a Woman's Job," *Greensboro Daily News*, June 15, 1921; and clipping enclosed in Branson to Johnson, June 20, 1921, BPW Records, Corr. with State Agencies, Box 10, Folder: UNC (Chapel Hill): General Correspondence, 1917–22.

32. For more on the gender politics of Beasley and Denson's appointment, see Krome-Lukens, "Reform Imagination," 175–80. After leaving the Board, Denson continued her long-standing work with women's clubs and cared for her mother. She obtained a law license in 1923, at age sixty, although it is unclear whether she ever practiced law. Mrs. W. T. Bost, "Teachers Entertained by Club Women," *Greensboro Daily News*, October 16, 1921; "Weddings—Announcements: Raleigh," *Greensboro Daily News*, January 22, 1928; "State Social Events," *Greensboro Daily News*, March 29, 1931; "State Social Events," *Greensboro Daily News*, April 24, 1932; "Eighty-Two Get Law License for State Practice," *Winston-Salem Journal*, August 25, 1923; "Funeral Planned for Mrs. Raney," *Greensboro Daily News*, March 8, 1952.

33. Roland Beasley to M. L. Kesler, June 21, 1919, BPW Records, General Corr. of the Board, Box 2, Folder: 1919; Minutes of the Board, March 22, 1919, BPW Records, Minutes of State Board of Charities and Public Welfare, 1917–21, vol. 2.

34. Beasley secured funding for this expansion from the 1921 legislature. "Explanation" [n.d., probably early 1921], in BPW Records, microfilmed minutes of State Board of Public Charities, Reel 1; *BCPW Report, 1920–22*, 12.

35. Beasley had created this division in early 1920 with temporary funding from the Red Cross. "Explanation." The first director had worked for the Board for only a few months before leaving for a position at UNC. UNC Trustees Minutes (Executive Committee), September 10, 1920, in UNC Trustees Minutes, Series 1, vol. 12, 247–49.

36. *BCPW Report, 1920–22*, 11, 40.

37. Lingle to Johnson, December 19, 1921, BPW Records, State Board Corr., Box 2, Folder: 1920–21; *BCPW Report, 1920–22*, 10–12; *BCPW Report, 1922–24*, 8.

38. Johnson reported that heads of other state agencies agreed. Johnson to McAlister, September 8, 1921 (copy of this letter sent to each member of the board), BPW Records, State Board Corr., Box 2, Folder: 1920–21.

39. On Shotwell's background, see "Trinity," *Charlotte Observer*, October 1, 1906; "Child Welfare Director Named," *Winston-Salem Journal*, September 25, 1921; 1916 and 1918 conference programs in CSS Papers, 2nd Accession, Box 1, Folder: Historical Material—Dr. Poe; "Social Events in North Carolina—Kinston," *Greensboro Daily News*, March 24, 1918; "Thrift Workers Meet Hearty Reception," *Winston-Salem Journal*, August 17, 1919; and "Miss Mary G. Shotwell Takes Up Her New Work," *Greensboro Daily News*, January 10, 1920.

40. *BCPW Report, 1920–22*, 26–27.

41. On the latter subject, Harry W. Crane was the speaker. *Raleigh Woman's Club Yearbook, 1922–23*, 22, in Denson Papers, Box 2, Folder: Yearbooks, Programs, By-laws.

42. "Miss Shotwell Named NYA Regional Director," *Greensboro Daily News*, March 15, 1941.

43. Emeth Tuttle had a master's degree. See Johnson to McAlister, September 1, 1926, BPW Records, State Board Corr., Box 2, Folder: 1924–26.

44. *BCPW Report, 1922–24*, 8. For another example, see "Miss Camp Joins Staff of Board of Public Welfare," *Public Welfare Progress* 6, no. 6 (June 1925): 1.

45. For example, after Emeth Tuttle resigned she taught case work at colleges wherever she and her new husband moved. Lucy Lay, the Board's publicity director, went on to a similar position for the National Conference of Social Work. See "Mrs. Emeth Cochran Passes at Asheboro," *Greensboro Daily News*, December 22, 1940; *BPCW Report, 1926–28*, 16.

46. "Research in Progress, July 1920–July 1921," *University of North Carolina Record*, no. 188 (August 1921): 52–53; "List of County Superintendents of Public Welfare as of November 30, 1920," *BCPW Report, 1919–20*, 65; Johnson to Sanders, April 21, 1921, BPW Records, Corr. with State Agencies, Box 10, Folder: UNC School of Public Welfare and Social Work, 1921–40.

47. *BCPW Report, 1920–22*, 11. On Sanders's participation in the study of Jackson, see Johnson to Mr. J. P. Cook [Jackson Training School], June 12, 1922, BPW Records, State Board Corr., Box 2, Folder: 1922–23. On Sanders's mountain investigation, see Johnson to Sanders, n.d. [early June 1921]; Sanders to Johnson, August 14, 1921; Sanders to Johnson, August 19,

1921; and Sanders to Johnson, August 22, 1921, all in BPW Records, Corr. with State Agencies, Box 10, Folder: UNC School of Public Welfare and Social Work, 1921–40.

48. Sanders to Johnson, December 11, 1921; Sanders to Johnson, May 19, 1922, both in BPW Records, Corr. with State Agencies, Box 10, Folder: UNC School of Public Welfare and Social Work, 1921–40.

49. On work in county organization, see notice of his resignation in Commissioner's Report to Board, October 9, 1923, Unprocessed BPW Records, Box 1, Folder 4: Reports of the State Board, 1919–25. On desire for work to count toward PhD, see Sanders to Johnson, February 19, 1922, BPW Records, Corr. with State Agencies, Box 10, Folder: UNC School of Public Welfare and Social Work, 1921–40. At the same time, Sanders was working part-time for the Conference for Social Service; see Johnson to McAlister, July 5, 1922, BPW Records, State Board Corr., Box 2, Folder: 1922–23.

50. "Carolina Alumni Parade Campus," *Winston-Salem Journal*, June 13, 1923; *University of North Carolina Alumni Review* 11, no. 9 (June 1923), 248; "Leonard Joins Charities Staff," *Winston-Salem Journal*, September 10, 1923; "Dr. Sanders, UNC Author, Dies at 75," *Greensboro Daily News*, August 10, 1973; Register of the Officers and Faculty of the University of North Carolina 1795–1945, compiled by the staff of the North Carolina Collection, https://docsouth.unc.edu/true/faculty/faculty.html.

51. Leonard to Harper, December 19, 1924, Unprocessed BPW Records, Box 1, Folder 8: State Board of Charities and Public Welfare, 1919–28.

52. Johnson to McAlister, September 1, 1926, BPW Records, State Board Corr., Box 2, Folder: 1924–26. For more information about Board staff, see staff lists in *BCPW Reports*, 1921–30; *BCPW Bulletins*, 1920–23; and Johnson's reports to the Board, Unprocessed BPW Records, Box 1, Folder 4: Reports of the State Board, 1919–25.

53. Some of the part-time welfare superintendents were actually school superintendents doing double duty. Data in these reports are sometimes inconsistent; other numbers in the same report indicated that thirty counties had no superintendent. Four counties lacked welfare boards altogether. *BCPW Report, 1919–20*, 12, 65–67, 70–75.

54. This law was actually a victory for the Board, which had narrowly averted an attempt to make superintendents optional, an attack that would have shattered the gains of 1919. Minutes of the Board, January 18, 1921, BPW Records, Minutes of State Board of Charities and Public Welfare, 1917–21, vol. 2; Beasley to McAlister, January 29, 1921; Beasley to McAlister, February 9, 1921; and other correspondence in BPW Records, State Board Corr., Box 2, Folder: 1920–21; "Rulings of the Attorney-General on Election of Superintendents of Public Welfare," *BCPW Bulletin* 4, no. 3 (July–September 1921): 8–10.

55. Pamphlet, "The Organization and Principles of Public Welfare Work in North Carolina" (State Board of Charities and Public Welfare, n.d. [1919]), at the North Carolina Collection, 6.

56. Most superintendents' experience was limited to involvement in churches, the Red Cross, and other service organizations; on experience and education, see "County Superintendents of Public Welfare, December 1, 1919," *BCPW Bulletin* 2, no. 4 (October–December 1919): 45–46; and typed tally sheet, n.d. [1922], Unprocessed BPW Records, Box 2, Folder 15: Tabulation of Questionnaires. To examine continuity of county welfare officials, I created a database based on: *BCPW Report, 1915*, 118–23; *BCPW Report, 1916*, 108–11; *BCPW Report, 1920*, 65–67; *Public Welfare Progress* 2, no. 3 (July–September 1919): 28–29; and *Public Welfare Progress* 2, no. 4 (October–December 1919): 45–46.

57. Brietz, "Case Studies of Delinquent Girls." Margaret Brietz was a UNC sociology student who was observing the workings of the welfare department as part of her master's thesis. Brietz did not indicate which city she was describing, naming it only as an industrial city in the foothills of the mountains with a population around 77,000 in 1926. Winston-Salem matches these characteristics, and her description of staff turnover matches BCPW records for Forsyth County. Rodwell also matches her description of the unnamed superintendent. See "Rodwell, Joseph L.," in 1920 US Census, Forsyth County, North Carolina, population schedule, Winston Twp., Winston-Salem City, First Ward, page 12B, enumeration district 85, dwelling 176, family 210; also *BCPW Report, 1919-20*, 65, and *BCPW Report, 1922-24*, 97.

58. Beasley, *Program of Work*; "Explanation."

59. For example, see "Mrs. Johnson to County Superintendents of Public Welfare," *BCPW Bulletin* 2, no. 3 (July–September 1919): 18–20. Every issue of the *Bulletin* was relevant to county superintendents, but some issues focused particularly on educating them about the basics. See *BCPW Bulletin* 2, no. 1 (January–April 1919); *BCPW Bulletin* 2, no. 4 (October–December 1919): 2–6.

60. *BCPW Report, 1919-20*, 6–7; *BCPW Report, 1920-22*, 15; Walker, *Social Work*, 138. On the development of professional social work, see Walkowitz, *Working with Class*; and Trattner, *From Poor Law to Welfare State*, 233–72. On rural social work, see Martinez-Brawley, ed., *Pioneer Efforts in Rural Social Work*.

61. "The School of Public Welfare," *University of North Carolina News Letter* (Chapel Hill), September 1, 1920.

62. E. C. Branson to John Sprunt Hill, September 9, 1919, E. C. Branson Papers, 1895–1933, Collection #2610, Southern Historical Collection, Wilson Library (hereafter Branson Papers), Series 1, Box 3, Folder 132; Branson to Hill, September 25, 1919, and Hill to Branson, September 27, 1919, Folder 134. For the origins of the school generally, see E. C. Branson, "A School of Public Welfare at the University of North Carolina," memo enclosed in Branson to H. W. Chase, December 3, 1919, Branson Papers, Series 1, Box 3, Folder 139.

63. The Red Cross first approached Branson in 1919 about using UNC as a new base for their regional summer training program. Dissatisfied with their current program at Emory, they described UNC as "by far the most forward-looking institution in the South along these lines." Beasley to Branson, November 24, 1919, BPW Records, Corr. with State Agencies, Box 10, Folder: UNC (Chapel Hill): General Correspondence, 1917–22; Minutes, June 15, 1920, UNC Trustees Minutes, vol. 12, 232; Brazil, *Howard W. Odum*, 346–50; Walker, *Social Work*, 138.

64. Odum's Institute for Research in Social Science helped launch UNC as a center of social science research. Some of the graduate students at IRSS worked for the Board directly, and others produced studies of interest to Johnson and her staff. Odum's *Journal of Social Forces* reviewed books with eugenics themes, and contributors occasionally mentioned eugenics as a solution to social problems, in the pattern of many social theorists at the time. On Odum, see Johnson and Johnson, *Research in Service to Society*, esp. 3–27; and Brazil, *Howard W. Odum*. On Odum's recruitment to UNC, see Branson Papers, Series 1, Box 3, Folders 138–41, Folder 144. On UNC studies of interest to the Board, see McGill thesis, 1925, in BPW Records, Corr. with State Agencies, Box 10, Folder: University of NC (CH): School of Public Administration, 1919–31; Mabel Boysworth to S. E. Leonard, April 16, 1925; and Sam Leonard to Mabel Boysworth, April 24, 1925, both in BPW Records,

Corr. with State Agencies, Box 10, Folder: UNC, 1923–40. For examples of eugenics in *Social Forces*, see V. V. Anderson, "The State Program for Mental Hygiene," *Social Forces* 1, no. 2 (January 1923): 92–100; Mildred Dennett Mudgett, "The Use of Advanced Students in Field Work," *Social Forces* 1, no. 4 (May 1923): 395–99; Ernest R. Groves, "The Family in Paper Cover," review of Paul Popenoe, *Eugenic Sterilization in California*, *Social Forces* 7, no. 4 (June 1929): 612–14; Benjamin Malzberg, "Notes on Sterilization and Social Control," *Social Forces* 8, no. 3 (March 1930): 398–401.

65. Odum, *Approach to Public Welfare*, 21–24; Jesse Frederick Steiner, "Education for Social Work in Rural Communities: Rural Sociology—Indispensable or Merely Desirable?" *Proceedings, National Conference of Social Work, 1927.*

66. Courses were organized in broad fields such as "Industry," "Fieldwork," "The Family and the Individual," and "Methods of Organization and Administration." On these courses and Odum's vision for the school's public role, see Odum, "University Cooperation in Public Welfare," *BCPW Bulletin* 3, no. 3 (July–September 1920): 38–43. On faculty and programs, see UNC Trustees Minutes, June 15, 1920, Series 1, vol. 12, 232; and "Catalogue of the University of North Carolina at Chapel Hill, 1922–23," *University of North Carolina Record*, no. 200 (March 1921): 179–85, 354–59. See also Johnson and Johnson, *Research in Service to Society*, 14; Brazil, *Howard W. Odum*, 352–53, 360.

67. Odum, "University Cooperation in Public Welfare," 43. The course was also open to Red Cross workers and other social workers, such as secretaries of Associated Charities, but admission standards for nonsuperintendents were higher, with a college degree or equivalent experience required. Many superintendents did not have a college degree; they were admitted to the course by virtue of their office. Printed "preliminary announcement" for summer public welfare institutes, n.d. [1920], BPW Records, Corr. with State Agencies, Box 10, Folder: University of NC (CH): School of Public Administration, 1919–31.

68. F. L. Wilson to Beasley, May 6, 1920, BPW Records, Corr. with State Agencies, Box 10, Folder: University of NC (CH): School of Public Administration, 1919–31.

69. Printed "preliminary announcement" for summer public welfare institutes, n.d. [1920]; Daily schedule of classes, 1920 summer school, BPW Records, Corr. with State Agencies, Box 10, Folder: University of NC (CH): School of Public Administration, 1919–31.

70. "Welfare Board to Hold School," *Winston-Salem Journal*, July 15, 1923.

71. On the importance of institute training and details of the 1922 program, see Kate Burr Johnson, "Institutes for Public Welfare," *Journal of Social Forces* 1, no. 1 (November 1922): 28–30. In 1924, the shorter two-week sessions drew forty county superintendents, plus another thirty-five attendees. The Board reported slightly lower numbers for 1924, at fifty-six attendees. This may have been the number of students who completed the course or the end-of-course examination. "Mr. Cline Studied at Welfare School," *Winston-Salem Journal*, July 22, 1924; Johnson to Mr. J. P. Cook, June 12, 1922, BPW Records, State Board Corr., Box 2, Folder: 1922–23; *BCPW Report, 1922–24*, 8; *BCPW Report, 1924–26*, 79, 99; *BCPW Report, 1926–28*, 77–79; "Appropriations by Last Legislature," *Danbury Reporter*, May 15, 1929.

72. The first set of standards, the product of meetings with committees of superintendents and university officials, required four years of practical experience plus one to three quarters of training at an accredited professional social work school for a "Grade A" certifi-

cate. Report of Special Institutes of Public Welfare, July 11–22 [1921], reprinted from North Carolina Club *News Letter*, 10, BPW Records, Corr. with State Agencies, Box 10, Folder: University of NC (CH): School of Public Administration, 1919–31; *Public Welfare Progress* 2, no. 4 (April 1922); Johnson to J. B. Buell, August 23, 1922, BPW Records, Corr. with Associations, Box 25, Folder: American Association of Social Workers, 1922–24; S. E. Leonard, "Certification of Superintendents of Public Welfare, *Social Forces* 1, no. 1 (November 1922): 30–31.

73. J. B. Buell to Johnson, October 24, 1922; Johnson to Buell, October 30, 1922; Harry L. Hopkins to Johnson, October 18, 1922; Johnson to Buell, November 10, 1922; Johnson to Buell, December 12, 1922, all in BPW Records, Corr. with Associations, Box 25, Folder: American Association of Social Workers, 1922–24.

74. "Establish Standards," *Public Welfare Progress* 4, no. 5 (September 1923): 1. Johnson also regularly enclosed copies of minimum qualifications for superintendents in her circular letters to county officials. See examples in BPW Records, Commissioner's Office, Box 173, Folder: Circular Letters, n.d., 1913–33.

75. In response, at least two newspapers demanded that the Board's approval power be revoked, and Johnson feared a fight in the legislature. Commissioner's Report to Board, October 9, 1923, 5, Unprocessed BPW Records, Box 1, Folder 4: Reports of the State Board, 1919–25.

76. For analysis of public welfare as a field that offered more professional opportunities and administrative control, in comparison to the field of public health, where women had less autonomy, see Krome-Lukens, "Reform Imagination," 238–44.

77. Beasley described complementary roles of superintendent and county boards as in a marriage: the superintendent as the head of the household and the county board as a devoted wife. "Organization and Principles of Public Welfare Work," 5. Similarly, UNC professor Eugene C. Branson assumed women's "social housekeeping . . . instincts" made them leaders in campaigns to educate the public but that paid agents would be men. E. C. Branson, "County Responsibility for Public Welfare," *BCPW Bulletin* 1, no. 2 (April–June 1918): 11. Of the eighty-nine county superintendents in November 1920, only five were women. On female superintendents, see Lingle to Beasley, June 5, 1919; McAlister to Beasley, July 14, 1919; Beasley to McAlister, July 15, 1919, all in BPW Records, State Board Corr., Box 2, Folder: 1919; *BCPW Report, 1919–20*, 65–67.

78. Johnson to [county commissioners and education boards], May 1929, BPW Records, Commissioner's Office, Box 173, Folder: Circular Letters, n.d., 1913–33.

79. Among the fifty *full*-time welfare superintendents, more than a third were women. *BCPW Report, 1924–26*, 82–84. See also *BCPW Report, 1930–32*, 59–61. The proportion of women continued to increase until 1944, when 64 percent of superintendents were women. *BCPW Report, 1942–44*, 112–14.

80. Of the nineteen workers, fourteen were women. Seven of these nineteen workers were Black, six women and one man. *BCPW Report, 1924–26*, 82–84. By 1941, 90 percent of caseworkers were women, most of them white. The caseworkers were overwhelmingly middle-class, with an average income of $1,210 to $1,360 a year, solidly within the range of the average income nationwide. Most held a college degree, and many had previous experience as teachers or clerical workers. Tillinghast, "Statistical Study of the Social Work Personnel," 41, table 22, "Distribution of Social Workers in NC County Departments of Public Welfare, by Class of Positions and Salary, November 1941."

81. *BCPW Report, 1920–22*, 13; "The NC Plan of Public Welfare," n.d. [1921], typed manuscript, Unprocessed BPW Records, Box 1, Folder 1: Development of Public Welfare; *BCPW Report, 1922–24*, 115.

82. Foundations with ties to the Rockefeller fortunes backed multiple projects in North Carolina. By far the best known are the public health campaigns spearheaded by the Rockefeller Sanitary Commission and the International Health Board, including efforts to combat malaria and hookworm. In addition to public health projects, Rockefeller money underwrote experimental public welfare initiatives and research in the social sciences. Between 1924 and 1940, the Laura Spelman Rockefeller Memorial and the Rockefeller Foundation funded five projects related to social welfare in North Carolina. Odum had already won the Rockefeller Foundation's financial support for the Institute for Research in Social Science, an interdisciplinary research center at UNC dedicated to solving the South's problems of rural poverty and economic stagnation. The Laura Spelman Rockefeller Memorial did not usually directly fund state agencies, and they were wary but willing to try. Ettling, *Germ of Laziness*; Walker, *Social Work*, 43–44, 178; Brazil, *Howard W. Odum*, 357, 369.

83. Odum to Ruml, May 15, 1924; and Ruml to Chase, August 16, 1924, both in Laura Spelman Rockefeller Memorial Fund Papers (Rockefeller Archive Center, Sleepy Hollow, New York; hereafter LSRM Records), Folder 786, Box 75, Series 3; and Copy of Resolutions of the Board, enclosed in William A. Blair to Beardsley Ruml, September 9, 1924, LSRM Records, Series 3, Box 75, Folder 786.

84. More counties had "asked to be considered for this demonstration, and Johnson hoped to add a fifth county in the eastern part of the state, but that plan did not materialize. On selection of the counties, see "A Four-County Demonstration in Public Welfare," n.d. [May 19, 1924], LSRM Records, Series 3, Box 75, Folder 786; "4 Counties Get Board's Aid," *Winston-Salem Journal*, December 15, 1924; *BCPW Report, 1922–24*, 13; "Choose Counties for Demonstration Work," *Public Welfare Progress* 5, no. 12 (December 1924): 1.

85. Lawrence, "Organization and Administration," 24–26, 31, 38. The counties did not agree to absorb the cost of welfare workers, but Odum—an eternal optimist—remained "hopeful" that the demonstration had laid a foundation for future work. "Preliminary Report of County Demonstrations," n.d. (February 14, 1927), LSRM Records, Series 3, Box 75, Folder 787, 30, 54–55.

86. Marjorie Bell, "A Brief Study of Social Work in Rural North Carolina," Study undertaken by the National Probation Association for the Committee on Undifferentiated Case Work of the Milford Conference, Enclosed in Howard Odum to Sydnor Walker, September 13, 1927, LSRM Records, Series 3, Box 62, Folder 661; *BCPW Report, 1924–26*, 127.

87. She also reported plowing fields, fixing tractors, and killing rattlesnakes. Bell, "Brief Study of Social Work in Rural North Carolina," 20–26.

88. Memorandum of interview, Walker with Johnson, Raleigh, November 8, 1927, LSRM Records, Series 3, Box 106, Folder 1076; Memo of interview with SHW and LO, with Mrs. Johnson, Miss Mitchell, Lt. Oxley, Raleigh, March 7, 1927, Subject: NC State Department of Public Welfare, LSRM Records, Series 3, Box 75, Folder 787; Final Report of NC SBCPW on Demonstration Under Grant from LSRM Fund, September 13, 1927, enclosed in Johnson to Ruml, September 20, 1927, LSRM Records, Series 3, Box 75, Folder 787.

89. *BCPW Report, 1922–24*, 127.

90. Johnson and Johnson, *Research in Service to Society*, 30–31.

91. William Louis Poteat, "Betterment of Rural Conditions Is Urged," *Public Welfare Progress* 6, no. 7 (July 1925): 1, 2. On the views of white women involved in interracial efforts, see Gilmore, *Gender and Jim Crow*, esp. 177–224.

92. *BCPW Report, 1920–22*, 90–91.

93. On the failure of Caswell and other Southern institutions to provide for the Black feebleminded, see Noll, *Feeble-Minded in Our Midst*, esp. 89–103.

94. On Efland, the reformatory for delinquent Black girls, see Sims, *Power of Femininity*. On Black social work, mutual aid, and racial uplift, see Higginbotham, *Righteous Discontent*; Gilmore, *Gender and Jim Crow*; White, *Too Heavy a Load*; Brown, "Womanist Consciousness"; Gordon, "Black and White Visions"; Carlton-LaNey, "African American Social Work"; Roberts, "Black Club Women and Child Welfare."

95. Countering more conservative white people, Stephenson also argued that helping uplift "this lowly race . . . does not in any way jeopardize race integrity," and once "race integrity [is] made inviolate, white people and negroes may cooperate in all matters that make for mutual progress." Gilbert T. Stephenson, "We Must Lift the Negro Up or He Will Drag Us Down," *Social Service Quarterly* 1, no. 1 (May–June 1913): 17–18.

96. *BCPW Report, 1924–26*, 16.

97. Odum to Ruml, May 15, 1924, LSRM Records, Series 3, Box 75, Folder 786.

98. According to some reports, Oxley was the only Black man in such a position with the US Army. See Carey B. Taylor, "Make Big Strides in Negro Welfare Work in North Carolina," *Winston-Salem Journal*, February 27, 1927. On Oxley and the racial politics of the Division of Work Among Negroes, see Burwell, "Lawrence Oxley and Locality Development."

99. "A Four-County Demonstration in Public Welfare," n.d. (May 19, 1924?), LSRM Records, Series 3, Box 75, Folder 786; Final Report of NC SBCPW on Demonstration Under Grant from LSRM Fund, September 13, 1927, enclosed in Johnson to Ruml, September 20, 1927, LSRM Records, Series 3, Box 75, Folder 787; *North Carolina's Social Welfare Program for Negroes*. For more on Oxley's strategies and details about his work in three counties, see Burwell, "Lawrence Oxley and Locality Development."

100. On Black organizers' willingness to cooperate with white leaders, see Carlton-LaNey, "African American Social Work," 313; on Oxley's work as advancing "community organization as a viable social work methodology," see Burwell, "Lawrence Oxley and Locality Development," 51.

101. Johnson and Oxley also created a statewide Black Advisory Committee, which occasionally met with the white state board. Director of Bureau of County Organization to Catharine Wilcox, January 7, 1924, BPW Records, Corr. with State Agencies, Box 10, Folder 6: University of North Carolina (Chapel Hill): 1923–40; *BCPW Report, 1924–26*, 109, 122, 124; Johnson to Blair, May 26, 1925, Johnson to Blair, July 6, 1925, and Johnson to Blair, January 18, 1926, all in BPW Records, Corr. of Board, Box 1, Corr.: Blair, William Allen, 1924–28; Burwell, "Lawrence Oxley and Locality Development," 59.

102. In general, the profession of social work was dominated by white people who worked with other white people, but Black social workers created their own distinctive models of social work, in addition to less professionalized forms of mutual support. Gary and Gary, "History of Social Work Education"; Carlton-LaNey, "African American Social Work."

103. At least one newspaper remarked with surprise when Oxley addressed white social workers at the 1925 white summer institute about his work. "Director Tells of Mothers' Aid," *Greensboro Record*, July 26, 1925.

104. The three-day institute in January 1927 brought over one hundred social workers to Winston-Salem Teachers' College, and similar numbers attended the 1928 session at the North College for Negroes in Durham. *BCPW Report, 1926–28*, 105–7. On North Carolina's institutes, see Burwell, "North Carolina Public Welfare Institutes." On debates about institutes versus other social work education models, see Gary and Gary, "History of Social Work Education."

105. *BCPW Report, 1926–28*, 105–7.

106. "A Deserved Honor," *Greensboro Record*, September 4, 1927; Taylor, "Make Big Strides"; "Negro Officer Is Honored by State Legion," *Greensboro Record*, September 4, 1927; *BCPW Report, 1924–26*, 119; "Negro Welfare 'on the Ether,'" *Greensboro Record*, August 25, 1926; "Negroes Address White Leaders' Conference," *Star of Zion* (Charlotte), July 29, 1926; "Lieut. Oxley's Appointment," *Africo-American Presbyterian* (Wilmington), December 2, 1926; "Social Welfare in North Carolina," *Star of Zion* (Charlotte), February 3, 1927; "Negro State-Wide Welfare Program," *Africo-American Presbyterian* (Wilmington), July 14, 1927.

107. "Worthy of Consideration," *Greensboro Daily News*, October 16, 1929; "Director Tells of Mothers' Aid"; "Miss Katherine Brady Elected President Student Volunteers," *Greensboro Daily News*, February 28, 1926. For more on the racial politics of the Division of Work Among Negroes, see Burwell, "Lawrence Oxley and Locality Development."

108. "Says Electrocution Does Not Meet Criminal Needs," *News and Observer*, December 20, 1928; *BCPW Report, 1924–26*, 101.

109. *BCPW Report, 1924–26*, 101–3; "More About Friends Meet," *Greensboro Record*, August 3, 1927; Taylor, "Make Big Strides."

110. Recent scholarship has emphasized some Black leaders' attraction to concepts of racial destiny. On the ways that Black leaders' sense of responsibility for the fate of the race led to the politicization of many areas of Black people's private lives, including reproduction, see Mitchell, *Righteous Propagation*. See also Dorr and Logan, "'Quality, Not Mere Quantity'"; Nuriddin, "Race, Sexuality, and the 'Progressive Physician'"; and Nuriddin, "Engineering Uplift."

111. White conservatives took an even dimmer view, believing, for example, that "crime is instinctive to the race." *BCPW Report, 1924–26*, 113; Taylor, "Make Big Strides."

112. L. A. Oxley, "Asheville," *Public Welfare Progress* 6, no. 12 (December 1925): 2.

113. "Old Negro Leading the Life of a Savage Is Discovered," *Watauga Democrat*, July 8, 1926.

114. Johnson, "The Rockefeller Grant," *Public Welfare Progress* 5, no. 9 (September 1924): 2; Final Report of the Board on Demonstration Under Grant, enclosed with Johnson to Ruml, September 20, 1927; Johnson to Ruml, February 18, 1927; and memorandum of interview with Walker and Oxley, with Mrs. Johnson, Miss Mitchell, Lieutenant Oxley, Raleigh, March 7, 1927, Subject: North Carolina State Department of Public Welfare, all in LSRM Records, Series 3, Box 75, Folder 787.

115. "Negro Welfare Program Falls Back upon State," *News and Observer*, January 18, 1931; Burwell, "Lawrence Oxley and Locality Development," 53.

116. "Work of Oxley Among Negroes," *Greensboro Record*, August 25, 1930; "Negro Welfare Program Falls Back upon State."

117. Johnson continued, "Case after case of social maladjustment can be traced back to defect or aberration of mind. Crime, immorality, dependency, in a large proportion of

cases, go back not to 'sin,' but to sickness or deficiency in the brain." *BCPW Report, 1922-24*, 11. A common text used for training was Mary Richmond's *Social Diagnosis* (1917), which included guidance for questioning and diagnosing types such as the "inebriate," "feeble-minded," and "neglected child." Psychiatry was integrated into social work training by the 1920s, although it created problems for the distinctive identity of the field. See Walkowitz, *Working with Class*, 57–85, 209; Trattner, *From Poor Law to Welfare State*, 253–72.

118. "If This Girl Has Children Will They Help This Land?" *Public Welfare Progress* 5, no. 3 (March 1924): 4; *BCPW Report, 1920–22*, 43; Kate Burr Johnson, "Public Welfare," in McMahon, ed., *Studies in Citizenship*, 91.

119. *BCPW Report, 1920–22*, 7, 10; *BCPW Report, 1922–24*, 9–10.

120. The Board published a quarterly *Bulletin* from 1918 to 1923. Beginning in 1921, they also published *Public Welfare Progress* (later *Public Welfare News*) every month to reach a combined audience of social workers and the general public.

121. "The Delinquent Child," *BCPW Bulletin* 4, no. 4 (October–December 1921): 15; *BCPW Report, 1926–28*, 35; Beasley, *Program of Work*, 7.

122. On "economic adjustment" as a result of mental level, see Glenn, "The Fehlers."

123. *BCPW Bulletin* 4, no. 4 (October–December 1921): 24.

124. The Mothers' Aid program was created and funded in 1923. See Saxon, *Social Services*, 14; and NC Public Laws 1923, chapter 260.

125. *BCPW Bulletin* 4, no. 4 (October–December 1921): 24.

126. For the best outlines of the racial dynamics of eugenics in the South, see Noll, *Feeble-Minded in Our Midst*; Dorr, *Segregation's Science*; and Lindquist Dorr, "Arm in Arm."

127. Larson, *Sex, Race, and Science*.

128. *Caswell Biennial Report, 1916–18*, 36–37; *BCPW Report, 1919–20*, 18; *BCPW Report, 1920–22*, 39; *BCPW Report, 1924–26*, 124; *BCPW Report, 1926–28*, 22–23; *BCPW Report, 1930–32*, 17.

129. *BCPW Report, 1924–26*, 101–3.

130. Lawrence Oxley, "Report of Bureau of Work Among Negroes (Six Months)," in Commissioner's Report to Board, July 1925, for fiscal year ending June 30, in Unprocessed BPW Records, Box 1, Folder 4: Reports of the State Board, 1919–25.

131. *BCPW Report, 1926–28*, 106–7; "Special Institute for Negro Welfare Workers," *Public Welfare Progress* 6, no. 12 (December 1925): 1; "Third Negro Institute Reflects Much Interest," *Public Welfare Progress* 9, no. 3 (March 1928): 1; "Crane to Address Negro Conference," *Daily Tar Heel*, February 18, 1930; "Crane Addresses Negro Institute Held in Raleigh," *Daily Tar Heel*, April 4, 1936.

132. The Board's reports usually listed sources of referrals for mental exams, but the charts do not indicate the race of either client or worker. They simply indicate that those making referrals included county superintendents, institutional heads, teachers, and other social workers. *BCPW Report, 1922–24*, 142–46; *BCPW Report, 1924–26*, 92–95; *BCPW Report, 1926–28*, 90–94; *BCPW Report, 1928–30*, 86–89.

133. "The Commissioner Says," *Public Welfare Progress* 5, no. 10 (October 1924): 4.

134. *BCPW Report, 1920–22*, 54a. For a similar example, see *BCPW Report, 1920–22*, 67.

135. "Our Child Problem in North Carolina," *BCPW Bulletin* 4, no. 4 (October–December 1921): 4.

136. *BCPW Report, 1920–22*, 6a, 39.

137. Saxon, *Social Services*, 14; Aydlett, "The North Carolina State Board," 22; *BCPW Report, 1928-30*, 13, 24-25, 40; *BCPW Report, 1922-24*, 21; Johnson, "Public Welfare," 89-90. On welfare programs for single mothers, see Gordon, *Pitied but Not Entitled*.

138. *BCPW Report, 1922-24*, 21; *BCPW Report, 1924-26*, 53, 57.

139. "The Defective Child," *BCPW Bulletin* 4, no. 4 (October-December 1921): 22.

140. *BCPW Report, 1920-22*, 8, 48.

141. For example, other states adopted North Carolina's reporting forms, and Mary Camp Sprinkle met with Tennessee officials in 1926 to discuss their desire to copy North Carolina's system. Commissioner's Report to Board, March [1922], Unprocessed BPW Records, Box 1, Folder 4: Reports of the State Board, 1919-25; and "Tennessee Working to Establish State System," *Public Welfare Progress* 7, no. 1 (January 1926): 3.

142. Johnson to Crowell, August 14, 1929, BPW Records, State Board Corr., Box 3, Folder: 1927-29.

143. "Mrs. Kate Burr Johnson," *North Carolina Clubwoman* (April 1935), 7, copy in FWC Records, Presidential Files, Kate Burr Johnson (Mrs. Clarence A.).

144. Johnson to Mrs. Herbert F. Seawell (Mrs. Ella McA. Seawell), November 8, 1929, BPW Records, State Board Corr., Box 3, Folder: 1927-29; John A. Ferrell to Johnson, January 27, 1930; Johnson to Ferrell, January 29, 1930; and Ferrell to Johnson, February 3, 1930, all in RF Records, RG 2, Series 236, Box 38, Folder 314: NC, A-Z, 1930.

145. William Louis Poteat, "The Social Significance of Heredity," Presidential Address to Southern Baptist Education Association, Memphis, TN, February 21, 1923, copy in Poteat Papers, Box 8, Folder 1078.

Chapter 5

1. "State Fair to Be Opened to Public on Tuesday," *Charlotte Observer*, October 15, 1922; "Current Observations by the Newspapers: 'Dispelling Prejudice' (From Charity and Children)," *Charlotte Observer*, October 27, 1922; "Heavy Price Is Paid for Insane," *Greensboro Daily Record*, May 10, 1927; "Welfare Board's Graphic Exhibit," *News and Observer*, October 18, 1922; *BCPW Report, 1920-22*, 53, 99-103; *BCPW Report, 1924-26*, 98. Eugenic-themed exhibits were popular at state and county fairs across the country. See Lovett, "'Fitter Families for Future Firesides.'"

2. On national patterns in sterilization laws, see Reilly, *Surgical Solution*, 67-68, 84-88; Kevles, *In the Name of Eugenics*, 110-12; and Dorr, *Segregation's Science*, 127-28. On the national reaction to *Buck v. Bell*, see Lombardo, *Three Generations, No Imbeciles*, 174-77.

3. "Solons Occupy Center of Stage," *Warren Record*, February 1, 1929; "Millner Sterilizing Act Passed by House on Its Final Reading," *Greensboro Daily News*, February 17, 1929.

4. This was Goddard's model at Vineland. See Zenderland, *Measuring Minds*, 105-42, 222-60. McNairy's comment was timely, since the legislature's 1917 revision of the welfare law renewed its emphasis on studying the causes and prevention of mental disease. *Caswell Biennial Report, 1916-18*, 6.

5. By mid-1920 McNairy claimed Caswell had a functioning psychological clinic and urged social workers to have testing done there, but he was probably doing the tests himself, on top of his other duties. He did not hire a medical director until 1922. *Caswell Biennial Report, 1920-22*, 7; Brown and Genheimer, *Haven on the Neuse*, 109.

6. NC Public Laws 1868–69, chapter 170, section 4. The state Board of Health also could have contended for leadership of the Bureau of Mental Health and Hygiene, particularly because syphilis was responsible for many cases of insanity. For one attempt by the head of the state health department to consolidate the Board of Charities and Public Welfare under his control, see BPW Records, State Board Corr., Box 3, Folder: 1927–29; Kate Burr Johnson to William Blair, March 21, 1929, BPW Records, State Board Corr., Box 1, Folder: Correspondence, W. A. Blair, 1929–32.

7. Beasley tried to have McDonald come earlier, but the war delayed their plans. See *BCPW Report, 1917–18*, 16–17; *BCPW Report, 1919–20*, 8, 28–34; Beasley to McAlister, February 13, 1920; and Beasley to McAlister, November 24, 1920, both in BPW Records, State Board Corr., Box 2, Folder: 1920–21; "Of Local Interest: Visiting Institutions," *Kinston Free Press*, March 1, 1920; and Speas, *History of the Voluntary Mental Health Movement*, 9. It appears that McDonald's report was not published in full. For excerpts of McDonald's report, see *BCPW Report, 1919–20*, 33–34. For an example of an NCMH survey of Georgia, see V. V. Anderson, "Mental Defect in a Southern State," *Mental Hygiene* 3 (October 1919): 527–65; for four examples of NCMH surveys from 1921 to 1924, including in Kentucky and Maryland, see Grob, ed., *Mental Hygiene*.

8. The Board's 1919 appropriation was $15,000. Beasley requested $25,000 but received only $20,000 in 1921. On requests and appropriations, see *BCPW Report, 1919–20*, 8; "Explanation" [n.d., probably early 1921], in BPW Records, microfilmed minutes of State Board of Public Charities, Reel 1; NC Public Laws 1921, chapter 86, section 23; *BCPW Report, 1920–22*, 40.

9. Crane's biographical details are compiled from "Crane, H. W.—Pedigree of Harry Wolven Crane Taken by K. M. Cowdery, 1915," ERO Records, Series VI, card file; and Charles Horton Cooley, "The Development of Sociology at Michigan," in *Sociological Theory and Social Research: Being Selected Papers of Charles Horton Cooley*, 12, http://www.brocku.ca/MeadProject/Cooley/Cooley_1930.html.

10. Amy Sue Bix notes that between 1910 and 1924, there were thirty-nine male students at the ERO's fieldworker training. Eleven subsequently taught at universities, some went to medical school, and at least six became psychological examiners during World War I. Bix writes, "It appears that only two men remained in eugenics work for a significant time after completing ERO classes": Karl Cowdery (in California) and Arthur Estabrook. Crane falls into the category of university teachers, but his subsequent academic research and applied work for the North Carolina Board of Charities and Public Welfare also qualify him as a longtime eugenics worker. Bix, "Experiences and Voices of Eugenics Field-Workers," 655.

11. "Crane, H. W.—Pedigree of Harry Wolven Crane Taken by K. M. Cowdery, 1915"; *Eugenical News* 1, no. 1 (January 1916): 2, 3; *Eugenical News* 1, no. 5 (May 1916): 33; *Eugenical News* 2, no. 4 (April 1917): 29; *Eugenical News* 2, no. 3 (March 1917): 21; *Eugenical News* 1, no. 6 (June 1916): 40; *Eugenical News* 1, no. 8 (August 1916): 58; *Eugenical News* 2, no. 9 (September 1917): 71.

12. Proctor and Evans, "E. B. Titchener, Women Psychologists, and the Experimentalists," 507; "Crane, Harry, Jr. and Crane, Mabel E.," in 1920 US Census, Franklin County, Ohio, population schedule, Precinct C, Columbus City, page 2B, enumeration district 266, dwelling 40, family 50. For Goudge's research, see Goudge, "A Simplified Method," and Goudge, "A Qualitative and Quantitative Study"; "Several Professors Attend Psychology Meet in New York," *Daily Tar Heel*, January 3, 1929.

13. Crane was the only permanent employee of the division during the 1920s, with other staff coming and going. Staff of the North Carolina Collection, *Register of the Officers and Faculty of the University of North Carolina 1795-1945* (1954); and "Historical Information," finding aid for Department of Psychology of the University of North Carolina at Chapel Hill Records, 1951-63, Southern Historical Collection; *BCPW Report, 1920-22*, 12; *Eugenical News* 3, no. 2 (February 1922): 13; Dr. Richard F. Richie, "Summary of Mental Hygiene Development in North Carolina," talk given at a meeting of the Charlotte Mental Hygiene Clinic Board, October 16, 1940, in BPW Records, Commissioner's Office, Subject File: Conference for Social Service, Box 169, Folder: n.d., 1913-33, NC CSS.

14. On Clifford Beers and the mental hygiene movement, see Trent, *Inventing the Feeble Mind*, 131, 172-73; and Zenderland, *Measuring Minds*, 224-25.

15. On the state board pushing the court system to use Crane's testing services, see Kate Burr Johnson to [solicitors in each of twenty districts], November 5, 1921, in BPW Records, Commissioner's Office, Box 173, Folder: Circular Letters, n.d., 1913-33.

16. *BCPW Report, 1920-22*, 40-41, 49; *BCPW Report, 1922-24*, 128, 144-45.

17. For Crane's estimates, see "The Feeble-Minded and the Law," *Charlotte Observer*, July 16, 1922. These estimates were often based on the commonly accepted principle that 2 percent of the population was feebleminded. For an estimate by McNairy, see "The Defective Child," *BCPW Bulletin* 4, no. 4 (October-December 1921): 20-21; for an estimate by Johnson, see "Mrs. Johnson's Clarion Call" (reprinted from the *Asheville Citizen*, October 2, 1927), *Public Welfare Progress* 8, no. 10 (October 1927): 2; for an official committee's estimate and discussion of how to determine the number of feebleminded, see *Report of the Committee on Caswell Training School*, 12.

18. Only five of the Black people Crane tested between 1922 and 1928 were female; the other sixty-one were male, perhaps because he was testing male inmates at a state institution. Of all the tests Crane and his staff conducted in this period (on Black and white people combined), 787 (52.8 percent) were of males and 702 (47.1 percent) were of females. *BCPW Report, 1920-22*, 41; *BCPW Report, 1922-24*, 146; *BCPW Report, 1924-26*, 94-95; *BCPW Report, 1926-28*, 93-94; *BCPW Report, 1930-32*, 87; "Majority of Psychologists Against Negro Admittance," *Daily Tar Heel*, January 15, 1939.

19. Johnson, like many welfare professionals at the time, believed that to properly address delinquency, dependency, and defectiveness, officials needed to classify individuals and house or treat them according to those classifications. She wanted to have Crane's staff administer mental and physical exams to all prisoners in order to send them to the right institution, viewing this testing as an important part of prison reform. See Johnson to McAlister, March 31, 1922, and Johnson to McAlister, July 5, 1922, both in BPW Records, State Board Corr., Box 2, Folder: General Correspondence, 1922-23.

20. *BCPW Report, 1922-24*, 138-39.

21. Rather than quote from the index cards, which I have not found and which may no longer exist, I am quoting from a case Crane published to argue for the need for qualitative notes as well as quantitative results of standardized mental tests. Crane, "Necessity of Psychometric Tests."

22. For the ERO's system, see Bix, "Experiences and Voices of Eugenics Field-Workers," esp. 643-44. On the number of entries, see *BCPW Report, 1922-24*, 139; *BCPW Report, 1924-26*, 89; *BCPW Report, 1926-28*, 86-87; *BCPW Report, 1928-30*, 82.

23. On information sharing, see *BCPW Report, 1922–24*, 139. On the importance of knowledge creation in the modern state, see Pearson, *Birth Certificate*; Pascoe, *What Comes Naturally*, esp. 131–59; and Scott, *Seeing Like a State*.

24. See, for example, "Dr. Banks McNairy Issues New Treatise on 'Eugenics,'" *Greensboro Daily News*, February 10, 1919; "Dr. M'Nairy Discusses Feeble-Minded People," *Greensboro Daily News*, June 16, 1923; W. H. Dixon, "Some Suggestions in Regard to State's Mental Defectives," *Public Welfare Progress* 7, no. 7 (July 1926): 1–2; "Dr. Dixon Outlines Methods of Training Used at Caswell," *Public Welfare Progress* 7, no. 12 (December 1926): 1; W. H. Dixon, "Census Shows Large Number Mental Defectives Clogging School System," *Public Welfare Progress* 8, no. 10 (October 1927): 1–2; W. H. Dixon, "Dr. Dixon Recommends Parole of Feeble-Minded," *Public Welfare Progress* 9, nos. 10–11 (October–November 1929): 1, 3.

25. McNairy joined the organization in 1917, became an officer in 1920, and was elected president in 1922. He presented research about his work at Caswell to the AASFM. *Journal of Psycho-Asthenics* 22 (1917–18): 53; *Journal of Psycho-Asthenics* 25 (1920–21): 184; *Journal of Psycho-Asthenics* 28 (June 1922–June 1923): 94; McNairy, "Some Phases of Construction, Organization, and Administration of an Institution for the Feebleminded in the South," *Journal of Psycho-Asthenics* 29 (June 1923–June 1924): 271–75; McNairy, "President's Conception of Our Task," *Journal of Psycho-Asthenics* 28 (1922–23): 94–99; W. H. Dixon, "Institutional Administration," *Journal of Psycho-Asthenics* 34 (1928–29): 62–68; "Dr. M'Nairy Discusses Feeble-Minded People"; Noll, *Feeble-Minded in Our Midst*, 53, 181n63.

26. In his first two years at Caswell, Newbold gave mental tests to seventy Caswell residents and fifty-seven noninstitutional residents. *Caswell Biennial Report, 1922–24*, 15.

27. William A. Newbold, "Endocrinology and Blood Chemistry," *Journal of Psycho-Asthenics* 29 (1925): 287–92.

28. Both Newbold and McNairy were forced out in mid-1925. For a brief period, the psychiatrist and medical director was Dr. J. T. Wright, who made fifty-five psychometric examinations during his first year; see *Caswell Biennial Report, 1924–26*, 28. But by 1927, the new medical director did not have psychological experience; see *Caswell Biennial Report, 1926–28*, 17, 19. The student who helped Crane was John Holman McFadden, another example of the close ties between state officials, institutional populations, and academic research. McFadden had training in psychological testing and continued graduate work in the field, probably basing some of his PhD dissertation on his work at Caswell. See McFadden, "Racial Differences Measured by the Downey-Will Temperament Test"; and McFadden, "Differential Responses of Normal and Feebleminded Subjects."

29. *BCPW Report, 1920–22*, 43–46; "Research in Progress, July 1921–July 1922," *UNC Record* no. 196 (July 1922): 60; "Crane Will Present Effects of Heredity," *Daily Tar Heel*, November 12, 1930; "Crane Will Attend National Meetings," *Daily Tar Heel*, May 2, 1939.

30. Margaret Brietz to Kate Burr Johnson, August 24, 1936, BPW Records, Corr. with Associations, Box 28C, Folder: NC Federation of Women's Clubs, 1926–47; Brietz, "Case Studies of Delinquent Girls," 1–4. For analysis of Brietz's work in terms of problems of modernity and delinquency, see Cahn, *Sexual Reckonings*; for discussion of Brietz's reliance on eugenic literatures, see Cahn, "Spirited Youth or Fiends Incarnate," esp. 217–18, 221.

31. Brietz, "Case Studies of Delinquent Girls," 163–70.

32. Brietz, "Case Studies of Delinquent Girls," 185–86. See also her description of Vivian Hart, 160.

33. *BCPW Report, 1922–24*, 135.

34. On family studies, see Rafter, ed., *White Trash*.

35. The "Swamp Island" study did not follow the methods of a eugenic family study, but I have grouped it here because it served a similar purpose in raising public awareness about degenerate families. For original publications, see "The Island District," *BCPW Bulletin* 4, no. 4 (October–December 1921): 28–30; State Board of Charities and Public Welfare, "Swamp Island: A Study of Conditions in an Isolated Section of North Carolina" (Capital Printing Company, 1922). For an analysis of the Swamp Island families in terms of imperialism, race degeneracy, and biopolitics, see Bickford, *Southern Mercy*, 27–59. There is a fourth family study that I have not been able to find: in 1923–24, George H. Lawrence (later a professor of social work at UNC, after finishing his PhD in 1928) was reportedly working on "The Rochell Family: A Study in Feeble-Mindedness." "Research in Progress, July 1923–July 1924," *UNC Record* no. 212 (July 1924): 90.

36. *BCPW Report, 1920–22*, 99–102. The Board referred to the family by pseudonyms, which I have maintained for the sake of clarity.

37. "Several Drunks—In One Case the Tables Are Turned," *Raleigh Times*, February 15, 1909; "Feeble Minded Prostitute Costs City $1,500 Yearly," *News and Observer*, December 5, 1922; Dix Hospital medical staff minutes and patient interviews (1916–17), North Carolina State Archives, cited in Caroline Waller, "Probable Moral Degenerates" (term paper), 2019, in author's possession; *BCPW report, 1920–22*, 98–103; "Terrible Winnie Is in Jail Again," *News and Observer*, October 10, 1922; North Carolina, Deaths, 1906-30, s.v. "Joe Francis" (1868–1925) and North Carolina, Death Certificates, 1906-76, s.v. "Ellender Frances" (1886–1925), cited in Waller, "Probable Moral Degenerates." I am grateful to Caroline Waller for sharing her research about this family with me.

38. *BCPW Report, 1920–22*, 98, 102–3.

39. Johnson also gave talks about the family, including one to a Rotary Club lunch. See "Feeble Minded Prostitute Costs City $1,500 Yearly." On the exhibit's travels, see "Chicago Will See Exhibit Defective 'Wake' Family," *Public Welfare Progress* 4, no. 6 (October 1923): 3; "Durham Woman's Club Studying Feebleminded," *Public Welfare Progress* 6, no. 12 (December 1925): 4; "Wake Family Charts Are Pursuing Useful Career," *Public Welfare Progress* 6, no. 10 (October 1925): 4; *BCPW Report, 1924-26*, 87–88; *BCPW Report, 1926-28*, 16; "Feeble-Minded on the Screen," *Public Welfare Progress* 5, no. 5 (May 1924): 3; "State Displays Child Welfare Exhibit," *Public Welfare Progress* 7, no. 12 (December 1926): 4.

40. [Calendar], August 28, 1929, in William M. Cochrane Papers, #5079 at Southern Historical Collection, Series 6, Folder 1666: Emeth Tuttle Cochrane, 1923–29; "Dealing in Human Misery," *Sun Record*, May 26, 1934, clipping in Cochrane Papers, Series 6, Folder 1669: Emeth Tuttle Cochrane, 1934.

41. "Heavy Price Is Paid for Insane," *Greensboro Daily Record*, May 10, 1927; "Student Groups See Wake County Charts," *Public Welfare Progress* 8, no. 12 (December 1927): 4; "Mental Defectives Traced by Charts," *Greensboro Daily News*, November 25, 1927; "Should Mental Defectives Marry?" *Concord Times*, December 1, 1927, 4.

42. The state official who met Rode was likely Roy M. Brown, field agent. While at UNC, Glenn also coauthored a study of uses of intelligence tests and worked on a three-year longitudinal study of the effects of environmental factors on mental and physical develop-

ment of children in a mill village. In addition to making up the last name "Fehler," it appears that Glenn used pseudonyms for all his subjects' names. Glenn, "The Fehlers," 1, 110–12; *BCPW Report 1922–24*, 135; "Research in Progress, July 1924–July 1925," *UNC Record* no. 226 (July 1, 1925): 67; J. F. Dashiell and W. D. Glenn, "A Re-Examination of a Socially Composite Group with Binet and with Performance Tests," *Journal of Educational Psychology* 16, no. 5 (May 1925): 335–40.

43. Glenn used the Stanford revision of the Binet-Simon test for seventy-five living family members but also gathered "various evidences of the degree of adjusting capacity" for a total of 360 individuals, suggesting that much of his evidence was hearsay. For mental tests, see Glenn, "The Fehlers," 151–54; "Research in Progress, July 1922–July 1923,"*UNC Record* no. 204 (July 1923), 57. On the Fehler family's poor "economic adjustment," see Glenn, "The Fehlers," 184–89. For stories of resisters, see Glenn, "The Fehlers," 48, 139. For "superior strain," see Glenn, "The Fehlers," 87.

44. Glenn, "The Fehlers," 8, 18–19, 61.

45. Glenn, "The Fehlers," esp. "Summary" and "Conclusions," 192–97, 206.

46. *BCPW Report, 1922–24*, 135–38; "Research in Progress, July 1922–July 1923," 57; "Mental Hygiene Important Part of Board's Activity," *Public Welfare Progress* 6, no. 1 (January 1925): 3. On publicity funds, see *BCPW Report, 1928–30*, 18. For an example of the Fehlers in a lecture, see Kate Burr Johnson, "State Welfare Program as It Relates to Mental Diseases and Crime," *Southern Medicine and Surgery* 89 no. 11 (November 1927): 771–76.

47. *Public Welfare Progress* 4, no. 1 (May 1923): 1. They also saw individual mental exams as fulfilling an educational role. See *BCPW Report, 1922–24*, 135.

48. On circulation, see "Five Years Ago," *Public Welfare Progress* 7, no. 10 (October 1926): 2. As the inaugural issue stated, the publication's purpose was not theoretical discussions of social welfare problems; rather, it was "frankly designed to elicit public attention." See *Public Welfare Progress* 1, no. 1 (October 1921). *Public Welfare Progress* was preceded by a quarterly bulletin, which ran from 1918 to 1923 and also featured articles about eugenics. For example, see "The Defective Child," *BCPW Bulletin* 4, no. 4 (October–December 1921): 20–21.

49. For an example of Crane's services, see "What the Superintendents Are Doing," *Public Welfare Progress* 2, no. 3 (March 1922): 1. For articles about Caswell, see "Dr. Dixon Outlines Methods of Training Used at Caswell"; "Results of Training Shown at Field Day," *Public Welfare Progress* 8, no. 6 (June 1927): 1. For articles by superintendents, see Albert Anderson, "Movement for Mental Hygiene Preventive," *Public Welfare Progress* 4, no. 8 (December 1923): 1, 4; W. H. Dixon, "Some Suggestions in Regard to State's Mental Defectives"; Dixon, "Census Shows Large Number Mental Defectives Clogging School System."

50. "A Common-Sense Measure," *Public Welfare Progress* 5, no. 8 (August 1924): 4; "The Governor Says" and "The Commissioner Says" boxes, *Public Welfare Progress* 5, no. 10 (October 1924): 4. For other examples, see "What'll You Do About It? Asks Dr. J K Hall," *Public Welfare Progress* 5, no. 5 (May 1924): 3; and Julian M. Baker, "Dr. Baker Addresses Welfare Conference," *Public Welfare Progress* 9, nos. 10–11 (October–November 1928): 1–2.

51. "Parenthood a Vocation Not a Right, Says Barr," *Public Welfare Progress* 4, no. 3 (July 1923): 3; "Reproduction of Unfit Costly," *Public Welfare Progress* 4, no. 1 (May 1923): 4; "Confusion of Terms," *Public Welfare Progress* 7, no. 1 (January 1926): 2.

52. "Eugenics Committee States Its Program," *Public Welfare Progress* 4, no. 6 (October 1923): 4; "Suppos'n," *Public Welfare Progress* 5, no. 4 (April 1924): 2. See also "Many Feeble-Minded Wait for Admission," *Public Welfare Progress* 5, no. 1 (January 1924): 7.

53. "What Is the State's Answer to This Fact?" *Public Welfare Progress* 4, no. 6 (October 1923): 1. In a similar article, Johnson told multiple stories of feebleminded children and young women and, as in the article several months earlier, repeated a refrain: "The Caswell Training School is full." See "'What Can We Do with Defectives' Is Question," *Public Welfare Progress* 5, no. 6 (June 1924): 3.

54. "What Would You Suggest?" *Public Welfare Progress* 7, no. 7 (July 1926): 2; W. H. Dixon, "Some Suggestions in Regard to State's Mental Defectives." For another example, see "Equality," *Public Welfare Progress* 5, no. 5 (May 1924): 2, where the editor called for adequate segregation at Caswell but also argued that "when real civilization is a little nearer, there will be general recognition of the fact that segregation alone can never solve the problem of mental deficiency."

55. Crane conducted a special study of girls at Samarcand from 1922 to 1924. He was unable to conduct any such studies between 1924 and 1926, so he probably drew his examples from his previous work at Samarcand. *BCPW Report, 1922–24*, 135; *BCPW Report, 1924–26*, 87.

56. "Did You Guess Right?" *Public Welfare Progress* 7, no. 7 (July 1926): 3; "Which One Would You Choose for the Brightest?" *Public Welfare Progress* 7, no. 7 (July 1926): 4; *BCPW Report, 1926–28*, 14.

57. "Feeble Minded Prostitute Costs City $1,500 Yearly"; William Louis Poteat, "Social Hygiene," [address to] Wake Forest College freshmen (1924), Poteat Papers, Box 9, Folder 1073; "Durham Woman's Club Studying Feebleminded," *Public Welfare Progress* 6, no. 12 (December 1925): 4; "Growing Interest in Feeble-Minded," *Public Welfare Progress* 7, no. 1 (January 1926): 1, 4; Kate Burr Johnson, speech before medical society, September 29, 1927, reprinted as Johnson, "State Welfare Program"; *BCPW Report, 1926–28*, 85–86; "North Carolina Club Women Meet in Charlotte Tuesday," *Greensboro Daily News*, April 28, 1929.

58. "Psychological Frat Sees Feeble-Minded Moving Picture Reel," *Daily Tar Heel*, February 16, 1929; "Crane Lectures P-TA," *Daily Tar Heel*, January 19, 1933.

59. NC Public Laws 1919, chapter 281, section 2. Members of the Conference for Social Service's eugenics committee had long called for the creation of a similar board, partly in order for physicians to help courts rule on mental competence in criminal trials. For example, see Dr. L. B. McBrayer, "The Problem of Feeble-Mindedness and Eugenics—Six Recommendations," *Social Service Quarterly* 1, no. 1 (May–June 1913): 16–17; and "Resolutions," *Social Service Quarterly* 5, no. 1 (January–March 1917): 4–7.

60. For commentary on the lack of sterilizations under the 1919 bill, see R. Eugene Brown to Ezra S. Gosney, February 14, 1938, Box 6, Folder 53, Association for Voluntary Sterilization Records, University of Minnesota Social Welfare History Archives; "Curb on Mental Defectives Now Provided by Law," *News and Observer*, February 17, 1929. For brief scholarly mentions of the law, see Noll, *Feeble-Minded in Our Midst*, 66; and Hoke, "Politics of Fertility," 34n18.

61. I have found no evidence that the "Board of Mental Hygiene" or the governor's office officially approved any sterilization cases or that the board met more than twice. McNairy called their first meeting for September 16, 1919, with a second "regular meeting" to be held on October 10, 1919. I have not been able to locate other records from this board.

C. Banks McNairy to [heads of institutions], September 1, 1919; untitled motion, n.d.; and McNairy to Dr. J. R. McCracken, September 29, 1919, all in Mental Hygiene Society Records, Box 1, Folder: Correspondence, 1919.

62. Minutes, Board of Directors of the State Hospitals, April 13, 1920, in Caswell Records, Executive Committee Reports, 220–23; NC Public Laws 1919, chapter 281, section 2.

63. Minutes, Board of Directors of the State Hospitals, April 13, 1920, in Caswell Records, Executive Committee Reports, 220–23. On national trends, see Trent, *Inventing the Feeble Mind*, chapter 6.

64. At this point, a hospital building was under construction but not ready for use. See Caswell Records, Executive Committee Reports, 253–66. Several dozen Caswell inmates were housed at the Raleigh mental hospital while burned-down dorms were replaced at Caswell. McNairy also reported sending other Caswell inmates to the Raleigh institution for "temporary care." *BCPW Report, 1919–20*, 49.

65. Minutes, Board of Directors of the State Hospitals, April 14, 1920, and December 16, 1920, in Caswell Records, Executive Committee Reports, 225, 231.

66. J. R. McCracken to W. S. Rankin, September 23, 1919, and McNairy to J. R. McCracken, September 20, 1919, both in Mental Hygiene Society Records, Box 1, Folder: Correspondence, 1919. On McCracken's support for eugenics policies, see J. R. M'Cracken, "What Is North Carolina Doing for Her Unfortunates," *Charlotte Observer*, May 25, 1919.

67. Hubert A. Royster, "An Account of the Surgical Service in the State Hospital for the Insane at Raleigh, 1922–32," *Southern Medicine and Surgery* 95 (April 1933): 319–21.

68. For a discussion of therapeutic sterilizations in psychiatric institutions, see Braslow, *Mental Ills and Bodily Cures*, 54–70.

69. Royster, "An Account of the Surgical Service." The hospital did not always provide a tally of surgeries in its biennial report, but from the tallies that do exist, the surgeries seem to be spread throughout this decade, and Royster, as a local member of the advisory board of surgeons, performed most of the abdominal surgeries. In the early 1930s, the hospital building was named after Royster in honor of his contributions. See *Biennial Report of the State Hospital at Raleigh, 1920–22*, 23; *Biennial Report of the State Hospital at Raleigh, 1922–24*, 24; *Biennial Report of the State Hospital at Raleigh, 1926–28*, 11; *Biennial Report of the State Hospital at Raleigh, 1930–32*, 6–7; *Biennial Report of the State Hospital at Raleigh, 1932–34*, 5. For a discussion of therapeutic sterilizations in psychiatric institutions, see Braslow, *Mental Ills and Bodily Cures*, 54–70. For an overview of surgical treatments at the Raleigh Hospital, see Kirby, "Footsteps to Sterilization." Thanks to John Kirby for sharing a copy of this article with me.

70. *Caswell Biennial Report, 1920–22*, 9–10; *BCPW Report, 1920–22*, 44–46. On McNairy's desire for a probation program and sterilization before release, see Minutes, Board of Directors of the State Hospitals, April 13, 1920; July 13, 1922; and April 30, 1923, in Caswell Records, Executive Committee Reports, 220–21, 292–93, and 318.

71. Minutes, Board of Directors of the State Hospitals, April 13, 1920, in Caswell Records, "Executive Committee Reports" (handwritten volume), 220; "Social Service Sessions Close," *News and Observer*, January 25, 1917; NC Public Laws 1923, chapter 34; on the first bill's passage as SB 69 and HB 239, see *Senate Journal, 1923*, 44, 70, 75; and *House Journal, 1923*, 102, 275, 424; "Find Caswell School in First Class Shape," *Greensboro Daily News*, February 24, 1923; "Refuse to Vote Money to Build Medical School," *Greensboro Record*, February 27, 1923.

72. The motion to table the bill came from William H. S. Burgwyn, a veteran politician whose politics tended toward the Progressive. For coverage of the bill, see "Say Sanitarium Kitchen Was Filthy," *Greensboro Record*, February 26, 1923; "The Day in the Legislature," *Winston-Salem Journal*, February 27, 1923; and on SB 70 and HB 290, see *Senate Journal, 1923*, 44, 70, 75; and *House Journal, 1923*, 102, 329, 523. On Burgwyn, see Juanita Ann Sheppard, "Burgwyn, William Hyslop Sumner, 1886–1977," in Powell, ed., *Dictionary of North Carolina Biography*, 279.

73. *BCPW report, 1922–24*, 140; "Would Make Ku Klux Klan Publish List of Members," *Charlotte Observer*, December 28, 1922; "Divorce Cannot Be Obtained for Insanity Pleas," *Winston-Salem Journal*, February 28, 1923; "Say Sanitarium Kitchen was Filthy"; "What'll You Do About It? Asks Dr. J. K. Hall"; *FWC Yearbook, 1924–25*, 130–31, cited in Sims, *Power of Femininity*, 117, 234n94; "Resolutions Adopted at State Convention," League of Women Voters *Monthly News* 2, no. 15 (April 1925). For similar language from Kate Burr Johnson, see "Charities Board Outlines State Policy in Regard to Caswell Training School," *Charlotte Observer*, August 7, 1925.

74. The Racial Integrity Act was not under judicial scrutiny until the 1967 case *Loving v. Virginia*. On these Virginia activists and cases, see Lindquist Dorr, "Arm in Arm"; Dorr, *Segregation's Science*, 127–28, 143–52; Landman, *Human Sterilization*, 83–84; and Laws of Virginia, 1924, chapter 394.

75. *North Carolina Manual, 1925*; "House Pushes Along Governor McLean's Consolidation Program; Braswell Bill Passes," *News and Observer*, March 1, 1925. Braswell likely introduced the bill at someone's request, but it is unclear from whom the request came. Unfortunately, the specifics of the bill (1925, SB 1098, HB 1070) are unknown, since no copy remains in legislative records at the state archive. "Braswell Measure Draws Session's Largest Crowd," *News and Observer*, February 28, 1925; *Session Records, 1925*; *House Journal, 1925*, 400, 450, 501, 530; *Senate Journal, 1925*, 408, 441.

76. "Legislature Now Thing of History," *News and Observer*, March 11, 1925; *Senate Journal, 1925*, 617; "Senators Horrified," *Greensboro Daily News*, March 14, 1925; "Senate Favors Sterilization," *News and Observer*, February 8, 1929; Hoke, "Politics of Fertility," 8.

77. Gatewood, *Preachers, Pedagogues, and Politicians*; *House Journal, 1925*, 291.

78. William Louis Poteat, "The Population and Its Prospects," 1924, Poteat Papers, Box 9, Folder 1008; Poteat, "The Old Method for the New World," 1920, Poteat Papers, Box 9, Folder 982; Hall, *William Louis Poteat*, esp. 129–56.

79. McNairy's firing came shortly after his work at Caswell was praised by a number of national experts who convened in Raleigh in May 1925 for the annual meeting of the American Association for the Study of the Feeble-Minded. Charles Davenport was one of the attendees. "Psychiatrists Visit Caswell," *News and Observer*, May 11, 1925; "Score Politics in Institutions," *News and Observer*, May 12, 1925. For an analysis of McNairy's dismissal as indicative of "inherent problems of southern institutions in general," caught between lack of funding and lack of political power, see Noll, *Feeble-Minded in Our Midst*, 56. For the Board's statement on McNairy's firing, see Minutes, Caswell Board of Trustees, July 31, 1925, in Caswell Records, Executive Committee Reports, 1911–32 (bound volume), 387–91.

80. *Report of the Committee on Caswell Training School*; "Dr. Rankin to Help in Caswell Survey," *Greensboro Daily News*, June 23, 1925; Gov. McLean to H. Galt Braxton, August 1, 1925, Tapp-Jenkins Papers (Manuscript Collection #312, East Carolina Special

Collections, Greenville, NC), Folder 312.1e; "Forming Caswell Advisory Board," *Greensboro Record*, July 30, 1925; "Hospital Is Given a Clean Bill After a Board Quiz," *Winston-Salem Journal*, July 23, 1926.

81. "Growing Interest in Feeble-Minded"; "Plan to Abate Feeble Minds," *Greensboro Record*, September 21, 1926; *Caswell Biennial Report, 1925–26*, 29; *Report of the Committee on Caswell Training School*, 19, 31, 26, 29, 35–37.

82. *Report of the Committee on Caswell Training School*, 20, 24. The report also noted that sociological definitions of feeblemindedness produced lower estimates than psychological definitions, and that until the last four or five years, the practice was to use estimates based on psychological definitions. *Report of the Committee on Caswell Training School*, 11–12.

83. *Report of the Committee on Caswell Training School*, 21–23, including quote from Stanley Powell Davies, *Social Control of the Feebleminded: A Study of Social Programs and Attitudes in Relation to the Problems of Mental Deficiency* (National Committee for Mental Hygiene, 1923).

84. *Report of the Committee on Caswell Training School*, 23.

85. *Report of the Committee on Caswell Training School*, 35; NC Public Laws, 1919, chapter 281.

86. *Report of the Committee on Caswell Training School*, 33.

87. Johnson, "State Welfare Program," 774; J. C. Baskervill, "Thinks Sterilization Law Should Be Enforced," *Concord Daily Tribune*, May 6, 1927. On interest in sterilization laws and *Buck v. Bell*, see Reilly, *Surgical Solution*, 67–68, 84–88; Kevles, *In the Name of Eugenics*, 110–12; Dorr, *Segregation's Science*, 127–28. For the national reaction to *Buck v. Bell*, Lombardo, *Three Generations, No Imbeciles*, 174–77.

88. *North Carolina Manual, 1929*, 565; Jake Wade, "Bill Providing for Sterilization Mental Defectives Introduced," *Winston-Salem Journal*, January 22, 1929.

89. Johnson was born and raised in Morganton, and her mother's family had built two antebellum houses there. Although her widowed mother died in 1905, Johnson had at least one cousin who remained in Morganton: Mary Avery, a clubwoman who chaired the Federation of Women's Club's public welfare department in 1927. Years later, after her retirement, Johnson lived with Avery in Raleigh. "Kate Burr Johnson," in William Starr Myers, ed., *Prominent Families of New Jersey*, vol. 1 (Clearfield, 2000), 575; Mary Avery to Johnson, January 21, 1927, BPW Records, Corr. with Associations, Box 28C, Folder: NC Federation of Women's Clubs, 1926–47; Dotty Cameron, "New W. C. Honorary Degree First College Sheepskin for Pioneer Office Holder," *News and Observer*, May 29, 1951; Mollie C. Davis, "Johnson, Kate Ancrum Burr," in Powell, ed., *Dictionary of North Carolina Biography*, vol. 3, 295–96.

90. The 1929 bill allowed sterilization or "asexualization," meaning that castration or ovariectomy was also an option. In naming these two types of operation, the 1929 bill was more explicit than the 1919 law, which used the looser phrasing "any surgical operation." *Senate Journal, 1929*, 43.

91. NC Public Laws 1929, chapter 34, sections 2, 3, and 5. In theory, this proviso left the decision about sterilization to families of noninstitutional residents. In practice, through institutional commitment laws and control over the approval process, state officials retained tools that left them with the final say in the matter.

92. "State Adopts Usable Law for Sterilization of Defectives," *Public Welfare Progress* 10, no. 3 (March 1929): 1. The *Buck v. Bell* decision probably also influenced the bill's

reception, although Millner's bill does not appear to be based on Virginia's statute. Millner's bill did not provide for notification or a hearing process for inmates, which Oliver Wendell Holmes had named as key procedural elements in his majority opinion in *Buck v. Bell.*

93. "Solons Occupy Center of Stage," *Warren Record,* February 1, 1929. The committee amended the bill to include more "safeguards." *Senate Journal, 1929,* 93; "Senate Favors Sterilization." On the subsequent debate, see also "Sterilization of Defectives Urged in Bill," *Greensboro Record,* February 7, 1929. On the bill's final passage in the Senate, see "Sterilizing Bill Passes in Senate," *News and Observer,* February 9, 1929; and "Senate Tables Police Pension Bill by 24 to 20," *Greensboro Record,* February 8, 1929.

94. Charles O'Hagan Laughinghouse, the state health officer, and Dr. Campbell, head of the State Hospital for the Insane at Morganton, had appeared before the Committee on Public Welfare. The state welfare board had also endorsed the bill. "Senate Favors Sterilization"; "Legislature Passes Sterilization Bill," *Marshall News-Record,* March 8, 1929.

95. "State Adopts Usable Law for Sterilization of Defectives"; "Senate Favors Sterilization"; *Senate Journal, 1929,* 93; *North Carolina Manual, 1929,* 33.

96. "Beasley Opposes Sterilizing Bill," *News and Observer,* February 10, 1929. On Beasley's post–welfare board career, first doing publicity with the International Petroleum Company of San Antonio and then as editor of the *Monroe Journal,* see Kate Burr Johnson to Miss Emma O. Lundberg, May 12, 1921, BPW Records, Commissioner's Office: Correspondence with Children's Bureau, Folder 6: Correspondence, 1919–23, 1926–30; and Beasley to McAlister, May 10, 1932, McAlister Papers, Folder 31: Roland F Beasley.

97. "Millner Sterilizing Act Passed by House on Its Final Reading," *Greensboro Daily News,* February 17, 1929; "Curb on Mental Defectives Now Provided by Law," *News and Observer,* February 17, 1929; "Sterilization Bill Is Enacted into Law when House Votes Favorably," *Goldsboro News,* February 17, 1929.

98. NC Public Laws, 1929, chapter 34. By the ERO's tally, North Carolina became the twenty-fourth state to have a sterilization law. "The North Carolina Sterilization Law," *Eugenical News* 15, no. 4 (April 1930): 57–59.

99. "The North Carolina Sterilization Law." One of the arguments against the 1924 Virginia law was that because the bill applied only to people in institutions, it did not pass the equal protection test—an argument that Holmes acknowledged in his *Buck v. Bell* ruling but ultimately rejected. In that sense, Millner's further-reaching bill may have satisfied some critics of the Virginia law. Lombardo, *Three Generations, No Imbeciles,* 167–70.

Chapter 6

1. For other discussions of the case, see Schoen, *Choice and Coercion,* 81–82; Brightman, Lenning, and McElrath, "State-Directed Sterilizations," 476, 478; Brophy and Troutman, "Eugenics Movement in North Carolina," 1920.

2. North Carolina was also spared weather-related catastrophes. Badger, *North Carolina and the New Deal,* 1–3; Abrams, *Conservative Constraints,* 3–5; Powell, *North Carolina Through Four Centuries,* 486; Tindall, *Emergence of the New South,* 354–90, 473–91.

3. Just under $17,500 went from the Emergency Fund to the BCPW for administrative purposes. The other major state-funded assistance took the form of institutions such as Caswell and mental hospitals. Abrams, *Conservative Constraints,* 10; *BCPW Report,*

1930–32, 8, 13, 52; Kirk, Cutler, and Morse, eds., *Emergency Relief in North Carolina*, 22–23; Powell, *North Carolina Through Four Centuries*, 489; *BCPW Report, 1928–30*, 9.

4. *BCPW Report, 1924–26*, 10; *BCPW Report, 1930–32*, 10, 12–13, 63, 76, 85; NC Public Laws 1929, chapter 34.

5. Like the previous educational campaigns, these campaigns drew from and were noted by national eugenics organizations. For example, *Public Welfare Progress* quoted well-known eugenicist Frank Lorimer, and the National Committee for Mental Hygiene praised a special issue on mental hygiene for its "excellence and instructiveness." See "State Adopts Usable Law for Sterilization of Defectives," *Public Welfare Progress* 10, no. 3 (March 1929): 1; for NCMH, see R. Eugene Brown, "Sterilization Law Is Being Used"; "Feeblemindedness"; and "Eugenics and Social Work," all in *Public Welfare Progress* 11, no. 4 (April 1930): 5–6; *BCPW Report, 1928–30*, 19.

6. "State Adopts Usable Law for Sterilization of Defectives"; "Eugenics and Social Work," *Public Welfare Progress* 10, no. 4 (April 1929): 6; "Dr. Harry Crane Takes Issue with Former President Medical Society on Sterilization," *News and Observer*, May 26, 1929; Johnson to heads of institutions, June 22, 1929, BPW Records, Commissioner's Office: Circular Letters, Box 173, Folder: Circular Letters, n.d., 1913–33.

7. In June 1930 the circulation of *Public Welfare Progress* was 4,000, with special issues sent to 4,500. In the next few years, the state continued to stress education about mental defects and sterilization at its public welfare institutes and publications. For Royster's presentation, see "Dr. Royster to Talk on Sterilization," *Public Welfare Progress* 10, no. 6 (June 1929): 1; and "Sterilization Is Way of Guiding Evolution," *Public Welfare Progress* 10, no. 7 (July 1929): 3; for circulation info, see *BCPW Report, 1928–30*, 19; for coverage of mental health and hygiene at institutes, see *BCPW Report, 1928–30*, 46; and *BCPW Report, 1930–32*, 79.

8. "$100 Now vs. Thousands for Future Care!" *Public Welfare Progress* 11, no. 1 (January 1930): 2; *BCPW Report, 1930–32*, 22, 26. On the reluctance of county commissioners to pay for operations, see also "The North Carolina Sterilization Law," *Eugenical News* 15, no. 4 (April 1930): 57–59.

9. Brown, "Sterilization Law Is Being Used"; "Welfare Workers Consider Sterilization of Patients," *Winston-Salem Journal*, December 8, 1929.

10. One of the men who was castrated was Junius Wilson, a deaf Black man who was institutionalized for over seven decades. See Burch and Joyner, *Unspeakable*. My analysis of sterilizations is derived from several sets of statistics that refer to different time periods, each with slightly different information. For the program's first year, see Brown, "Sterilization Law Is Being Used." For a report up to June 1932 that includes petitions denied, see *BCPW Report, 1930–32*, 76. For two later reports that do *not* separate the data at the establishment of the Eugenics Board in February 1933, see Brown, *Eugenical Sterilization in North Carolina* (1935), 13, 16–20; and *First Biennial Report of the Eugenics Board, 1934–36*. See also R. Eugene Brown, "Nature Thwarted by Civilization," *News and Observer*, October 29, 1933. It is also worth noting that other sterilizations likely happened that were not recorded in the Board's records. For example, see the discrepancy between numbers in *BCPW Report, 1930–32*, 76; and Royster, "An Account of the Surgical Service in the State Hospital for the Insane at Raleigh, 1922–32," *Southern Medicine and Surgery* 95 (April 1933): 319–21.

11. "Welfare Workers Consider Sterilization of Patients," *Winston-Salem Journal*, December 8, 1929; "Let's Use the Law," *Public Welfare Progress* 10, no. 11 (November 1929): 1.

On similar depictions of white mountain families in Virginia, see Catte, *Pure America*, 111–46; on reformers' views of Appalachians, see Irvine, "Reclaiming Appalachia."

12. "Welfare Workers Consider Sterilization of Patients"; "Let's Use the Law." No record exists of whether this couple were sterilized or their children were removed from their custody. Sometime between 1929 and 1932 one woman from Buncombe County and one woman from the Rutherford County home were sterilized. There was also a sterilization operation approved but not reported as completed for a person from Burke County. The husband or wife in Dosher's case may have been among these three cases from mountain counties. *BCPW Report, 1930–32*, 76. Dosher had first entered social work as a student at UNC's School of Public Welfare in the 1920s, and she joined the state board as field agent for Mothers' Aid in July 1927. She went on to direct the Division of County Organization and served as a district relief supervisor under FERA. See Kate Burr Johnson to Howard Odum, March 22, 1928, LSRM Records, Series 3, Box 75, Folder 787: UNC-State Board of Charities 1927–28; *BCPW Report, 1926–28*, 16; *BCPW Report, 1930–32*, 4; *BCPW Report, 1932–34*, 14; *BCPW Report, 1934–36*, 12.

13. My account of the Samarcand case draws in particular on Cahn, *Sexual Reckonings*. See also Zipf, *Bad Girls at Samarcand*; Bickford, *Southern Mercy*; Leidholdt, *Battling Nell*.

14. For descriptions of Samarcand in the 1920s and early 1930s, see Cahn, *Sexual Reckonings*, esp. 47–48; Zipf, *Bad Girls at Samarcand*, 44–62.

15. Leidholdt, *Battling Nell*, 164, quoting article in *News and Observer*, November 20, 1926; Zipf, *Bad Girls at Samarcand*, 138, 143–44.

16. McNeill to Nell Battle Lewis, April 30, 1931, Nell Battle Lewis Papers (PC #255 at State Archives of North Carolina, Raleigh; hereafter Lewis Papers), Correspondence 1931–39, Folder: Correspondence—1931; "Firemen and Policy Needed to Subdue Riot Staged by Lumberton Girl Prisoners," *Greensboro Daily News*, April 16, 1931; Bess Davenport Thompson, "Twelve Samarcand Girls Get State Prison Terms," *News and Observer*, May 21, 1931; Zipf, *Bad Girls at Samarcand*, 107, 120–22; Cahn, *Sexual Reckonings*, 48.

17. Nell Battle Lewis to Kate Burr Johnson, May 26, 1931, Lewis Papers, Correspondence 1931–39, Folder: Correspondence—1931; Nell Battle Lewis, "Samarcand Not Different from World of Humanity," *News and Observer*, November 20, 1926. For Lewis's political views, including pro-labor and anti–death penalty views, see Leidholdt, *Battling Nell*.

18. Mrs. Thomas E. Williams to Nell Battle Lewis, March 24, 1931, Lewis Papers, Correspondence 1931–39, Folder: Correspondence—1931. During the trial Lewis formally represented only Virginia Hayes, but she took on the defense arguments for all the girls. On the roles of defense attorneys Lewis, George McNeil, and special counsel W. R. Clegg, see Nell Battle Lewis to George W. McNeill, April 24, 1931, Lewis Papers, Correspondence 1931–39, Folder: Correspondence—1931; and Thompson, "Twelve Samarcand Girls Get State Prison Terms."

19. Lewis to Mr. George W. McNeill, April 24, 1931, and Lewis to Mr. David C. Sinclair Jr., April 29, 1931, both in Lewis Papers, Correspondence 1931–39, Folder: Correspondence—1931; Bess Davenport Thompson, "Defense Holds Samarcand Girls Victims State Neglect," *News and Observer*, May 20, 1931; Thompson, "Twelve Samarcand Girls Get State Prison Terms"; *BCPW Report 1930–32*, 77–78; Zipf, *Bad Girls at Samarcand*, 108, 133, 140.

20. Lewis to David C. Sinclair, April 29, 1931, and Lewis to Kate Burr Johnson, May 26, 1931, both in Lewis Papers, Correspondence 1931–39, Folder: Correspondence—1931; Thompson, "Defense Holds Samarcand Girls Victims State Neglect"; Thompson, "Twelve

Samarcand Girls Get State Prison Terms." For more on the fire, the staff's investigation, and conditions at Samarcand, see Zipf, *Bad Girls at Samarcand*, 109–11; Leidholdt, *Battling Nell*, 164, 166.

21. The court-appointed defense lawyer McNeill agreed with Lewis about their mental capacity. Lewis to Harry Crane, April 25, 1931; Crane to Lewis, April 28, 1931; Lewis to Crane, April 29, 1931; Crane to Lewis, April 30, 1931; and McNeill to NBL, April 30, 1931, all in Lewis Papers, Correspondence 1931–39, Folder: Correspondence—1931; Thompson, "Defense Holds Samarcand Girls Victims State Neglect."

22. Two of the girls' cases were nol-prossed, and two were given suspended sentences. Thompson, "Defense Holds Samarcand Girls Victims State Neglect"; Thompson, "Twelve Samarcand Girls Get State Prison Terms."

23. "The Samarcand Fire," *Greensboro Record*, March 18, 1931; "What's the Trouble," *Greensboro Record*, April 17, 1931; "Our Reform System," *Greensboro Daily News*, April 25, 1931 (reprinted from *Wilmington Star*); Thompson, "Defense Holds Samarcand Girls Victims State Neglect"; Lewis to Mrs. Janie Carlyle Hargroves, Lumberton, April 29, 1931, and Lewis to Rev. H. L. Canfield, May 24, 1931, both in Lewis Papers, Correspondence 1931–39, Folder: Correspondence—1931. For analysis of the girls' public image in the context of appropriate Southern womanhood, see Cahn, *Sexual Reckonings*, 44, 48–52; and Zipf, *Bad Girls at Samarcand*, 87–130.

24. "12 Young Girls from Samarcand Are Given Terms in State Prison," *Greensboro Daily News*, May 21, 1931; Thompson, "Twelve Samarcand Girls Get State Prison Terms"; "Needs Looking Into," *Greensboro Daily News*, May 22, 1931.

25. See table III and table VIII, which together indicate that at least two ovariectomy operations were performed at Samarcand in 1930, in Brown, *Eugenical Sterilization in North Carolina* (1935), 17, 20. On Robson, see Brown, *Eugenical Sterilization in North Carolina* (1935), 18.

26. Cahn, *Sexual Reckonings*, 45. While Zipf (*Bad Girls at Samarcand*) argues that the Samarcand trial was a significant moment in the redefinition of wayward white girls (from redeemable to unfit), I see the shift happening earlier but less completely, given the harsh reaction to Lydia Spruill's behavior in 1919 and the generally sympathetic reaction to the Samarcand girls in 1931.

27. Zipf, *Bad Girls at Samarcand*, 60; Case File of Mrs. W. H. Kimball, Case Records, 16–19, *Brewer v. Valk* Records, NC Supreme Court Records (North Carolina State Archives, Raleigh, NC), 33S-363 (hereafter *Brewer v. Valk* Records).

28. "Survey of Statutory Changes in North Carolina in 1929," *North Carolina Law Review* 7, no. 4 (June 1929): 392–95; on Wettach's authorship of this article, see Brief of Appellee, *Brewer v. Valk*, Supreme Court of NC, Fall Term 1932, no. 378, renumbered Spring Term, no. 363, 16, *Brewer v. Valk* Records; "The North Carolina Sterilization Law"; "Sterilization Laws," *Eugenical News* 16, no. 8 (August. 1931): 129. For an overview of how the courts treated sterilization laws, see Brophy and Troutman, "Eugenics Movement in North Carolina." See also Haller, *Eugenics*, 130–41. For one version of the ERO's model statute, see Laughlin, *Eugenical Sterilization*, 446–51.

29. NC Public Laws, 1933, chapter 224.

30. Case File of Mrs. W. H. Kimball, Case Records, 16–19, *Brewer v. Valk* Records.

31. "Oldham, Mary," in 1920 US Census, Forsyth County, North Carolina, population schedule, Broadbay Twp. no. 2, page 15B, enumeration district 90, dwelling 294, family 304; *Brewer v. Valk* Records.

32. June Brewer and Mary Oldham, September 20, 1920, Forsyth County, North Carolina, US, Marriage Index, 1741–2004, North Carolina State Archives, Raleigh, North Carolina; "Brewer, Junius A.," in 1920 US Census, Forsyth County, North Carolina, population schedule, Winston Twp., Winston Salem City, Ward 4, page 5A, enumeration district 103, dwelling 72, family 84; Junius Brewer in 1911, 1913, 1915, 1916, and 1921 Winston-Salem City Directories; "Oldham, Mary," 1920 US Census; Case File of Mrs. W. H. Kimball, Case Records, 16–19, *Brewer v. Valk* Records.

33. Testimony of Mary Chalmers and A. W. Cline, Case Records, 11–13, 16, *Brewer v. Valk* Records; Case File of Mrs. W. H. Kimball, Case Records, 16–19, *Brewer v. Valk* Records; *Brewer v. Valk*, 204 NC 378 (1932).

34. Testimony of Mary Chalmers and A. W. Cline, Case Records, 11–13, 15, *Brewer v. Valk* Records; Case File of Mrs. W. H. Kimball, Case Records, 16–19, *Brewer v. Valk* Records; Julian M. Pleasants, "Richard Thurmond Chatham," in Powell, ed., *Dictionary of North Carolina Biography*.

35. Psychological Record, Case Records, 14–15, *Brewer v. Valk* Records; Brief of Appellants, 8, *Brewer v. Valk* Records.

36. Testimony of A. W. Kline, Mrs. Letha Brown, and Mary Chalmers, Case Records, 12–13, 15, *Brewer v. Valk* Records.

37. On W. T. Wilson, see "William Thomas Wilson," in *History of North Carolina*, vol. 5: *North Carolina Biography*, 22. Wilson went on to serve as mayor of Winston-Salem from 1935 to 1939; see City of Winston-Salem, "W. T. Wilson," https://www.cityofws.org/1132/WT-Wilson.

38. This is the block bounded by Main, Liberty, 3rd, and 4th streets. For locations of offices, see Winston-Salem City Directory for 1932, 523–24, 607–9. On Cline's encounters, see Testimony of A. W. Cline, Case Records, 12–13, *Brewer v. Valk* Records.

39. Brief of Appellants, *Brewer v. Valk*, 2, *Brewer v. Valk* Records; Petition for Appointment of Guardian of Mary Brewer, Case Records, 8–9, *Brewer v. Valk* Records; Record of Hearing, April 29, 1932, Forsyth County Superior Court, Case Records, 11–19, *Brewer v. Valk* Records; Notice of Hearing, April 16, 1932, Case Records, 10, *Brewer v. Valk* Records.

40. "Petition for Appointment," filed with Forsyth County Court, May 21, 1932, *Brewer v. Valk* Records; *The Chanticleer, 1928*, 54; Justin Miller to Cale K. Burgess, November 14, 1933, Papers of Dean Justin Miller, 1929–34 (Duke University, David M. Rubenstein Rare Book and Manuscript Library, Deans Papers, School of Law Records, 1914–2010s; hereafter, Miller Papers), Box 1, Folder: B Correspondence, 1931–34.

41. Georgetown Law Library Special Collections, Bradway, John S. (John Saeger), https://aspace.ll.georgetown.edu/public/agents/people/256; Durden, "Rebuilding of Duke University's Law School," 332, 338.

42. On the Human Betterment Foundation, see Kline, *Building a Better Race*; Stern, *Eugenic Nation*; and "USC Removes Name of Rufus von KleinSmid, a Eugenics Leader, from Prominent Building," *Los Angeles Times*, June 11, 2020. For Bradway's civic memberships, see Memorandum [from Bradway] to Dean Miller, September 22, 1933, John S. Bradway Papers (Duke University, David M. Rubenstein Rare Book and Manuscript Library; hereafter, Bradway Papers), Box 32, Folder: Memos to Dean Miller; Bradway to Miller, November 1, 1932, Miller Papers, Folder: Legal Aid Clinic, 1932–34 (1 of 2); "Crane Speaks in Durham," *Daily Tar Heel*, March 3, 1933; "County Expects Juvenile Court," *Daily Tar Heel*, March 3, 1934. On Bradway's later interest in social reform and mental hygiene, see

Bradway Papers, Box 18, Folder: NC Mental Hygiene Society; list of CSS members, 1934–35, Bradway Papers, Box 18, Folder: NC CSS 1; Dr. Richard F. Richie, "Summary of Mental Hygiene Development in North Carolina," talk at meeting of Charlotte Mental Hygiene Clinic Board on October 16, 1940, NC Conference for Social Service, BPW Records, Subject Files: NC CSS, Box 169, Folder: n.d., 1913–33; Bradway, "Legality of Human Sterilization."

43. Bradway reported conflicting numbers, but the higher tallies include many cases the clinic turned away because the clients were not eligible. Durden, "Rebuilding of Duke University's Law School," 343–44; John M. Lindsey, "Introduction," in John S. Bradway, "Duke University Legal Aid Materials," ii, vi–x, John Saeger Bradway Collection, (Coll. 32), National Equal Justice Library Collection, Georgetown Law Library; Memorandum [from Bradway] to Dean Miller, September 27, 1933, and Memorandum [from Bradway] to Dean Miller, January 17, 1934, both in Bradway Papers, Box 32, Folder: Memos to Dean Miller; Bradway to Miller, May 15, 1932, Bradway to Miller, September 24, 1932, and Legal Aid Clinic *News Letter* 2, No. 3, February 1, 1933, all in Miller Papers, Folder: Legal Clinic, 1932–34 (1 of 2); Bradway memo to faculty, February 1, 1933, Bradway to Miller, March 29, 1933, and Minutes, staff meeting, April 28, 1933, all in Miller Papers, Folder: Legal Clinic, 1932–34 (2 of 2).

44. On Bradway, see finding aid for John S. Bradway Papers, http://library.duke.edu/rubenstein/findingaids/uabradjs/. On Hutchins as Forsyth County attorney in 1932, see "Secret Inquest Gets Approval from Judge," *Greensboro Daily News*, July 9, 1932. On Hutchins's career, see Hubbell, *Hubbell's Legal Directory for Lawyers and Businessmen*, 369. On Hutchins's correspondence with Bradway, see C. A. Walker to Bradway, November 12, 1929, Bradway Papers, Red Volume 42, Section 3; "Hutchins Put on Committee," *Winston-Salem Journal*, December 15, 1929.

45. The supreme court opinion quoted Brewer's October 1932 complaint to the effect that Wilson's request for sterilization was *also* on April 29, 1932, but they were mistaken about the date. Other records indicate clearly that Wilson made this request to the commissioners, but a brief by the appellant (Valk et al.) said that Wilson made the request to the commissioners on August 1, 1932. See *Brewer v. Valk*; Brief of Appellants, 3–4; Petition, August 1, 1932, Case Records, 22–23; Resolution of Board of County Commissioners, August 1, 1932, Case Records, 24; W. T. Wilson, [Sterilization] Order to Dr. A. Valk, August 2, 1932, Case Records, 25–26, all in *Brewer v. Valk* Records.

46. Since the court had ruled that Brewer was not competent to represent herself, in legal filings after April 29, Hester had Lucy Oldham (as "next friend") represent her "incompetent" daughter. This created a situation of some irony, since Brewer had at least some schooling and could read and write, while Oldham was illiterate.

47. See *Brewer v. Valk*; Brief of Appellee, *Brewer v. Valk* Records. In this sense, Brewer's plea challenged procedural due process rather than substantive due process. Thanks to Jedediah Purdy for alerting me to this distinction.

48. Judge A. M. Stack signed a temporary injunction on October 6, 2013, followed by a hearing and a permanent injunction two days later. *Brewer v. Valk* Records.

49. Lawyers for both sides had filed briefs with the state supreme court within two weeks after the injunction. After the preliminary injunction was issued on October 6, 1932, the defendants waived their right to a ten-day period in which they could show cause why the restraining order should not become permanent and voluntarily appeared for a hearing

on the morning of October 8, 1932. At that hearing, the injunction was made permanent and the defendants were "forever enjoined from sterilizing the said Mary Brewer" or performing "any operation ... which might impair her procreative organs." Lawyers for Wilson and Valk filed their intent to appeal with the supreme court only two days later, on October 10, and filed their brief on October 14. Lawyers for the appellee filed their brief on October 19, 1932; Brief of Appellee and Brief of Appellants, *Brewer v. Valk* Records.

50. Bulletins of Duke University School of Law, 1930–36; "A Friendly Favor," *Time*, July 24, 1950, 14; Bradway memo to faculty, February 1, 1933, Miller Papers, Folder: Legal Clinic, 1932–34 (2 of 2).

51. The brief, a response to a supreme court justice's question during oral arguments, argued that Oldham had standing to file a suit on Brewer's behalf against Wilson, the court-appointed guardian. Supplemental Brief joined in by counsel for appellee and counsel for appellant, *Brewer v. Valk* Records. This was not the only time that year Bradway's students argued both sides of a case. In another case regarding landownership, the chief justice of the state supreme court asked Bradway for help, and Bradway assigned Lassiter and one other student to write amicus briefs for each side of the case. John Bradway to Justin Miller, October 1, 1932, Miller Papers, Folder: Legal Aid Clinic, 1932–34 (1 of 2).

52. In doing so, they referred to the US Supreme Court decision in *Buck v. Bell*, which rested in part on Virginia's "very careful provisions" to protect "the patients from possible abuse," and judged that North Carolina's law fell short in this regard since it "makes no provision for notice and hearing." *Brewer v. Valk*.

53. The court sided with the appellant-defendants in saying that sterilization fell within the realm of police powers of the state, rather than the appellee-plaintiff's claim (made almost in passing) that sterilization would cause "irreparable physical and mental hurt and loss." Thus, the decision supported the appellant-defendants' argument that the law did not violate substantive due process, while ruling with the appellee-plaintiff that the law was unconstitutional on procedural due process grounds. *Brewer v. Valk*.

54. Bradway mentioned "Mr. Brown's invitation" to "prepare an amendment and urge it upon the committee," presumably referring to R. Eugene Brown, the assistant to the commissioner of public welfare and the director of the Division of Institutions. Brown would go on to be secretary of the Eugenics Board. John S. Bradway to Robert H. Wettach, February 24, 1933, in "Documents Concerning Amendments of N.C. Public Laws of 1929, Chapter 34: Sterilization of Persons Mentally Defective," Law Library Rare Books, University of North Carolina at Chapel Hill.

55. "Suggestions in Re Sterilization Bill"; John S. Bradway to Robert H. Wettach, February 13, 1933; and John S. Bradway to Robert H. Wettach, February 24, 1933, all in "Documents Concerning Amendments."

56. "Report of Sub-Committee No. 4 of Mental Examinations and Sterilization of the Social Code Committee of the North Carolina Conference for Social Service," [n.d.]; and copy of HB 675 in John S. Bradway to Robert H. Wettach, February 24, 1933, both in "Documents Concerning Amendments"; 1933 HB 675, Session Records, 1933; *House Journal, 1933*, 258.

57. Bradway noted that R. Eugene Brown had invited them to prepare an amendment to Thompson's bill. John S. Bradway to Robert H. Wettach, February 24, 1933, "Documents Concerning Amendments"; drafts of bill in "Documents Concerning Amendments"; Brown, *Eugenical Sterilization in North Carolina* (1935), 8.

58. HB 1013, Session Records, 1933. The text is virtually identical to the edited sixth revision of Bradway's bill in "Documents Concerning Amendments."

59. *House Journal, 1933,* 274, 295, 446, 494, 513, 580; *Senate Journal, 1933,* 228, 370, 384, 405, 427, 446, 459.

60. NC Public Laws, 1933, chapter 224, esp. sections 4 and 20. For analysis of the procedural protections in the 1933 law in the context of *Buck v. Bell* and other case law, see Brophy and Troutman, "Eugenics Movement in North Carolina."

61. Brown, *Eugenical Sterilization in North Carolina* (1935), 8.

62. See "Voluntary Eugenical Sterilization: A Draft of a Model Statute for Regulating the Voluntary Sexual Sterilization of Certain Natural Classes," *Eugenical News* 16, no. 4 (April 1931): 54–56. Dorr notes similar patterns in Virginia's 1924 sterilization law, designed by Aubrey Strode, which "allowed lawmakers to act on the commonsense wisdom of the stockyard and the ledger book, as well as the esoteric laws of the genetics laboratory. Strode's language familiarized lay legislators with the normal science of the day." Dorr, *Segregation's Science*, 128.

63. R. Eugene Brown to Bradway, July 25, 1933; Bradway to Brown, September 20, 1933; Bradway to Brown, September 22, 1933, all in Bradway Papers, Box 34, Folder: Misc. 1933–35; Bradway to E. S. Gosney, October 23, 1933; Bradway to Paul N. [Popenoe], October 12, 1933; Bradway to Hon. Clark N. Higbee, October 18, 1933; Bradway to Brown, December 4, 1933; and Bradway to Brown, January 13, 1934, all in Bradway Papers, Box 34, Folder: Sterilization Law, 1933.

64. Brief of Appellants, 8, *Brewer v. Valk* Records. I have searched US Census records for 1940 for all members of the family, as well as city directories in Winston-Salem, 1932–36, for all members of the family. I can find no record of a death certificate for Mary or June Brewer in North Carolina or adjacent states. Their son was at Jackson Training School; see "Brewer, Junius," in 1940 US Census, Cabarrus County, North Carolina, population schedule, Township 11, Baptist Church, Stonewall Jackson Training School for Boys, page 5A, enumeration district 13–28. For Samarcand sterilization totals, see *Biennial Report of the Eugenics Board of North Carolina, 1938–40,* 17.

65. On *Buck v. Bell* as an inside job, see Lombardo, *Three Generations, No Imbeciles.*

66. Although I have not found evidence to this effect, some of the lawyers in the case may have also been involved in contemporary legal efforts, led by the ACLU and the NAACP, to challenge narrow readings of the Fourteenth Amendment and extend the federal Bill of Rights to local and state cases. Brewer's initial plea and the supreme court decision cited both the Fourteenth Amendment to the US Constitution and Section 1, Article 17, of the North Carolina Constitution. Thanks to Laura F. Edwards for making me aware of this context. For examples of citations of *Brewer* on due process, see petitioner's reply brief in *David Hyun v. Herman R. Landon District Director, Immigration and Naturalization Service,* 1956 (WL 88916, US Appellate Brief, Supreme Court of US; no. 201, October Term, 1955, March 15, 1956); and *Robert King, Ann King, Margaret Shaley, and A. William King v. Pender County, Marianne Orr, and Robert Orr,* 2013 (WL 3358996, NC Appeals, no. COA 13–618. June 25, 2013).

Chapter 7

1. Case 19, in Benson, "Sterilization," 47–49. Benson used case records of Orange County welfare officials to describe twenty-one sterilization cases, some involving entire families.

He does not give dates for Pearl's case, but the cases for which he provides details took place between 1933 and 1936.

2. *BCPW Report, 1932–34*, 7.

3. A. Laurance Aydlett, "More Than Six Million Dollars Is Spent on Government Programs of Assistance Last Year," *Public Welfare News* 1, no. 12 (September 1939): 1–3; "Yelton Explains Public Assistance Outlook for North Carolina During Next Two Years" [text of a radio address over WPTF, February 28, 1939], *Public Welfare News* 1, no. 6 (March 1939): 1.

4. Tindall, *Emergence of the New South*, 488.

5. In 1929, total state expenditures were $555 million; in 1942 they were $1.1 billion; and in 1948 they were $2.3 billion. Revenues came from federal contributions but also from increased taxes, particularly state sales taxes on commodities. Tindall, *Emergence of the New South*, 490.

6. On the tension between federal ideals for New Deal programs and local politics, see Tani, *States of Dependency*.

7. R. Eugene Brown, unknown publication, quoted in Benson, "Sterilization," 89.

8. Bost's roles included president of a parent-teacher association, trustee of the North Carolina College for Women, and membership on executive councils of the League of Women Voters and the Raleigh Community Chest. She also fostered connections with state and national social work organizations. Bost's professional memberships included the National Conference for Social Work, the American Public Welfare Association (for which she served on the board of directors), the State Commission for the Blind, the North Carolina Mental Hygiene Society, the Interracial Commission, and the North Carolina Conference for Social Service. Nell Battle Lewis, "Incidentally," *News and Observer*, June 2, 1951; Harriette Hammer Walker, "Mrs. Bost Filling Important Post in State's Improvement," *Charlotte Observer*, October 12, 1930; Harriette Hammer Walker, "Mrs. W. Thomas Bost Is Worthy Successor to Mrs. Kate Burr Johnson as State Public Welfare Commissioner," *Greensboro Daily News*, October 12, 1930; Margarette Wood Smethurst, "Carolina Cavalcade," *News and Observer*, August 2, 1954; "Mrs. W. T. Bost Is Elected to Succeed Mrs. Johnson," *Public Welfare Progress* 11, no. 3 (March 1930): 1, 5; "Mrs. W. T. Bost," *Charlotte Observer*, July 23, 1939; "Welfare Board to Tackle Job of Picking New Chief," *News and Observer*, February 16, 1944; "We're Sorry, Mrs. B., Good Work!" *News and Observer*, February 20, 1944; "Tar Heel Micro-Biographies," *Greensboro Daily News*, December 10, 1944; Thomas S. Morgan, "Annie Kizer Bost," and A. M. Burns, "William Thomas ('Tom') Bost," both in Powell, ed., *Dictionary of North Carolina Biography*.

9. Biles, *South and the New Deal*, 33; Abrams, *Conservative Constraints*, 11; Kirk, Cutler, and Morse, eds., *Emergency Relief*, 23–24. On the decision to create the GOR as a separate agency from the Board of Charities and Public Welfare, and the influence of both the Board's statutory and traditional political independence and a 1930 report on state government by the Brookings Institution, which suggested this change, see Dobelstein, "Public Welfare," 136–40.

10. *BCPW Report, 1926–28*, 16; *BCPW Report, 1930–32*, 4; *BCPW Report, 1932–34*, 14; Kirk, Cutler, and Morse, eds., *Emergency Relief*, 23.

11. The total for 1932–33 was $60,898.60, compared to a total of $102,247.46 for 1928–29, with a state allocation that year of $41,699.72. The following two years saw significant drops in state funding, to $33,631.10 and $30,513.50. There was a slight uptick in 1931–32, as the state fulfilled its promise to the Laura Spelman Rockefeller Memorial to take over funding

of the Division of Work Among Negroes, but in January 1933 the severity of the crisis meant that the state budget bureau faced shortfalls and had to recalculate all state appropriations mid-year. Funds from philanthropic groups, namely the Rosenwald Fund and the Rockefeller Foundation, also fell. *BCPW Report, 1928–30*, 16–17; *BCPW Report, 1930–32*, 10, 13–15, 51; *BCPW Report, 1932–34*, 15, 20, 44; Dobelstein, "Public Welfare," 141.

12. Link, *Paradox of Southern Progressivism*, 372–74, 378–79; Tindall, *Emergence of the New South*, 409–14. On the importance of the AAA for North Carolina, see Abrams, *Conservative Constraints*, 55–81, 254–55; and Badger, *North Carolina and the New Deal*, 13–29.

13. FERA ultimately distributed over $3 billion. Some of the federal funds were supposed to be matched by state funds, but Ehringhaus refused to contribute to unemployment relief. As a result, the federal government covered 94 percent of the cost, with local governments contributing the rest. Tindall, *Emergence of the New South*, 473; Kennedy, *Freedom from Fear*, 170–71; Abrams, *Conservative Constraints*, 116; Badger, *North Carolina and the New Deal*, 47; Federal Works Agency, *Final Statistical Report*, 278–79.

14. Ehringhaus was responding in part to FERA criteria, which required certain standards for state agencies administering FERA funds, but he was also likely driven by political considerations. Kate Burr Johnson had firmly maintained the political independence of the Board of Charities and Public Welfare during her long tenure. Annie Kizer Bost did not have so many strong political connections, but she had shown since her appointment in 1930 that she intended to follow Johnson's precedent. Ehringhaus's decision to put millions of dollars in the hands of a new appointee was in part retaliation against welfare officials' long-standing apolitical stance. On FERA standards and political fights over control of New Deal funds, see Badger, *North Carolina and the New Deal*, 40–44. On politics, see Dobelstein, "Public Welfare," 136–43; Badger, *North Carolina and the New Deal*, 47–48; and Abrams, *Conservative Constraints*. On NC ERA generally, see Link, *Paradox of Southern Progressivism*, 375.

15. O'Berry may have been one of only two women in the country to hold such a position. On O'Berry's presidency of the FWC, 1927–29, see Weathers, *Century to Celebrate*, 33. On survey and on O'Berry's position, see Wilkerson-Freeman, "From Clubs to Parties," 320, 327, 330; Badger, *North Carolina and the New Deal*, 42; Kirk, Cutler, and Morse, eds., *Emergency Relief*, 23; and Link, *Paradox of Southern Progressivism*, 382.

16. Link, *Paradox of Southern Progressivism*, 375; Tindall, *Emergence of the New South*, 473; Badger, *North Carolina and the New Deal*, 40–41. On the limited impact of ERA and CWA relief in North Carolina, given endemic poverty and political pushback, see Badger, *North Carolina and the New Deal*, 44–47; and Abrams, *Conservative Constraints*, 113–60, 254–62. On types of relief nationally (direct cash relief, in-kind relief, and work relief), see Kennedy, *Freedom from Fear*, 172; Federal Works Agency, *Final Statistical Report*, 20–22, 105; Kirk, Cutler, and Morse, eds., *Emergency Relief*, 31; and Abrams, *Conservative Constraints*, 117. On gaps in relief under FERA, see Abrams, *Conservative Constraints*, 125–28. On Crane's rent, see "Crane, Harry W.," in 1930 US Census, Durham County, North Carolina, population schedule, Durham Township, Ward 5, page 2B, enumeration district 32-16, dwelling 41, family 42. For crude estimates of per capita income (these estimates are merely an average of all forms of income spread over the total population, and income inequality was extreme in 1933), see US Bureau of Economic Analysis, Personal income per capita, retrieved from FRED, Federal Reserve Bank of St. Louis, https://fred.stlouisfed.org/series/A792RC0Q052SBEA; Saez and Zucman, "Wealth Inequality." Thanks to Adams Bailey for his help with this data.

17. In 1933–34, the Board reported spending state funds of $27,170 on staff and administration, plus $32,310 in relief for dependent children and Mothers' Aid. Meanwhile, NC ERA spent $19.7 million that year, including $13.3 million in direct relief. Badger paints the Board of Charities and Public Welfare as obstinate in its desire to maintain the county-unit system despite the federal government's belief that it was "basically inadequate." Badger sees the welfare board as part of the "forces of localism," backed by Odum, who were "too entrenched to be displaced." Badger, *North Carolina and the New Deal*, 48.

18. In the fall of 1934, to save funds and increase efficiency, the ERA consolidated its work into thirty-one districts. Kirk, Cutler, and Morse, eds., *Emergency Relief*, 23, 29.

19. *BCPW Report, 1932–34*, 49–50; "Over Hundred at Welfare School," *News and Observer*, June 22, 1933; Kirk, Cutler, and Morse, eds., *Emergency Relief*, 25; *BCPW Report, 1930–32*, 57. In 1934, the institute apparently returned to its former length. *BCPW Report, 1932–34*, 12–13.

20. O'Berry's refusal to indulge in patronage politics had antagonized state Democratic leaders. Unlike the ERA, the WPA was a federal agency, and the power of appointments shifted to congressional leaders rather than the governor. Badger, *North Carolina and the New Deal*, 42–44, 48; Abrams, *Conservative Constraints*, 124–25, 131–36.

21. More people, however, remained jobless—by one estimate 53,000 cases, who still depended primarily on local funds now that assistance for direct relief had dried up. Abrams, *Conservative Constraints*, 137–38, 142.

22. *BCPW Report, 1934–36*, 8–9, 17, 19, 115–16; Aydlett, "North Carolina State Board of Public Welfare," 26; Abrams, *Conservative Constraints*, 146; *BCPW Report, 1936–38*, 7–8.

23. Aydlett, "North Carolina State Board of Public Welfare," 26. On the ways North Carolina's resistance to change "limited the New Deal," see Abrams, *Conservative Constraints*, 153–54, 254–62.

24. It was not at first clear that the welfare board would have control of OAA; the Labor Department was also an option. See "Real Pensions Measure Pends," *Greensboro Record*, January 16, 1937. For the laws establishing the Social Security infrastructure, see NC Public Laws 1937, chapters 135, 288, 295, 319, and 436.

25. North Carolina's payments under these Social Security programs were relatively low because of the state's low investment. State and county governments had to come up with half of OAA funds and two-thirds of ADC funds, while the federal government provided the rest. As a result, in OAA payments, North Carolina ranked thirty-ninth among the states, and on ADC payments, forty-third. Aydlett, "North Carolina State Board of Public Welfare," 27–28; Abrams, *Conservative Constraints*, 156–57; *BCPW Report, 1936–38*, 88.

26. On challenges to the Board's independence in 1937, including a copy of the proposed legislation, see correspondence between Brown and McAlister, McAlister Papers, Folder 59. For the final version of the bills, see NC Public Laws 1937, chapter 288, section 2, and chapter 319, sections 2 and 5; and Aydlett, "North Carolina State Board of Public Welfare," 27.

27. Ultimately, North Carolina's per capita relief amounts, including both direct payments and WPA spending, remained near the bottom of the nation. *BCPW Report, 1934–36*, 7–9, 12, 19; Aydlett, "North Carolina State Board of Public Welfare," 28; *BCPW Report, 1936–38*, 7–8, 88, 163; Bost to McAlister, August 29, 1936, BPW Records, State Board Corr., Box 3, Folder: 1932–36; Abrams, *Conservative Constraints*, 156–57; Badger, *North Carolina and the New Deal*, 47.

28. Abrams, *Conservative Constraints*, 161–89; Tindall, *Emergence of the New South*, 540–74. On developments in public health during the New Deal that maintained racial segregation, see Thomas, *Deluxe Jim Crow*.

29. Oxley also fielded many requests from other states about how North Carolina was handling Black poverty. *BCPW Report, 1928–30*, 93–94; *BCPW Report, 1930–32*, 10, 98, 101–2; *BCPW Report, 1932–34*, 87.

30. *BCPW Report, 1930–32*, 10, 98–102. Oxley resigned in 1934 and was replaced by William Randolph Johnson, an experienced social worker. "Johnson Named to Charities Board," *Watauga Democrat*, April 5, 1934.

31. Federal funds went directly to child welfare, the Division of Mental Hygiene, and the Division of Institutions and Corrections. *BCPW Report, 1934–36*, 27; *BCPW Report, 1938–40*, 20, 173–74, 179–81.

32. Abrams, *Conservative Constraints*, 156–57, 175; US Census Bureau, *1940 Census of the Population*, vol. 2: *Characteristics of the Population*, part 5, 266 (table 4). On the adverse effects of the New Deal for African Americans in North Carolina, see Abrams, *Conservative Constraints*, 161–89.

33. The division was renamed "Mental Hygiene" between 1932 and 1934. *BCPW Report, 1930–32*, 84; *BCPW Report, 1932–34*, 78–80; *BCPW Report, 1934–36*, 95, 97–99, 102; North Carolina Commission for the Study of the Care of the Insane and Mental Defectives, *Study of Mental Health in North Carolina*, 70–72, 253–56; "Dr. J. Wallace Nygard Resigns from Mental Hygiene Division to Take Up Work with U.S. Justice Department," *Public Welfare News* 2, no. 1 (October 1939): 3–4; "Scout Leaders Meet in Seminar First of Month," *Daily Tar Heel*, November 9, 1932; "Crane Speaks in Durham," *Daily Tar Heel*, March 3, 1933; "Psychologist Returns from Inspection Tour," *Daily Tar Heel*, October 21, 1933; "Psychology Professor to Speak in Charlotte," *Daily Tar Heel*, November 9, 1934; "New Society Picks Groves as President," *Daily Tar Heel*, January 24, 1937.

34. The Eugenics Board was not part of the Board of Charities and Public Welfare by statute. Rather, as Bost wrote in 1936, "it so happened" that because R. Eugene Brown was its executive secretary, the Eugenics Board's work was carried out in the welfare office he led, the Division of Institutions and Corrections. *BCPW Report, 1934–36*, 12; NC Public Laws 1933, chapter 224.

35. R. Eugene Brown, "Nature Thwarted by Civilization," *News and Observer*, October 29, 1933; Brown, *Eugenical Sterilization in North Carolina* (1938).

36. North Carolina Commission for the Study of the Care of the Insane and Mental Defectives, *Study of Mental Health in North Carolina*, 335–36; "State Department Offices Take Most of Fifth Floor of Latest Addition to Capitol Buildings," *Public Welfare News* 1, no. 3 (December 1938): 4; *BCPW Report, 1934–36*, 102–3; "Eighteen Months of Operation of Public Assistance Program Show Eligibles Above Estimate," *Public Welfare News* 1, no. 4 (January 1939): 1. On the number of entries, see *BCPW Report, 1922–24*, 139; *BCPW Report, 1924–26*, 89; *BCPW Report, 1926–28*, 86–87; *BCPW Report, 1928–30*, 82; *BCPW Report, 1930–32*, 85; *BCPW Report, 1932–34*, 78; *BCPW Report, 1934–36*, 102–3; *BCPW Report, 1936–38*, 119–20.

37. The 1937 Social Security legislation made appointment of a county welfare superintendent the job of the thirty-member county welfare board, but the state board still had the power to approve or deny the appointment. They set minimum qualifications, including a bachelor's degree, a year at a school of social work, and a minimum of one year's

experience in social work. Still, they were plagued by the challenge of "securing qualified workers." With similar standards in place in 1936, the state's chapter of the American Association of Social Workers had only thirty-nine members, only twenty-four of whom were actively engaged in social work. The lack of qualified workers was of consistent concern to federal agencies. On association membership, see North Carolina Commission for the Study of the Care of the Insane and Mental Defectives, *Study of Mental Health in North Carolina*, 318; on 1936 standards, see *BCPW Report, 1934-36*, 19; on 1938 standards, see *BCPW Report, 1936-38*, 163; on concerns about qualified workers, see Badger, *North Carolina and the New Deal*, 47-48.

38. Almost all the others received training at another institution in the Southeast, such as Tulane University or the Atlanta University School of Social Work. Calculations here are based on Tillinghast, "Statistical Study," 29, table 15, "Distribution of Social Workers in NC County Departments of Public Welfare, by Class of Positions and School of Social Work Attended, November 1941."

39. "State Welfare Commissioner Reviews Some of Activities of Department During Year 1938," *Public Welfare News* 1, no. 3 (December 1938): 2; *BCPW Report 1934-36*, 19, 115; "Miss Cassatt Will Conduct Series of One-Day Training Institutes," *Public Welfare News* 1, no. 4 (January 1939): 2; *BCPW Report, 1936-38*, 19-20.

40. *Biennial Report of the Eugenics Board, 1934-36*, 9.

41. Brown headed UNC's public welfare program from 1936 to 1945. For course titles and information, see syllabi in Folder 8, Roy M. Brown Papers, 1924-56 (Collection #3883), Southern Historical Collection, Wilson Library, University of North Carolina at Chapel Hill; "Don't Look Now," *Daily Tar Heel*, December 11, 1936; "The Graduate School: Division of Public Welfare and Social Work," *University of North Carolina Record*, no. 332 (April 1938): 22; and "The Graduate School," *University of North Carolina Record*, no. 318 (March 1937): 148, both in the North Carolina Collection, Wilson Library, UNC–Chapel Hill.

42. Some changes were required to comply with ADC regulations, notably that use of the fund become mandatory for every county; that the residence requirement be shortened from three years to one; that the maximum age be raised from fourteen to sixteen; and that close relatives besides mothers must be eligible. The scale of the program also changed significantly. In the last year of Mothers' Aid, the state spent about $30,000, and in the first year of ADC, over $800,000 in relief funds went to over 22,000 children, with a usual grant of ten to sixteen dollars per family per month. *BCPW Report, 1934-36*, 37; *BCPW Report, 1936-38*, 13, 48-50, 70. On the CCC, see *BCPW Report, 1936-38*, 197-201.

43. *BCPW Report 1934-36*, 115; *BCPW Report, 1936-38*, 7. On the renewed focus on families during the Depression, see Kline, *Building a Better Race*, 95-123. On "paupers," see *BCPW Report, 1936-38*, 110. On ADC families being discontinued for not cooperating, see *BCPW Report, 1936-38*, 50. On denial rates, see *Public Assistance Statistics*, vol. 2, 1937-38, 16-21.

44. On interactions between families and social workers, see *BCPW report, 1934-36*, 116; Hopkins, *Spending to Save*, 101-2, quoted in Kennedy, *Freedom from Fear*, 174; Hoke, "Politics of Fertility," 27-29; Schoen, *Choice and Coercion*. On cases referred, see *BCPW Report, 1932-34*, 82-83. On the desire for traveling clinics, see North Carolina Commission for the Study of the Care of the Insane and Mental Defectives, *Study of Mental Health in North Carolina*, 367.

45. Tillinghast, "Statistical Study," 41, table 22, "Distribution of Social Workers in NC County Departments of Public Welfare, by Class of Positions and Salary, November 1941." On social workers' class status and identity in Northern urban environments, see Walkowitz, *Working with Class*.

46. This figure is based on reports that from mid-1934 to mid-1940, operations were performed for an average of just over 85 percent of all approved petitions, and that a mean of 150 operations were performed each year between 1935 and 1940. There were only four operations performed in 1933, since the Eugenics Board met for the first time in October 1933. The number of operations performed soon jumped, with 61 in 1934 and 178 in 1935. *Biennial Report of the Eugenics Board, 1942–44*, 9–10. For a comprehensive analysis of factors influencing the Eugenics Board's review of sterilization cases over four decades, see Schoen, *Choice and Coercion*, 75–103.

47. The Eugenics Board kept track of only "negro" and "white" racial categories. Calculations are based on statistics published in *Biennial Report of the Eugenics Board, 1942–44*, 9–10. Other reports in this time period indicate similar demographic patterns. See, for example, *Biennial Report of the Eugenics Board, 1938–40*, 16–18. For overviews of sterilization under the Eugenics Board, see Schoen, *Choice and Coercion*, 75–138; Hoke, "Politics of Fertility."

48. Although most Eugenics Boards records are restricted, the state has published at least one redacted example of minutes. See Eugenics Board Minutes, October 25, 1950, https://www.doa.nc.gov/jsv/ojsv-5252011-dncr-handout-b-pdf/open.

49. Calculations based on data in *Biennial Report of the Eugenics Board, 1942–44*, 9.

50. These sterilizations were listed as noninstitutional cases in Eugenics Board Reports. See Brown, *Eugenical Sterilization in North Carolina* (1935), 18.

51. North Carolina Commission for the Study of the Care of the Insane and Mental Defectives, *Study of Mental Health in North Carolina*, 302; Brown, *Eugenical Sterilization in North Carolina* (1935), 12.

52. In 1934–38, 211 Raleigh inmates were sterilized, compared to Royster's report of 127 in 1922–32 and 94 for 1929 to mid-1935. See *Report of the State Hospital at Raleigh, 1934–36*, 26; *Report of the State Hospital at Raleigh, 1936–38*, 115; Royster, "An Account of the Surgical Service," 320–21; Brown, *Eugenical Sterilization in North Carolina* (1935), 20.

53. Of the 408 Black people sterilized, 261 were at Goldsboro. *Biennial Report of the Eugenics Board, 1942–44*, 12; North Carolina Commission for the Study of the Care of the Insane and Mental Defectives, *Study of Mental Health in North Carolina*; *Caswell Biennial Report, 1934–36*, 7.

54. Most state laws applied specifically to inmates of state institutions, but a handful of other states at the time allowed for sterilization of people living in county institutions or outside of institutions: Michigan (petitions could come from any sheriff or superintendent of the poor); New Hampshire (inmates of county institutions, citing economic burdens to the state); South Dakota (any feebleminded person); Vermont (idiots, imbeciles, feebleminded, or insane, including noninstitutional residents); and Wisconsin (residents of county institutions). See Welborn, "Eugenical Sterilization," 7–57; Lutz Kaelber, "Eugenics: Compulsory Sterilization in 50 States," https://www.uvm.edu/~lkaelber/eugenics/.

55. *BCPW Report, 1936–38*, 20. For additional analysis of geographic factors in later years, see Gartner, Krome-Lukens, and Delamater, "Implementation of Eugenic Sterilization."

56. Welborn, "Eugenical Sterilization"; Benson, "Sterilization." Benson conducted his thesis under the direction of Ernest R. Groves, who suggested the topic. At the time, Groves was a member of the commission that surveyed mental health conditions in the state. North Carolina Commission for the Study of the Care of the Insane and Mental Defectives, *Study of Mental Health in North Carolina*.

57. Benson, "Sterilization," 24–25; *University of North Carolina Record* no. 212 (July 1924): 90; Lawrence, "Organization and Administration of Public Welfare in Orange County"; "Report of Sub-Committee No. 4 of Mental Examinations and Sterilization of the Social Code Committee of the North Carolina Conference for Social Service," n.d., "Documents Concerning Amendments"; Register of the Officers and Faculty of the University of North Carolina 1795–1945, compiled by the staff of the North Carolina Collection, https://docsouth.unc.edu/true/faculty/faculty.html; *BCPW Report, 1934–36*, 25.

58. Benson, "Sterilization," 70; Welborn, "Eugenical Sterilization," 102.

59. For example, see Benson, "Sterilization," 36–38, 40–41, 50. In addition, Welborn noted that 55.5 percent had been confined to an institution at least once before sterilization; most of these commitments were to Samarcand, the state training school for delinquent white girls. Eleven percent were to maternity homes. Welborn also argued that sterilization reduced the incidence of sex delinquency. This information supports Johanna Schoen's argument that sexual misbehavior was a frequent reason for female sterilization. Interestingly, only three cases had been confined to Caswell, the state's only facility for the feebleminded, and three cases to the state's hospitals for the insane. It should be noted that Welborn based her research on questionnaires voluntarily returned by county welfare offices, and she did not receive completed questionnaires for 20.1 percent of the noninstitutional cases that occurred during her period of study (she received completed questionnaires for 183 of the 229 cases). Welborn, "Eugenical Sterilization," 110–12, 116, 119, 129; Schoen, *Choice and Coercion*, 92–96.

60. Welborn, "Eugenical Sterilization," 110–12, 116, 119, 129; Brown, *Eugenical Sterilization in North Carolina* (1935), 28–29, 34–35.

61. Brown, *Eugenical Sterilization in North Carolina* (1935), 3 (quoting *Eugenics*, March 1930), 9; North Carolina Commission for the Study of the Care of the Insane and Mental Defectives, *Study of Mental Health in North Carolina*, 301.

62. Benson, "Sterilization," 28–30, 36–38, 40, 43–44, 46; *BCPW Report, 1936–38*, 7.

63. From 1929 to 1944, 89 percent of operations outside institutions were on women, compared to 69 percent of operations in state institutions. Woodside, *Sterilization in North Carolina*, 41–43; *Biennial Report of the Eugenics Board, 1942–44*, 11–12. On gender and sterilization, see Schoen, *Choice and Coercion*, esp. 76, 95.

64. On average relief costs, see *BCPW Report, 1936–38*, 155; 206–7; and *Public Assistance Statistics*, vol. 2, 1937–38. Welborn reported that from 1933 to 1939, the average cost of a sterilization operation was $21.40 and the most frequent cost was $30. Benson reported that one salpingectomy and associated hospital bills cost $31.65. In some hospitals the cost was higher; in the Kinston hospital where Caswell inmates were sterilized, the cost was seventy-five dollars. Another report in 1935 indicated that each sterilization cost about twenty-eight dollars, including a two-week hospital stay. Welborn, "Eugenical Sterilization," 137; Benson, "Sterilization," 33–4; North Carolina Commission for the Study of the Care of the Insane and Mental Defectives, *Study of Mental Health in North Carolina*, 286; "Sterilization Gets Start in Orange County," *Chapel Hill Weekly*, December 13, 1935.

65. Mrs. W. B. Aycock to Superintendents of Public Welfare, May 21, 1937, BPW Records, Commissioner's Office, Box 173: Circular Letters, n.d., 1913–46, Folder: Circular Letters, 1933–39; Woodside, *Sterilization in North Carolina*, 43.

66. For examples, see Benson, "Sterilization."

67. *First Biennial Report of Eugenics Board*, 9–10; Sanders, *Juvenile Courts*; Woodside, "Sterilization in North Carolina," chapter 5.

68. In the end, officials decided it was not worth sterilizing the father, partly because his wife would be sterilized and his operation would thus be "unnecessary." Benson, "Sterilization," 36–38. On individuals' opposition to sterilization, see Schoen, *Choice and Coercion*, 125–28; and Hoke, "Politics of Fertility," 27–29.

69. *First Biennial Report of Eugenics Board*, 7–8; Brown, *Eugenical Sterilization in North Carolina* (1935), 16.

70. On the question of consent and ways that some people resisted by making use of the prescribed hearing process, see Schoen, *Choice and Coercion*, 125–27. In 1938–40, the Eugenics Board reported that families signed consent forms in 93.5 percent of cases; see *Biennial Report of the Eugenics Board, 1938–40*, 7. For the 1935 amendment and other changes to sterilization laws, see *Biennial Report of the Eugenics Board, 1934–36*, 8; Brown, *Eugenical Sterilization in North Carolina* (1938); NC Public Laws 1935, chapter 463 (appeals and consent); NC Public Laws 1937, chapter 243 (allowed a welfare superintendent to prosecute a petition for an inmate on parole from an institution); and NC Public Laws 1937, chapter 221 (allowed for admission of patients to hospitals solely for a sterilization operation).

71. Benson, "Sterilization," 49–53. On elective sterilizations, see Schoen, *Choice and Coercion*, 112–24.

72. Thurman D. Kitchin, "President's Address," *Transactions* 76 (1929), 58–63; "Sea Breeze Theatre" and "Merry-Go-Round at Sea Breeze," *Beaufort News*, May 5, 1938. For an overview of objections, see Woodside, *Sterilization in North Carolina*, chapter 5.

73. "New Laws Bring Social Reform," *News and Observer*, May 25, 1933; "The Welfare Problem," *Charlotte Observer*, November 7, 1934; "Sterilization of the Incompetents," *Roanoke Beacon* (Plymouth, NC), March 15, 1935; "Views and Reviews," *Roxboro Courier*, June 27, 1935; "Scientific Intelligence," *Daily Tar Heel*, March 29, 1935. On general public support for sterilization, see "Sterilization Law Explained," *Charlotte Observer*, May 1, 1935.

74. North Carolina Commission for the Study of the Care of the Insane and Mental Defectives, *Study of Mental Health in North Carolina*, 66, 257–58, 300–302, 363–65. On membership, see Memo, May 17, 1935, RF Records, RG 1.1, 236A, Folder 44.

75. *BCPW Report, 1934–36*, 11, 73, 124; *BCPW Report, 1937–38*, 139; North Carolina Commission for the Study of the Care of the Insane and Mental Defectives, *Study of Mental Health in North Carolina*, 274–77, 300, 363–64.

76. On public sentiment, see A. Gregg's diary, October 21, 1936, RF Records, RG 1.1, 236A, Folder 45. For newspaper coverage, see Nell Battle Lewis, "Detailed Survey Completed of Mental Health Problems," *News and Observer*, February 7, 1937; "Mental Health," *Elizabeth City Daily Independent*, January 23, 1937; "A North Carolina 47th," *News and Observer*, February 8, 1937; "State Lags with Treating Insane," *Henderson Daily Dispatch*, January 18, 1938. On Caswell, see "Legislative Record," *News and Observer*, March 3, 1937; 1937 Supplement to the North Carolina Code of 1935, chapter 96, article 12, section 5912(1). On the sterilization bill, see HB 776, "To Prohibit the Marriage of Persons with Contagious Diseases or

Imbecility," cited in "Legislative Record," *News and Observer*, March 5, 1937; "An Act to Regulate Marriage with Respect to Venereal Disease, Tuberculosis, and Imbecility," reprinted in *Biennial Report of the NC State Board of Health, 1936-38*, 57–58. On a unified board, see A. Gregg's diary, June 21, 1938, and Bryant to Gregg, January 11, 1939, both in RF Records, RG 1.1, 236A, Folder 46; Bryant to Judge Marshall T. Spears, Chairman, Board of Inquiry to Investigate State Hospital at Morganton, July 8 1942; and Bryant to Gregg, March 18, 1943, both in RF Records, RG 1.1, 236A, Folder 47.

77. Annie Kizer Bost, circular letter, April 12, 1932, in CSS Papers, Acc. 1, Box 13, Folder: [no title].

78. Ella (Mrs. W. B.) Waddill, President's Report to CSS (emphasis in original), 1932, 10, 14, 20–22, CSS Papers, Acc. 2, Box 1, Folder: Historical—President's Report—1932—Mrs. W. B. Waddill.

79. On North Carolina's birth control programs and the movement leading to them, see Schoen, *Choice and Coercion*; and Rogoff, *Gertrude Weil*, 81–82, 198–200. On Conference discussions, see NC CSS, Resolutions and Recommendations, May 1, 1934; Bradway to Newbold, November 1 and November 8, 1934; Minutes, Meeting of Integrating Committee, NC CSS, October 31, 1934; and Minutes, Business Meeting, Winston-Salem, May 7, 1935, CSS, all in Bradway Papers, Box 18, Folder: NC Conference for Social Service 1.

80. See, for example, Minutes, Meeting of Integrating Committee, NC CSS, October 31, 1934; and List of Members, CSS, 1934–35, both in Bradway Papers, Box 18, Folder: NC Conference for Social Service 1; W. C. Jackson to Members of the Committee on the Administration on Public Social Service, April 2, 1934, Bradway Papers, Box 18, Folder: NC Conference for Social Service 2; and Minutes, Board of Directors, October 22, 1936, CSS, Bradway Papers, Box 18, Folder: NC Conference for Social Service 3.

81. Gulledge, *North Carolina Conference for Social Service*, 62, 71, 73; R. Eugene Brown, "Interest in State Mental Hygiene Society Developed Years Before Organization," *Public Welfare Progress* 6, no. 4 (December 1943): 17.

82. "Some Remarks on Neuropsychiatry in NC, with References to the Veterans Administration," delivered by Raymond S. Crispell at NC Neuropsychiatric Association Meeting, Greensboro, NC, October 17, 1952, copy in RF Records, RG, 1.1, 236A, Folder 47.

83. On the Human Betterment League, see Wilds, "And the North Carolina Morons"; Charter, Human Betterment League, n.d. [1947], Human Betterment League of North Carolina, Inc., Records, 1947–88, Collection #4519, Southern Historical Collection, Wilson Library, Series 1, Folder 24, Charter (Original) and Minutes, 1947–72.

84. Eileen Boris, "Ellen Black Winston: Social Science for Social Welfare," in Gillespie and McMillen, eds., *North Carolina Women*.

85. Schoen links this decline in institutional sterilizations to growing skepticism among psychiatrists who worked at state institutions. Schoen, *Choice and Coercion*, 100.

86. Schoen, *Choice and Coercion*, 105–11, 128–29.

87. Tani, *States of Dependency*; Amsterdam, *Roaring Metropolis*; Biles, *South and the New Deal*.

88. Badger, *North Carolina and the New Deal*, esp. 47–49.

89. Several historians have chronicled the tension between welfare officials and the state ERA during its tenure from 1933 to 1935. See Dobelstein, "Public Welfare in the American System," 136–43; Badger, *North Carolina and the New Deal*, 47–48; Abrams, *Conservative Constraints*; Wilkerson-Freeman, "From Clubs to Parties."

90. Scholars of social welfare have helpfully analyzed social programs as divided into two channels, one better-supported channel with programs entitling white men to certain benefits and one channel for other people. See Gordon, ed., *Women, the State, and Welfare*; Skocpol, *Protecting Soldiers and Mothers*; Fraser and Gordon, "Contract Versus Charity"; Fraser and Gordon, "A Genealogy of Dependency"; Mink, *Wages of Motherhood*; Mettler, *Dividing Citizens*; Schneider and Ingram, *Deserving and Entitled*. For a similar two-track system in child welfare policy, see Ladd-Taylor, *Fixing the Poor*, 14–15.

Epilogue

1. On the US welfare system generally, see Gordon, *Pitied but Not Entitled*; on the federal–state system, see Tani, *States of Dependency*.

2. On the interaction of public policies and social constructions of groups, see Schneider and Ingram, *Deserving and Entitled*.

3. On the importance of administrative structures and contingent factors in determining policy outcomes, see Berkowitz, "Social Welfare History in the Age of Diversity"; on path dependence and policy as a moment of choice, see Pierson, "Increasing Returns" and "Study of Policy Development." On social critiques and tensions between reform and professionalism in social work and the social sciences, see Trolander, *Professionalism and Social Change*; Haskell, *Emergence of Professional Social Science*; Silverberg, ed., *Gender and American Social Science*; Carlton-LaNey and Burwell, "Introduction: African American Community Practice Models." On North Carolina's political climate, see Abrams, *Conservative Constraints*, esp. 158–59. On alternative political or analytical possibilities, see essays in Cox and Gardner, *Reassessing the 1930s South*.

4. For the series that sparked public interest, see Kevin Begos et al., "Against Their Will," *Winston-Salem Journal*, December 2002; Begos et al., *Against Their Will*. For an account of the fight for compensation by a journalist who covered the story, see Railey, *Rage to Redemption*.

5. For this analysis, I reviewed nearly a hundred newspaper articles between 2010 and 2015 in a variety of state and national news sources. Most articles mention some sort of demographic data, but the emphasis is on race and class. When articles discuss the "poor black women" who were targets of the program in later years, they do not discuss these women in terms of their gender. Some articles do not mention the sex of victims at all. See, for example, Rob Christensen and Jim Morrill, "Deadline for Commenting on Eugenics Rules Is Looming," *News and Observer Under the Dome* blog, October 19, 2013. One exception to the rule is an article that spends a few paragraphs dealing with the question of gender: Lara Torgeson, "N.C. Eugenics Survivors Seek Justice: The Ultimate Betrayal," *Independent Weekly*, March 24, 2010.

6. On racial demographics and the politics of sterilization programs after 1944, see Schoen, *Choice and Coercion*, 105–11; Boris, "Ellen Black Winston."

7. Railey, *Rage to Redemption*, 152; Bakst, "North Carolina's Forced-Sterilization Program," 2; Daren Bakst, "Compensate N.C.'s Sterilization Victims," *News and Observer*, May 19, 2011. For a pro-life perspective, see Nora Sullivan, "Eugenics Compensation Bill Reintroduced in North Carolina," LifeNews.com, January 31, 2013, www.lifenews.com/2013/01/31/eugenics-compensation-bill-reintroduced-in-north-carolina/. For other analyses of North Carolina's confrontation with its eugenics past, see Trent, *Inventing the*

Feeble Mind; Schoen, *Choice and Coercion*; Schoen, "Reassessing Eugenic Sterilization"; Brophy and Troutman, "Eugenics Movement in North Carolina."

8. On Georgia, see Lombardo, "Disability, Eugenics, and the Culture Wars." On Virginia, see "About Us," Justice for Sterilization Victims Project, accessed May 2, 2017, www.forcedsterilization.org/about-us/; Bill Sizemore, "Va. 2nd State to Pay Victims of Forced Sterilization," *Detroit Free Press*, March 27, 2015; Mark Bold, "It's Time for California to Compensate Its Forced-Sterilization Victims," *Los Angeles Times*, March 5, 2015; "Unfit to Breed," WRIC.com, January 10, 2014; Alicia Petska, "General Assembly May Finally Move on Virginia Eugenics Reparations," *Lynchburg News Advance*, February 14, 2015; and Jenna Portnoy, "Va. General Assembly Agrees to Compensate Eugenics Victims," *Washington Post*, February 27, 2015.

9. "NC Lawmakers Pass Ban on Abortions Because of Downs Syndrome," WRAL News, June 10, 2021, www.wral.com/story/nc-lawmakers-pass-ban-on-abortions-because-of-down-syndrome/19719655/. For an analysis of the lessons of eugenics, which are not simple, see Paul, *Politics of Heredity*, 95–115; and Paul, "Reflections on the Historiography." Many scholars have drawn parallels between eugenics and potential applications of new genetic technologies, including CRISPR. For example, see O'Brien, *Eugenics, Genetics, and Disability*; McCabe and McCabe, "Are We Entering a 'Perfect Storm'"; Comfort, *Science of Human Perfection*; Panofsky, *Misbehaving Science*; and Stern, *Telling Genes*.

Bibliography

Manuscript Collections
Chapel Hill, NC
  University of North Carolina at Chapel Hill
    Alexander W. McAlister Papers. Collection #4318, Southern Historical Collection, Wilson Library
    Alfred Moore Scales Papers. Collection #4037, Southern Historical Collection, Wilson Library
    Board of Trustees of the University of North Carolina Records, Series 1: Minutes. Collection #40001, University Archives, Wilson Library
    Charles L. Coon Papers, 1775–1831. Collection #177, Southern Historical Collection, Wilson Library
    E. C. Branson Papers, 1895–1933. Collection #2610, Southern Historical Collection, Wilson Library
    Howard Washington Odum Papers, 1908–82. Collection #3167, Southern Historical Collection, Wilson Library
    Human Betterment League of North Carolina, Inc., Records, 1947–88. Collection #4519, Southern Historical Collection, Wilson Library
    Law Library Rare Books
    Roy M. Brown Papers, 1924–56. Collection #3883, Southern Historical Collection, Wilson Library
    Tuttle Family Papers, 1842–1903. Collection #04233-z, Southern Historical Collection, Wilson Library
    William M. Cochrane Papers. Collection #5079, Southern Historical Collection, Wilson Library
Durham, NC
  Duke University
    David M. Rubenstein Rare Book and Manuscript Library
      John S. Bradway Papers
      Papers of Dean Justin Miller, 1929–34, Deans Papers, School of Law Records, 1914–2010s
      University Archives Photography Collection, 1961–2011, UA.01.15.0009
    Goodson Law Library
      Duke University School of Law Photograph Collection, ID 2011.A
Greenville, NC
  East Carolina University Special Collections
    Sybil Hyatt Papers. Manuscript Collection #778
    Tapp-Jenkins Papers. Manuscript Collection #312

Kinston, NC
   Caswell Center
      Unprocessed records, Caswell Center
   Kinston-Lenoir Public Library
      Sybil Hyatt Papers
Minneapolis, MN
   University of Minnesota
      Association for Voluntary Sterilization Records, University of Minnesota Social Welfare History Archives
Philadelphia, PA
   American Philosophical Society Library
      Charles B. Davenport Papers, Mss.B.D27
      Eugenics Record Office Records, Mss.Ms.Coll.77
Raleigh, NC
   North Carolina Federation of Women's Clubs Headquarters
      North Carolina Federation of Women's Clubs Records
   State Archives of North Carolina
      Board of Public Welfare Records, Social Services Record Group
         BPW Records, Commissioner's Office: Circular Letters
         BPW Records, Commissioner's Office, Subject File: Conference for Social Service
         BPW Records, Minutes of State Board of Charities and Public Welfare
         BPW Records, Minutes of the State Board of Public Charities
         Commissioner's Office: Correspondence with Associations and Committees, 1918–58
         Commissioner's Office: Correspondence with State Agencies, Boards, and Commissions, 1917–58
         Commissioner's Office: General Correspondence of the Board, 1891–1922
         Commissioner's Office: Secretary's Diaries, 1905–17
         Commissioner's Office: State Board Correspondence, 1897–1947
         Unprocessed Board of Charities and Public Welfare papers. MARS ID 97.101, Old Records Center
      Delia Hyatt Papers. PC #1529
      Denson Family Papers. PC #1230
      Nell Battle Lewis Papers. PC #255
      North Carolina Conference for Social Service Records. Org. 100
      North Carolina Mental Health Association (NC Mental Hygiene Society, 1913–55) Records. Org. 117
      North Carolina Supreme Court Records
      Papers of Governor Thomas Walter Bickett
      Session Records, North Carolina Senate and House of Representatives, 1919, 1923, 1925, 1929, 1933
      Woman's Club of Raleigh Records
Sleepy Hollow, NY
   Rockefeller Center Archive
      Laura Spelman Rockefeller Memorial Records
      Rockefeller Foundation Records

Washington, DC
   Georgetown University
      John Saeger Bradway Collection (Coll. 32), National Equal Justice Library Collection. Georgetown Law Library
Winston-Salem, NC
   Wake Forest University
      William Louis Poteat Papers, 1856–1938. MS 91, Z. Smith Reynolds Library Special Collections and Archives

Newspapers, Periodicals, and Yearbooks

Africo-American Presbyterian (Wilmington, NC)
Asheville Citizen
Beaufort (NC) News
Board of Charities and Public Welfare Bulletin
Bulletin of the North Carolina State Board of Health
Carolina and the Southern Cross
Carolina Times (Durham, NC)
Chanticleer (Duke University)
Chapel Hill Weekly
Charlotte Evening Chronicle
Charlotte Medical Journal
Charlotte Observer
Daily Tar Heel (Chapel Hill, NC)
Duke Law School Bulletin
Eugenical News
Everything Weekly (Greensboro, NC)
Greensboro Daily News
Greensboro Patriot
Greensboro Record
Henderson Daily Dispatch
Hill Directory Co.'s City Directories
Journal of Psycho-Asthenics
Journal of Social Forces
Kinston Free Press
Mebane Leader
Mental Hygiene
News and Observer (Raleigh, NC)
News-Record (Marshall, NC)
North Carolina League of Women Voters Monthly News
Proceedings of the National Conference of Charities and Correction
Proceedings of the Southern Sociological Congress
Public Welfare News
Public Welfare Progress
Raleigh State Journal
Social Forces
Social Service Quarterly
Southern Pines Pilot
Southern Medicine and Surgery
Star of Zion (Charlotte, NC)
Survey
Transactions of the Medical Society of North Carolina
Transactions of the North Carolina Health Officers' Association
University of North Carolina Alumni Review
University of North Carolina News Letter (Chapel Hill, NC)
University of North Carolina Record
Warren Record (Warrenton, NC)
Winston-Salem Journal

Published Government Reports and Documents

Annual Reports of the North Carolina Board of Public Charities, 1899–1916.
Beasley, Roland F. "Program of Work for County Superintendents of Public Welfare, Including Instructions in Method and Procedure of Keeping Records." State Board of Charities and Public Welfare, 1919.

Biennial Report of the North Carolina State Board of Health, 1920–22.
Biennial Reports of the Caswell Training School for Mental Defectives, 1915–34.
Biennial Reports of the Eugenics Board of North Carolina, 1934–50.
Biennial Reports of the North Carolina Board of Charities and Public Welfare, 1917–38.
Biennial Reports of the North Carolina School for the Feeble-Minded, 1911–14.
Biennial Reports of the State Hospital at Raleigh, 1920–34.
Brown, R. Eugene. *Eugenical Sterilization in North Carolina: A Brief Survey of the Growth of Eugenical Sterilization and a Report of the Work of the Eugenics Board of North Carolina Through June 30, 1935*. Eugenics Board of North Carolina, 1935.
———. *Eugenical Sterilization in North Carolina: Purpose, Statutory Provisions, Forms and Procedure*. Eugenics Board of North Carolina, 1938.
Federal Works Agency, Work Projects Administration. *Final Statistical Report of the Federal Emergency Relief Administration*. US Government Printing Office, 1942.
Journal of the House of Representatives of the General Assembly of North Carolina, 1911, 1917, 1919, 1923, 1925, 1929, 1933.
Journal of the Senate of the General Assembly of North Carolina, 1911, 1917, 1919, 1923, 1925, 1929, 1933.
Kirk, J. S., Walter A. Cutler, and Thomas W. Morse, eds. *Emergency Relief in North Carolina, 1932–35*. Edwards and Broughton, 1936.
Martin, Sanford, and R. B. House, eds. *Public Letters and Papers of Thomas Walter Bickett, Governor of North Carolina, 1917–21*. Edwards and Broughton, 1923.
McNairy, C. Banks, and Mary Schwarberg. "Information Concerning the Caswell Training Center, Kinston, North Carolina." Edwards and Broughton, n.d.
North Carolina Commission for the Study of the Care of the Insane and Mental Defectives. *A Study of Mental Health in North Carolina: Report to the North Carolina Legislature*. Edwards Brothers, 1937.
North Carolina Constitution of 1868, Article XI, Section 7.
North Carolina Manual, 1919, 1925, 1929. North Carolina Historical Commission.
North Carolina State Board of Charities and Public Welfare. "Swamp Island: A Study of Conditions in an Isolated Section of North Carolina." Capital Printing Company, 1922.
North Carolina's Social Welfare Program for Negroes. Special Bulletin no. 8. North Carolina State Board of Charities and Public Welfare, 1926.
"The Organization and Principles of Public Welfare Work in North Carolina." North Carolina Board of Charities and Public Welfare, 1919.
Public Assistance Statistics. North Carolina Board of Charities and Public Welfare, Division of Public Assistance.
Public Documents, Session 1917. Edwards and Broughton, 1920.
Public Laws and Resolutions of the State of North Carolina Passed by the General Assembly. North Carolina General Assembly, 1868–69, 1911, 1913, 1915, 1917, 1919, 1921, 1923, 1929, 1933, 1935, 1937.
Public Welfare Progress. North Carolina Board of Charities and Public Welfare, 1921–30.
Report of the Committee on Caswell Training School in Its Relation to the Problem of the Feeble-Minded of the State of North Carolina. Capital Printing Company, 1926.
US Census Bureau, 1900 Census of the Population, vol. 1: Population, Part 1.

US Census Bureau, 1940 Census of the Population, vol. 2: Characteristics of the Population, Part 5.

US Census Bureau, *Insane and Feeble-Minded in Institutions, 1910: General Tables*. US Government Printing Office, 1914.

US Census Bureau, Federal Population Census Schedules, 1860, 1870, 1880, 1900, 1910, 1920, 1930, 1940.

Other Published Sources

Abrams, Douglas Carl. *Conservative Constraints: North Carolina and the New Deal*. University Press of Mississippi, 1992.

Alphonso, Gwendoline. "From Need to Hope: The American Family and Poverty in Partisan Discourse, 1900–2012." *Journal of Policy History* 27, no. 4 (2015): 582–635.

Amsterdam, Daniel. *Roaring Metropolis: Businessmen's Campaign for a Civic Welfare State*. University of Pennsylvania Press, 2016.

Aydlett, A. Laurance. "The North Carolina State Board of Public Welfare." *North Carolina Historical Review* 24, no. 1 (January 1947): 1–33.

Ayers, Edward L. *The Promise of the New South: Life After Reconstruction*. Oxford University Press, 1992.

Badger, Anthony. *North Carolina and the New Deal*. North Carolina Department of Cultural Resources, Division of Archives and History, 1981.

Baker, Andrew C. "Race and Romantic Agrarianism: The Transnational Roots of Clarence Poe's Crusade for Rural Segregation in North Carolina." *Agricultural History* 87, no. 1 (January 2013): 93–114.

Bakst, Daren. "North Carolina's Forced-Sterilization Program: A Case for Compensating the Living Victims." John Locke Foundation, 2011.

Bashford, Allison, and Phillipa Levine, eds. *The Oxford Handbook of the History of Eugenics*. Oxford University Press, 2010.

Battle, Kemp Plummer. *The Early History of Raleigh, the Capital City of North Carolina; and an Account of the Centennial Celebration, Prepared by the Chairman of the Publication Committee, at the Request of the Board of Managers*. Edwards and Broughton, 1893.

Baynton, Douglas C. *Defectives in the Land: Disability and Immigration in the Age of Eugenics*. University of Chicago Press, 2016.

Bederman, Gail. *Manliness and Civilization: A Cultural History of Gender and Race in the United States, 1890–1917*. University of Chicago Press, 1995.

Begos, Kevin, Danielle Deaver, John Railey, and Scott Sexton. *Against Their Will: North Carolina's Sterilization Program*. Gray Oak Books, 2012.

Benson, J. McLean. "Sterilization, with Special Reference to Orange County, North Carolina." Master's thesis, University of North Carolina at Chapel Hill, 1936.

Berg, Allison. *Mothering the Race: Women's Narratives of Reproduction, 1890–1930*. University of Illinois Press, 2002.

Berkowitz, Edward D. "Social Welfare History in the Age of Diversity." *Journal of Policy History* 33, no. 4 (2021): 429–40.

Bickford, Annette Louise. *Southern Mercy: Empire and American Civilization in Juvenile Reform, 1890–1944*. University of Toronto Press, 2016.

Biles, Roger. *The South and the New Deal*. University Press of Kentucky, 1994.
Bix, Amy Sue. "Experiences and Voices of Eugenics Field-Workers: 'Women's Work' in Biology." *Social Studies of Science* 27, no. 4 (August 1997): 625–68.
Boles, John B., and Bethany L. Johnson, eds. *Origins of the New South: Fifty Years Later: The Continuing Influence of a Historical Classic*. Louisiana State University Press, 2003.
Boris, Eileen. "Ellen Black Winston: Social Science for Social Welfare." In *North Carolina Women: Their Lives and Times*, edited by Michele Gillespie and Sally G. McMillen. University of Georgia Press, 2015.
Bowers, William L. *The Country Life Movement in America, 1900–1920*. Kennikat Press, 1974.
Brabble, Jessica Marie. "Save the Babies: Progressive Women and the Fight for Child Welfare in the United States, 1912–1929." Master's thesis, Virginia Polytechnic Institute and State University, 2021.
Bradway, John S. "The Legality of Human Sterilization in North Carolina." *North Carolina Medical Journal* 11, no. 5 (May 1950): 250–52.
Braslow, Joel T. *Mental Ills and Bodily Cures: Psychiatric Treatment in the First Half of the Twentieth Century*. University of California Press, 1997.
Brazil, Wayne D. *Howard W. Odum: The Building Years, 1884–1930*. Garland, 1988.
Brice, Tanya Smith. "Undermining Progress in Early 20th Century North Carolina: General Attitudes Towards Delinquent African American Girls." *Journal of Sociology and Social Welfare* 34 (March 2007): 131–53.
Brietz, Margaret C. "Case Studies of Delinquent Girls in North Carolina." Master's thesis, University of North Carolina at Chapel Hill, 1927.
Briggs, Laura. *Reproducing Empire: Race, Sex, Science, and U.S. Imperialism in Puerto Rico*. University of California Press, 2002.
Brightman, Sarah, Emily Lenning, and Karen McElrath. "State-Directed Sterilizations in North Carolina: Victim-Centredness and Reparations." *British Journal of Criminology* 55, no. 3 (May 2015): 474–93.
Bristow, Nancy K. *Making Men Moral: Social Engineering During the Great War*. New York University Press, 1996.
Broberg, Gunnar, and Nils Roll-Hansen, eds. *Eugenics and the Welfare State: Sterilization Policy in Denmark, Sweden, Norway, and Finland*. Michigan State University Press, 1996.
Brophy, Alfred L., and Elizabeth Troutman. "The Eugenics Movement in North Carolina." *North Carolina Law Review* 94, no. 6 (2016), Article 2.
Brown, Elizabeth M., and Sarah Shaw Genheimer. *Haven on the Neuse: A History of Caswell Center, Kinston, North Carolina, 1911–1964*. Vantage Press, 1969.
Brown, Elsa Barkley. "Womanist Consciousness: Maggie Lena Walker and the Independent Order of Saint Luke." *Signs* 14, no. 3 (1989): 610–33.
Brown, Roy M. *Public Poor Relief in North Carolina*. University of North Carolina Press, 1928.
Brundage, W. Fitzhugh. "Introduction." In *The Folly of Jim Crow: Rethinking the Segregated South*, edited by Stephanie Cole and Natalie J. Ring. Texas A&M University Press, 2012.
Bruno, Frank J. *Trends in Social Work, 1874–1956: A History Based on the Proceedings of the National Conference of Social Work*. Columbia University Press, 1957.

Bullard, Katharine S. *Civilizing the Child: Discourses of Race, Nation, and Child Welfare in America*. Lexington Books, 2014.
Burch, Susan, and Hannah Joyner. *Unspeakable: The Story of Junius Wilson*. University of North Carolina Press, 2015.
Burwell, N. Yolanda. "Lawrence Oxley and Locality Development." *Journal of Community Practice* 2, no. 4 (1996): 49–69.
———. "North Carolina Public Welfare Institutes for Negroes 1926–46." *Journal of Sociology and Social Welfare* 21, no. 1 (March 1994): 55–66.
Cahn, Susan K. *Sexual Reckonings: Southern Girls in a Troubling Age*. Harvard University Press, 2007.
———. "Spirited Youth or Fiends Incarnate: The Samarcand Arson Case and Female Adolescence in the American South." In *Other Souths: Diversity and Difference in the U.S. South, Reconstruction to Present*, edited by Pippa Holloway. University of Georgia Press, 2008.
Canaday, Margot. *The Straight State: Sexuality and Citizenship in Twentieth-Century America*. Princeton University Press, 2009.
Canaday, Margot, Nancy F. Cott, and Robert O. Self. *Intimate States: Gender, Sexuality, and Governance in Modern U.S. History*. University of Chicago Press, 2021.
Carlson, Elof Axel. *The Unfit: The History of a Bad Idea*. Cold Spring Harbor Laboratory Press, 2001.
Carlton-LaNey, Iris. "African American Social Work Pioneers' Response to Need." *Social Work* 44, no. 4 (July 1999): 311–21.
Carlton-LaNey, Iris, and N. Yolanda Burwell. "Introduction: African American Community Practice Models: Historical and Contemporary Responses." *Journal of Community Practice* 2, no. 4 (1996): 1–6.
Castles, Katherine Lynn. "Little 'Tardies': Mental Retardation, Race, and Class in American Society, 1945–1965." PhD dissertation, Duke University, 2006.
Catte, Elizabeth. *Pure America: Eugenics and the Making of Modern Virginia*. Belt Publishing, 2021.
Chamberlain, Chelsea D. "Challenging Custodialism: Families and Eugenic Institutionalization at the Pennsylvania Training School for Feeble-Minded Children at Elwyn." *Journal of Social History* 55, no. 2 (2021): 484–509.
Chambers, Clarke A. "Women in the Creation of the Profession of Social Work." *Social Service Review* 60, no. 1 (March 1986): 1–33.
Cole, Stephanie, and Natalie J. Ring, eds. *The Folly of Jim Crow: Rethinking the Segregated South*. Texas A&M University Press, 2012.
Comfort, Nathaniel. *The Science of Human Perfection: How Genes Became the Heart of American Medicine*. Yale University Press, 2012.
Cooke, Kathy J. "The Limits of Heredity: Nature and Nurture in American Eugenics Before 1915." *Journal of the History of Biology* 31, no. 2 (Summer 1998): 263–78.
Cott, Nancy F. "Marriage and Women's Citizenship in the United States, 1830–1934." *American Historical Review* 103, no. 5 (December 1998): 1440–74.
Cotten, Sallie Southall. *History of the North Carolina Federation of Women's Clubs, 1901–1925*. Edwards and Broughton, 1925.
Cox, Fred M. "Alexander Johnson." In *Biographical Dictionary of Social Welfare in America*, edited by Walter I. Trattner. Greenwood Press, 1986.

Cox, Karen L., and Sarah E. Gardner. *Reassessing the 1930s South*. Louisiana State University Press, 2018.
Crane, Harry W. "The Necessity of Psychometric Tests in the Study of Maladjustments." *Journal of Applied Psychology* 15, no. 3 (June 1931): 304–9.
Crow, Jeffrey J. "An Apartheid for the South." In *Race, Class, and Politics in Southern History: Essays in Honor of Robert F. Durden*, edited by Jeffrey J. Crow, Paul D. Escott, and Charles L. Flynn Jr. Louisiana State University Press, 1989.
Cuddy, Lois A., and Claire M. Roche, eds. *Evolution and Eugenics in American Literature and Culture, 1880–1940: Essays on Ideological Conflict and Complicity*. Bucknell University Press, 2003.
Cullen, David. "Back to the Future: Eugenics—A Bibliographic Essay." *Public Historian* 29, no. 3 (Summer 2007): 163–75.
Currell, Susan, and Christina Cogdell, eds. *Popular Eugenics: National Efficiency and American Mass Culture in the 1930s*. Ohio University Press, 2006.
Dashiell, J. F., and W. D. Glenn. "A Re-Examination of a Socially Composite Group with Binet and with Performance Tests." *Journal of Educational Psychology* 16, no. 5 (May 1925): 335–40.
Degler, Carl. *In Search of Human Nature: The Decline and Revivalism of Darwinism in American Social Thought*. Oxford University Press, 1991.
Dobelstein, Andrew. "Public Welfare in the American System: The North Carolina Experience." PhD dissertation, Duke University, 1973.
Dorey, Annette K. Vance. *Better Baby Contests: The Scientific Quest for Perfect Childhood Health in the Early Twentieth Century*. McFarland & Company, 1999.
Dorr, Gregory Michael. *Segregation's Science: Eugenics and Society in Virginia*. University of Virginia Press, 2008.
Dorr, Gregory Michael, and Angela Logan. "'Quality, Not Mere Quantity, Counts': Black Eugenics and the NAACP Baby Contests." In *A Century of Eugenics in America: From the Indiana Experiment to the Human Genome Era*, edited by Paul A. Lombardo. Indiana University Press, 2011.
Dowbiggin, Ian Robert. *Keeping American Sane: Psychiatry and Eugenics in the United States and Canada, 1880–1940*. Cornell University Press, 2018.
Downs, Gregory P. "University Men, Social Science, and White Supremacy in North Carolina." *Journal of Southern History* 65, no. 2 (May 2009): 267–304.
Durden, Robert F. "The Rebuilding of Duke University's School of Law, 1925–1947, Part I." *North Carolina Historical Review* 66, no. 3 (July 1989): 321–52.
Ehrenreich, John H. *The Altruistic Imagination: A History of Social Work and Social Policy in the United States*. Cornell University Press, 1985.
English, Daylanne K. *Unnatural Selections: Eugenics in American Modernism and the Harlem Renaissance*. University of North Carolina Press, 2004.
Engs, Ruth Clifford. *The Eugenics Movement: An Encyclopedia*. Greenwood Press, 2005.
Ettling, John. *The Germ of Laziness: Rockefeller Philanthropy and Public Health in the New South*. Harvard University Press, 1981.
Evans, Peter, Dietrich Rueschemeyer, and Theda Skocpol, eds. *Bringing the State Back In*. Cambridge University Press, 1985.
Feimster, Crystal. *Southern Horrors: Women and the Politics of Rape and Lynching*. Harvard University Press, 2009.

Filene, Peter G. "An Obituary for 'The Progressive Movement.'" *American Quarterly* 22 (Spring 1970): 20–34.
Fitzpatrick, Ellen F. *Endless Crusade: Women Social Scientists and Progressive Reform.* Oxford University Press, 1990.
Flynt, Wayne. "'Feeding the Hungry and Ministering to the Broken Hearted': The Presbyterian Church in the United States and the Social Gospel, 1900–1920." In *Religion in the South*, edited by Charles Reagan Wilson. University Press of Mississippi, 1985.
———. *Southern Religion and Christian Diversity in the Twentieth Century.* University of Alabama Press, 2016.
Frankel, Noralee, and Nancy S. Dye, eds. *Gender, Class, Race, and Reform in the Progressive Era.* University Press of Kentucky, 1991.
Fraser, Nancy, and Linda Gordon. "Contract Versus Charity: Why Is There No Social Citizenship in the United States?" *Socialist Review* 22 (1992): 45–68.
———. "A Genealogy of Dependency: Tracing a Keyword of the U.S. Welfare State." *Signs* 19, no. 2 (Winter 1994): 309–36.
Gallagher, Wendy. *Breeding Better Vermonters: The Eugenics Project in the Green Mountain State.* University Press of New England, 1999.
Gartner, Danielle R., Anna L. Krome-Lukens, Paul L. Delamater. "Implementation of Eugenic Sterilization in North Carolina: Geographic Proximity to Raleigh and Its Association with Female Sterilization During the Mid-20th Century." *Southeastern Geographer* 60, no. 3 (2020): 254–74.
Gary, Robenia Baker, and Lawrence E. Gary. "The History of Social Work Education for Black People, 1900–1930." *Journal of Sociology and Social Welfare* 21, no. 1 (March 1994): 67–81.
Gatewood, Willard B. *Preachers, Pedagogues, and Politicians: The Evolution Controversy in North Carolina, 1920–1927.* University of North Carolina Press, 1966.
Gendzel, Glen. "What the Progressives Had in Common." *Journal of the Gilded Age and Progressive Era* 10, no. 3 (July 2011): 331–39.
Gibson, Campbell. "Population of the 100 Largest Cities and Other Urban Places in the United States: 1790 to 1990." Working Paper No. POP-WP027. US Census Bureau, June 1998.
Gilmore, Glenda. *Gender and Jim Crow: Women and the Politics of White Supremacy in North Carolina, 1896–1920.* University of North Carolina Press, 1996.
———. *Who Were the Progressives?* Palgrave, 2002.
Glenn, William. "The Fehlers: A Social and Psychometric Study of a Cacogenic Family." PhD dissertation, University of North Carolina at Chapel Hill, 1930.
Goddard, H. H. *Feeble-Mindedness: Its Causes and Consequences.* Macmillan, 1914.
———. *Sterilization and Segregation.* Russell Sage Foundation, 1913.
Gordon, Linda. "Black and White Visions of Welfare: Women's Welfare Activism, 1890–1945." *Journal of American History* 78, no. 2 (September 1991): 559–90.
———. *Pitied but Not Entitled: Single Mothers and the History of Welfare.* Harvard University Press, 1994.
———. "Social Insurance and Public Assistance: The Influence of Gender in Welfare Thought in the United States, 1890–1935." *American Historical Review* 97, no. 1 (February 1992): 19–54.

———, ed. *Women, the State, and Welfare*. University of Wisconsin Press, 1990.
Goudge, Mabel Ensworth. "A Qualitative and Quantitative Study of Weber's Illusion." *American Journal of Psychology* 29 (1918): 81–119.
———. "A Simplified Method of Conducting McDougall's Spot-Pattern Test." *Journal of Educational Psychology* 6 (1915): 73–84.
Gould, Stephen Jay. *The Mismeasure of Man*, rev. ed. Norton, 1996.
Grantham, Dewey. *Southern Progressivism: The Reconciliation of Progress and Tradition*. University of Tennessee Press, 1983.
Green, Elna, ed. *Before the New Deal: Social Welfare in the South, 1830–1930*. University of Georgia Press, 1999.
———. "Gendering the City, Gendering the Welfare State: The Nurses' Settlement of Richmond, 1900–1930." *Virginia Magazine of History and Biography* 113, no. 3 (2005): 276–311.
———. "National Trends, Regional Differences, Local Circumstances: Social Welfare in New Orleans, 1870s–1920s." In *Before the New Deal: Social Welfare in the South, 1830–1930*, edited by Elna Green. University of Georgia Press, 1999.
———. *This Business of Relief: Confronting Poverty in a Southern City, 1740–1940*. University of Georgia Press, 2003.
Grob, Gerald N., ed. *Mental Hygiene in Twentieth Century America: Four Studies, 1921–1924*. Arno Press, 1980.
Gulledge, Virginia. *The North Carolina Conference for Social Service: A Study of Its Development and Methods*. The Conference, 1942.
Guyer, Michael F. *Being Well-Born: An Introduction to Eugenics*. Bobbs-Merrill, 1916.
Hale, Grace Elizabeth. *Making Whiteness: The Culture of Segregation in the South, 1890–1940*. Vintage Books, 1998.
Haley, Sarah. *No Mercy Here: Gender, Punishment, and the Making of Jim Crow Modernity*. University of North Carolina Press, 2016.
Hall, Amy Laura. *Conceiving Parenthood: American Protestantism and the Spirit of Reproduction*. William B. Eerdmans, 2008.
Hall, Jacquelyn Dowd. "O. Delight Smith's Progressive Era: Labor, Feminism and Reform in the Urban South." In *Visible Women: New Essays on American Activism*, edited by Nancy Hewitt and Suzanne Lebsock. University of Illinois Press, 1993.
———. *Revolt Against Chivalry: Jessie Daniel Ames and the Women's Campaign Against Lynching*. Columbia University Press, 1979.
Hall, Jacquelyn Dowd, and Anne Firor Scott. "Women in the South." In *Interpreting Southern History: Historiographical Essays in Honor of Sanford W. Higginbotham*, edited by John B. Boles and Evelyn Thomas Nolen. Louisiana State University Press, 1987.
Hall, Jacquelyn Dowd, Mary Murphy, James Leloudis, Robert Korstad, Lu Ann Jones, and Christopher B. Daly. *Like a Family: The Making of a Southern Cotton Mill World*. W. W. Norton, 1987.
Hall, Randal L. *William Louis Poteat: A Leader of the Progressive-Era South*. University Press of Kentucky, 2000.
Haller, Mark. *Eugenics: Hereditarian Attitudes in American Thought*. Rutgers University Press, 1963.

Hanchett, Thomas W. *Sorting Out the New South City: Race, Class, and Urban Development in Charlotte, 1875–1975*, 2nd ed. University of North Carolina Press, 2020.
Handy, Robert T. *The Social Gospel in America, 1870–1920*. Oxford University Press, 1966.
Harper, Keith. *The Quality of Mercy: Southern Baptists and Social Christianity, 1890–1920*. University of Alabama Press, 1996.
Harvey, Paul. "Religion in the American South Since the Civil War." In *A Companion to the American South*, edited by John B. Boles. Blackwell, 2002.
Haskell, Thomas L. *The Emergence of Professional Social Science: The American Social Science Association and the Nineteenth-Century Crisis of Authority*. University of Illinois Press, 1977.
Herbin-Triant, Elizabeth A. "Southern Segregation South Africa–Style: Maurice Evans, Clarence Poe, and the Ideology of Rural Segregation." *Agricultural History* 87, no. 2 (2013): 170–93.
———. *Threatening Property: Race, Class, and Campaigns to Legislate Jim Crow Neighborhoods*. Columbia University Press, 2019.
Hickey, Georgina. *Hope and Danger in the New South City: Working-Class Women and Urban Development in Atlanta, 1890–1940*. University of Georgia Press, 2003.
Higginbotham, Evelyn Brooks. *Righteous Discontent: The Women's Movement in the Black Baptist Church, 1880–1920*. Harvard University Press, 1993.
Higham, John. *Strangers in the Land: Patterns of American Nativism, 1860–1925*, 2nd ed. Rutgers University Press, 1988.
History of North Carolina, vol. 5: *North Carolina Biography*. Lewis Publishing, 1919.
Hofstadter, Richard. *The Age of Reform: From Bryan to F.D.R.* Knopf, 1955.
Hoke, Kathleen E. "The Politics of Fertility: Coercive Sterilization and Public Health Birth Control in North Carolina, 1929–1960." Master's thesis, University of North Carolina–Greensboro, 1991.
Holloway, Pippa. *Sexuality, Politics, and Social Control in Virginia, 1920–1945*. University of North Carolina Press, 2006.
Hood, Davyd Foard. *To the Glory of God: Christ Church, 1821–1996*. Marblehead, 1997.
Hopkins, Harry L. *Spending to Save: The Complete Story of Relief*. W. W. Norton, 1936.
Hubbell, J. H. *Hubbell's Legal Directory for Lawyers and Businessmen*. Rumford Press, 1922.
Hunter, Tera. *To 'Joy My Freedom: Southern Black Women's Lives and Labors After the Civil War*. Harvard University Press, 1997.
Ingram, Tammy. *Dixie Highway: Road Building and the Making of the Modern South, 1900–1930*. University of North Carolina Press, 2014.
Irvine, Tina A. "Reclaiming Appalachia: Mountain Reform and the Preservation of White Citizenship, 1890–1929." PhD dissertation, University of Pennsylvania, 2019.
Jacobson, Matthew Frye. *Whiteness of a Different Color: European Immigrants and the Alchemy of Race*. Harvard University Press, 1998.
Johnson, Guy Benton, and Guion Griffis Johnson. *Research in Service to Society: The First Fifty Years of the Institute for Research in Social Science at the University of North Carolina*. University of North Carolina Press, 1980.
Johnson, Joan Marie. "The Colors of Social Welfare in the New South: Black and White Clubwomen in South Carolina, 1900–1930." In *Before the New Deal: Social*

Welfare in the South, 1830–1930, edited by Elna Green. University of Georgia Press, 1999.

———. *Southern Ladies, New Women: Race, Region, and Clubwomen in South Carolina, 1890–1930*. University Press of Florida, 2004.

Johnson, Kimberley. *Reforming Jim Crow: Southern Politics and State in the Age Before Brown*. Oxford University Press, 2010.

Jones, Lu Ann. *Mama Learned Us to Work: Farm Women in the New South*. University of North Carolina Press, 2002.

Katz, Michael B. *In the Shadow of the Poorhouse: A Social History of Welfare in America*, rev. ed. Basic Books, 1996.

———. *The Price of Citizenship: Redefining the American Welfare State*, updated ed. University of Pennsylvania Press, 2008.

Kayser, John A. "The Early History of Racially Segregated, Southern Schools of Social Work Requesting or Receiving Funds from the Rockefeller Philanthropies and the Responses of Social Work Educators to Racial Discrimination." Grant-in-Aid Report to the Rockefeller Archive Center, 2005.

Kennedy, David M. *Freedom from Fear: The American People in Depression and War, 1929–1945*. Oxford University Press, 1999.

Kevles, Daniel J. *In the Name of Eugenics: Genetics and the Uses of Human Heredity Genetics and the Uses of Human Heredity*. Alfred A. Knopf, 1985.

———. "Testing the Army's Intelligence: Psychologists and the Military in World War I." *Journal of American History* 55, no. 3 (December 1968): 565–81.

Kirby, Jack Temple. "Clarence Poe's Vision of a Segregated 'Great Rural Civilization.'" *South Atlantic Quarterly* 68, no. 1 (Winter 1969): 27–38.

———. *Darkness at the Dawning: Race and Reform in the Progressive South*. Lippincott, 1972.

Kirby, John. "Footsteps to Sterilization: Psychiatry and Surgery at the North Carolina State Hospital for the Insane at Raleigh, 1922–1932." *Journal of Graduate Liberal Studies* 11, no. 1 (Fall 2005): 79–90.

Kline, Wendy. *Building a Better Race: Gender, Sexuality, and Eugenics from the Turn of the Century to the Baby Boom*. University of California Press, 2001.

Kotch, Seth. *Lethal State: A History of the Death Penalty in North Carolina*. University of North Carolina Press, 2019.

Koven, Seth, and Sonya Michel, eds. *Mothers of a New World: Maternalist Politics and the Origins of Welfare States*. Routledge, 1993.

Koven, Seth, and Sonya Michel. "Womanly Duties: Maternalist Politics and the Origins of Welfare States in France, Germany, Great Britain, and the United States, 1880–1920." *American Historical Review* 95 (October 1990): 1076–108.

Krome-Lukens, Anna L. "The Reform Imagination: Gender, Eugenics, and the Welfare State in North Carolina, 1900–1940." PhD dissertation, University of North Carolina at Chapel Hill, 2014.

Kuby, William. *Conjugal Misconduct: Defying Marriage Law in the Twentieth-Century United States*. Cambridge University Press, 2018.

Kuhn, Clifford. *Contesting the New South Order: The 1914–1915 Strike at Atlanta's Fulton Mills*. University of North Carolina Press, 2001.

Kunzel, Regina G. *Fallen Women, Problem Girls: Unmarried Mothers and the Professionalization of Social Work, 1890–1945.* Yale University Press, 1993.

Ladd-Taylor, Molly. *Fixing the Poor: Eugenic Sterilization and Child Welfare in the Twentieth Century.* Johns Hopkins University Press, 2017.

———. *Mother-Work: Women, Child Welfare, and the State, 1890–1930.* University of Illinois Press, 1994.

———. "Saving Babies and Sterilizing Mothers: Eugenics and Welfare Politics in the Interwar United States." *Social Politics* 4, no. 1 (Spring 1997): 136–53.

———. "The 'Sociological Advantages' of Sterilization: Fiscal Policies and Feeble-Minded Women in Interwar Minnesota." In *Mental Retardation in America: A Historical Reader*, edited by Steven Noll and James W. Trent Jr. New York University Press, 2004.

Landman, Jacob Henry. *Human Sterilization: The History of the Sexual Sterilization Movement.* Macmillan, 1932.

Lantzer, Jason S. "The Indiana Way of Eugenics: Sterilization Laws, 1907–74." In *A Century of Eugenics: From the Indiana Experiment to the Human Genome Era*, edited by Paul A. Lombardo. Indiana University Press, 2011.

Largent, Mark A. *Breeding Contempt: The History of Coerced Sterilization in the United States.* Rutgers University Press, 2008.

———. "'The Greatest Curse of the Race': Eugenic Sterilization in Oregon, 1909–1983." *Oregon Historical Quarterly* 103, no. 2 (2002): 188–209.

Larson, Edward J. "'In the Finest, Most Womanly Way': Women in the Southern Eugenics Movement." *American Journal of Legal History* 39 (April 1995): 119–47.

———. *Sex, Race, and Science: Eugenics in the Deep South.* Johns Hopkins University Press, 1995.

Larson, Edward J., and Leonard J. Nelson III. "Involuntary Sexual Sterilization of Incompetents in Alabama: Past, Present, and Future." *Alabama Law Review* 42, no. 2 (Winter 1992): 399–444.

Laughlin, Harry H. *Eugenical Sterilization in the United States.* Psychopathic Laboratory of the Municipal Court of Chicago, 1922

Lawrence, George H. "The Organization and Administration of Public Welfare in Orange County, North Carolina." Master's thesis, University of North Carolina at Chapel Hill, 1928.

Leidholdt, Alexander S. *Battling Nell: The Life of Southern Journalist Cornelia Battle Lewis, 1893–1956.* Louisiana State University Press, 2009.

Leloudis, James L. *Schooling the New South: Pedagogy, Self, and Society in North Carolina, 1880–1920.* University of North Carolina Press, 1996.

Lindquist Dorr, Lisa. "Arm in Arm: Gender, Eugenics, and Virginia's Racial Integrity Acts of the 1920s." *Journal of Women's History* 11, no. 1 (Spring 1991): 143–66.

Lingle, Walter L. *Memories of Davidson College.* John Knox Press, 1947.

Link, Arthur S. "The Progressive Movement in the South, 1870–1914." *North Carolina Historical Review* 23, no. 1 (April 1946): 172–95.

Link, Arthur S., and Richard L. McCormick. *Progressivism.* Harlan Davidson, 1983.

Link, William A. *Frank Porter Graham: Southern Liberal, Citizen of the World.* University of North Carolina Press, 2021.

———. *North Carolina: Change and Tradition in a Southern State*, 2nd ed. Wiley-Blackwell, 2018.

———. *The Paradox of Southern Progressivism, 1880–1930*. University of North Carolina Press, 1992.

Lombardo, Paul, ed. *A Century of Eugenics in America: From the Indiana Experiment to the Human Genome Era*. Indiana University Press, 2011.

———. "Disability, Eugenics, and the Culture Wars." *St. Louis University Journal of Health Law and Policy* 2, no. 57 (2008–9): 57–80.

———. "From Better Babies to the Bunglers: Eugenics on Tobacco Road." In *A Century of Eugenics in America: From the Indiana Experiment to the Human Genome Era*, edited by Paul Lombardo. Indiana University Press, 2011.

———. *Three Generations, No Imbeciles: Eugenics, the Supreme Court, and* Buck v. Bell. Johns Hopkins University Press, 2008.

Lovett, Laura L. *Conceiving the Future: Pronatalism, Reproduction, and the Family in the United States, 1890–1938*. University of North Carolina Press, 2007.

———. "'Fitter Families for Future Firesides': Florence Sherbon and Popular Eugenics." *Public Historian* 29, no. 3 (Summer 2007): 69–85.

Lubove, Roy. *The Professional Altruist: The Emergence of Social Work as a Career, 1880–1930*. Harvard University Press, 1965.

Lowery, Malinda Maynor. *Lumbee Indians in the Jim Crow South: Race, Identity, and the Making of a Nation*. University of North Carolina Press, 2010.

Luker, Ralph. *The Social Gospel in Black and White: American Racial Reform, 1885–1912*. University of North Carolina Press, 1991.

Marshall, Thomas Humphrey. *Citizenship and Social Class, and Other Essays*. Cambridge University Press, 1950.

Martinez-Brawley, Emilia E., ed. *Pioneer Efforts in Rural Social Welfare: Firsthand Views Since 1908*. Pennsylvania State University Press, 1980.

Matthews, Scott L. *Capturing the South: Imagining America's Most Documented Region*. University of North Carolina Press, 2018.

McCabe, Linda L., and Edward R. B. McCabe. "Are We Entering a 'Perfect Storm' for a Resurgence of Eugenics? Science, Medicine, and Their Social Context." In *A Century of Eugenics in America: From the Indiana Experiment to the Human Genome Era*, edited by Paul A. Lombardo. Indiana University Press, 2011.

McCrady, Edward, and Samuel A'Court Ashe, *Cyclopedia of Eminent and Representative Men of the Carolinas of the Nineteenth Century*. Brant & Fuller, 1902.

McCulloch, James E., ed. *The Call of the New South: Addresses Delivered at the Southern Sociological Congress, Nashville, Tennessee, May 7–10, 1912*. Southern Sociological Congress, 1912.

———, ed. *Democracy in Earnest: Southern Sociological Congress, 1916–1918*. Southern Sociological Congress, 1918.

McDowell, John Patrick. *The Social Gospel in the South: The Woman's Home Mission Movement in the Methodist Episcopal Church, South, 1886–1939*. Louisiana State University Press, 1982.

McFadden, John Holman. "Differential Responses of Normal and Feebleminded Subjects of Equal Mental Age, on the Kent-Rosanoff Free Association Test and the Stanford

Revision of the Binet-Simon Intelligence Test." PhD dissertation, University of North Carolina at Chapel Hill, 1930.

———. "Racial Differences Measured by the Downey-Will Temperament Test." Master's thesis, University of North Carolina at Chapel Hill, 1922.

McGerr, Michael. *A Fierce Discontent: The Rise and Fall of the Progressive Movement in America, 1870–1920*. Oxford University Press, 2003.

McMahon, Mrs. Phil, ed. *Studies in Citizenship for North Carolina Women*. North Carolina League of Women Voters, 1926.

McRae, Elizabeth Gillespie. *Mothers of Massive Resistance: White Women and the Politics of White Supremacy*. Oxford University Press, 2018.

Mettler, Suzanne. *Dividing Citizens: Gender and Federalism in New Deal Public Policy*. Cornell University Press, 1998.

———. "The Stratification of Social Citizenship: Gender and Federalism in the Formation of Old Age Insurance and Aid to Dependent Children." *Journal of Policy History* 11, no. 1 (1999): 31–58.

Michelmore, Molly. *Tax and Spend: The Welfare State, Tax Politics, and the Limits of American Liberalism*. University of Pennsylvania Press, 2012.

Mink, Gwendolyn. *The Wages of Motherhood: Inequality in the Welfare State, 1917–1942*. Cornell University Press, 1995.

Mitchell, Michelle. *Righteous Propagation: African Americans and the Politics of Racial Destiny After Reconstruction*. University of North Carolina Press, 2004.

Muncy, Robyn. *Creating a Female Dominion in American Reform, 1890–1935*. Oxford University Press, 1991.

Myers, William Starr, ed. *Prominent Families of New Jersey*, vol. 1. Clearfield, 2000.

Nackenoff, Carol, and Julie Novkov, eds. *Statebuilding from the Margins: Between Reconstruction and the New Deal*. University of Pennsylvania Press, 2014.

Neal, Margaret Clark. *North Carolina Conference for Social Service: The Record of Twenty-Five Years, 1912–1937*. Typed manuscript, North Carolina Collection, Wilson Library, University of North Carolina at Chapel Hill.

Noll, Steven. "A Far Greater Menace: Feebleminded Females in the South, 1900–1940." In *Hidden Histories of Women in the New South*, edited by Virginia Bernhard et al. University of Missouri Press, 1994.

———. *Feeble-Minded in Our Midst: Institutions for the Mentally Retarded in the South, 1900–1940*. University of North Carolina Press, 1995.

———. "The Public Face of Southern Institutions for the 'Feeble-Minded.'" *Public Historian* 27, no. 2 (Spring 2005): 25–41.

Nuriddin, Ayah. "Engineering Uplift: Black Eugenics as Black Liberation." In *Nature Remade: Engineering Life, Envisioning Worlds*, edited by Luis A. Campos et al. University of Chicago Press, 2021.

———. "Race, Sexuality, and the 'Progressive Physician': African American Doctors, Eugenics, and Public Health, 1900–1940." Master's thesis, University of Maryland, College Park, 2014.

O'Brien, Gerald. *Eugenics, Genetics, and Disability in Historical and Contemporary Perspective: Implications for the Social Work Profession*. Oxford University Press, 2023.

Odem, Mary E. *Delinquent Daughters: Protecting and Policing Adolescent Female Sexuality in the United States, 1885–1920*. University of North Carolina Press, 1995.
Odum, Howard W. *An Approach to Public Welfare and Social Work*. University of North Carolina Press, 1926.
———. *Systems of Public Welfare*. University of North Carolina Press, 1925.
Ordover, Nancy. *American Eugenics: Race, Queer Anatomy, and the Science of Nationalism*. University of Minnesota Press, 2003.
Orleck, Annelise. *Storming Caesar's Palace: How Black Mothers Fought Their Own War on Poverty*. Beacon Press, 2005.
Painter, Nell Irvin. *Standing at Armageddon: The United States, 1877–1919*. W. W. Norton, 1987.
Panofsky, Aaron. *Misbehaving Science: Controversy and the Development of Behavior Genetics*. University of Chicago Press, 2014.
Pascoe, Peggy. *Relations of Rescue: The Search for Female Moral Authority in the American West, 1874–1939*. Oxford University Press, 1990.
———. *What Comes Naturally: Miscegenation Law and the Making of Race in America*. Oxford University Press, 2009.
Paul, Diane. *Controlling Human Heredity, 1865 to the Present*. Humanities Press, 1995.
———. *The Politics of Heredity: Essays on Eugenics, Biomedicine, and the Nature-Nurture Debate*. State University of New York Press, 1998.
———. "Reflections on the Historiography of American Eugenics: Trends, Fractures, Tensions." *Journal of the History of Biology* 49 (2016): 641–58.
Pearson, Susan J. *The Birth Certificate: An American History*. University of North Carolina Press, 2021.
Perdue, Theda. "Southern Indians and Jim Crow." In *The Folly of Jim Crow: Rethinking the Segregated South*, edited by Stephanie Cole and Natalie J. Ring. Texas A&M University Press, 2012.
Pernick, Martin S. *The Black Stork: Eugenics and the Death of "Defective" Babies in American Medicine and Motion Pictures Since 1915*. Oxford University Press, 1996.
Perry, Nicole. *Policing Sex in the Sunflower State: The Story of the Kansas State Industrial Farm for Women*. University Press of Kansas, 2021.
Pickens, Donald K. *Eugenics and the Progressives*. Vanderbilt University Press, 1968.
Pierson, Paul. "Increasing Returns, Path Dependence, and the Study of Politics." *American Political Science Review* 94, no. 2 (2000): 251–67.
———. "The Study of Policy Development." *Journal of Policy History* 17, no. 1 (2005): 35–51.
Piven, Frances Fox, and Richard A. Cloward. *Regulating the Poor: The Functions of Public Welfare*, updated ed. Vintage Books, 1993.
Platt, Anthony. *The Child Savers: The Invention of Delinquency*. University of Chicago Press, 1977.
Polansky, Lee S. "I Certainly Hope That You Will Be Able to Train Her: Reformers and the Georgia Training School for Girls." In *Before the New Deal: Social Welfare in the South, 1830–1930*, edited by Elna Green. University of Georgia Press, 1999.
Poole, Mary. *The Segregated Origins of Social Security: African Americans and the Welfare State*. University of North Carolina Press, 2006.
Powell, William S., ed. *Dictionary of North Carolina Biography*. University of North Carolina Press, 1979–96.

———. *North Carolina Through Four Centuries*. University of North Carolina Press, 1989.
Price, Gregory N., William Darity Jr., and Rhonda V. Sharpe. "Did North Carolina Economically Breed-Out Blacks During Its Historical Eugenic Sterilization Campaign?" *American Review of Political Economy* 15, no. 1 (June 2020).
Proctor, Robert W., and Rand Evans. "E. B. Titchener, Women Psychologists, and the Experimentalists." *American Journal of Psychology* 127, no. 4 (2014): 501–26.
Rabinowitz, Howard N. *The First New South, 1865–1920*. Harlan Davidson, 1992.
Rafter, Nicole Hahn. *Partial Justice: Women, Prisons, and Social Control*. Transaction, 1990.
———, ed. *White Trash: The Eugenic Family Studies, 1877–1919*. Northeastern University Press, 1988.
Railey, John. *Rage to Redemption in the Sterilization Age: A Confrontation with American Genocide*. Cascade Books, 2015.
Ready, Milton. *The Tar Heel State: A History of North Carolina*. University of South Carolina Press, 2005.
Reilly, Philip R. *The Surgical Solution: A History of Involuntary Sterilization in the United States*. Johns Hopkins University Press, 1991.
Richmond, Mary. *Social Diagnosis*. Russell Sage Foundation, 1917.
Ring, Natalie J. *The Problem South: Region, Empire, and the New Liberal State, 1880–1930*. University of Georgia Press, 2012.
Ritterhouse, Jennifer. *Growing Up Jim Crow: How Black and White Southern Children Learned Race*. University of North Carolina Press, 2006.
Roberts, Dorothy E. "Black Club Women and Child Welfare: Lessons for Modern Reform." *Florida State University Law Review* 32, no. 3 (Spring 2005): 957–72.
———. *Killing the Black Body: Race, Reproduction, and the Meaning of Liberty*. Pantheon Books, 1997.
Rodgers, Daniel T. "In Search of Progressivism." *Reviews in American History* 10, no. 4 (December 1982): 113–32.
Rogoff, Leonard. *Gertrude Weil: Jewish Progressive in the New South*. University of North Carolina Press, 2017.
Rose, Sarah F. *No Right to Be Idle: The Invention of Disability, 1840s–1930s*. University of North Carolina Press, 2017.
Rosen, Christine. *Preaching Eugenics: Religious Leaders and the American Eugenics Movement*. Oxford University Press, 2004.
Rosenberg, Gabriel. "No Scrubs: Livestock Breeding, Eugenics, and the State in the Early Twentieth-Century United States." *Journal of American History* 107, no. 2 (September 2020): 362–87.
Royster, Hubert A. "An Account of the Surgical Service in the State Hospital for the Insane at Raleigh, 1922–1932." *Southern Medicine and Surgery* 95 (1933): 320–21.
Ruswick, Brent. *Almost Worthy: The Poor, Paupers, and the Science of Charity in America, 1877–1917*. Indiana University Press, 2013.
Saez, Emmanuel, and Gabriel Zucman. "Wealth Inequality in the United States Since 1913: Evidence from Capitalized Income Tax Data." *Quarterly Journal of Economics* 131, no. 2 (May 2016): 519–78.
Sallee, Shelley. *The Whiteness of Child Labor Reform in the New South*. University of Georgia Press, 2004.

Sanders, Wiley B. *Juvenile Courts in North Carolina*. University of North Carolina Press, 1948.

Saxon, John L. *Social Services in North Carolina*. University of North Carolina School of Government, 2008.

Schneider, Anne L., and Helen M. Ingram. *Deserving and Entitled: Social Constructions and Public Policy*. State University of New York Press, 2004.

Schoen, Johanna. *Choice and Coercion: Birth Control, Sterilization, and Abortion in Public Health and Welfare*. University of North Carolina Press, 2005.

———. "From the Footnotes to the Headlines: Sterilization Apologies and Their Lessons." *Sexuality Research and Social Policy* 3, no. 3 (September 2006): 7–22.

———. "Reassessing Eugenic Sterilization: The Case of North Carolina." In *A Century of Eugenics in America: From the Indiana Experiment to the Human Genome Era*, edited by Paul A. Lombardo. Indiana University Press, 2011.

Schultz, Mark. *The Rural Face of White Supremacy: Beyond Jim Crow*. University of Illinois Press, 2007.

Scott, Anne Firor. *Natural Allies: Women's Associations in American History*. University of Illinois Press, 1991.

———. *The Southern Lady: From Pedestal to Politics, 1830–1930*. University Press of Virginia, 1995.

Scott, James C. *Seeing Like a State: How Certain Schemes to Improve the Human Condition Have Failed*. Yale University Press, 1998.

Selden, Steven. *Inheriting Shame: The Story of Eugenics and Racism in America*. Teachers College Press, 1999.

Sharpless, Rebecca, and Melissa Walker. "Inside the Farmhouse: Ruth Allen and Margaret Jarman Hagood Confront Rural Realities." In *Reassessing the 1930s South*, edited by Karen L. Cox and Sarah E. Gardner. Louisiana State University Press, 2018.

Shaw, Margaret Elizabeth. "The Development of the North Carolina Federation of Women's Clubs." Master's thesis, University of North Carolina at Chapel Hill, 1925.

Shivers, Lyda Gordon. "The Social Welfare Movement in the South: A Study in Regional Culture and Social Organization." PhD dissertation, University of North Carolina at Chapel Hill, 1935.

Silverberg, Helene, ed. *Gender and American Social Science: The Formative Years*. Princeton University Press, 2021.

Sims, Anastatia. *The Power of Femininity in the New South: Women's Organizations and Politics in North Carolina, 1880–1930*. University of South Carolina Press, 1997.

Singal, Daniel. *The War Within: From Victorian to Modernist Thought in the South, 1919–1945*. University of North Carolina Press, 1982.

Skocpol, Theda. *Protecting Mothers and Soldiers: The Political Origins of Social Policy in the United States*. Belknap Press of Harvard University Press, 1992.

Smith, J. Douglas. *Managing White Supremacy: Race, Politics, and Citizenship in Jim Crow Virginia*. University of North Carolina Press, 2002.

Speas, Ethel. *History of the Voluntary Mental Health Movement in North Carolina*. North Carolina Mental Health Association, 1961.

Stein, Melissa. "Nature Is the Author of Such Restrictions: Science, Ethnological Medicine, and Jim Crow." In *The Folly of Jim Crow: Rethinking the Segregated*

South, edited by Stephanie Cole and Natalie J. Ring. Texas A&M University Press, 2012.

Stern, Alexandra Minna. *Eugenic Nation: Faults and Frontiers of Better Breeding in Modern America*. University of California Press, 2005.

———. "Making Better Babies: Public Health and Race Betterment in Indiana, 1920–1935." *American Journal of Public Health* 92, no. 5 (2002): 742–52.

———. *Telling Genes: The Story of Genetic Counseling in America*. Johns Hopkins University Press, 2012.

———. "'We Cannot Make a Silk Purse Out of a Sow's Ear': Eugenics in the Hoosier Heartland." *Indiana Magazine of History* 103, no. 1 (March 2007): 3–38.

Storrs, Landon R. Y. *Civilizing Capitalism: The National Consumers' League, Women's Activism, and Labor Standards in the New Deal Era*. University of North Carolina Press, 2000.

Stubblefield, Anna. "Beyond the Pale: Tainted Whiteness, Cognitive Disability, and Eugenic Sterilization." *Hypatia* 22, no. 2 (Spring 2007): 162–81.

Sylla, Richard. "Long-Term Trends in State and Local Finance: Sources and Uses of Funds in North Carolina, 1800–1977." In *Long-Term Factors in American Economic Growth*, edited by Stanley L. Engerman and Robert E. Gallman. University of Chicago Press, 1986.

Szymanski, Ann-Marie. "Beyond Parochialism: Southern Progressivism, Prohibition, and State-Building." *Journal of Southern History* 69, no. 1 (February 2003): 107–36.

Tani, Karen. *States of Dependency: Welfare, Rights, and American Governance, 1935–1972*. Cambridge University Press, 2016.

Thomas, Karen Kruse. *Deluxe Jim Crow: Civil Rights and American Health Policy, 1935–1954*. University of Georgia Press, 2011.

Tillinghast, Anne Williams. "A Statistical Study of the Social Work Personnel in the North Carolina County Departments of Public Welfare, November 1941." Master's thesis, University of North Carolina at Chapel Hill, 1943.

Tindall, George Brown. *The Emergence of the New South, 1913–1945*. Louisiana State University Press, 1967.

Trattner, Walter I., ed. *Biographical Dictionary of Social Welfare in America*. Greenwood Press, 1986.

———. *From Poor Law to Welfare State: A History of Social Welfare in America*, 6th ed. Free Press, 1999.

Trent, James W., Jr. *Inventing the Feeble Mind: A History of Intellectual Disability in the United States*, 2nd ed. Oxford University Press, 2017.

Trolander, Judith. *Professionalism and Social Change: From the Settlement House to Neighborhood Centers, 1886 to the Present*. Columbia University Press, 1987.

Turda, Marius. "Race, Science, and Eugenics in the Twentieth Century." In *The Oxford Handbook of the History of Eugenics*, edited by Allison Bashford and Phillipa Levine. Oxford University Press, 2010.

Turner, Elizabeth Hayes. *Women, Culture, and Community: Religion and Reform in Galveston, 1880–1920*. Oxford University Press, 1997.

Vogt, Sara. "Bodies of Surveillance: Disability, Femininity, and the Keepers of the Gene Pool, 1910–1925." PhD dissertation, University of Illinois at Chicago, 2012.

Walker, Sydnor H. *Social Work and the Training of Social Workers*. University of North Carolina Press, 1928.

Walkowitz, Daniel. "The Making of a Feminine Professional Identity: Social Workers in the 1920s." *American Historical Review* 95, no. 4 (October 1990): 1051–75.

———. *Working with Class: Social Workers and the Politics of Middle-Class Identity*. University of North Carolina Press, 1999.

Ware, Susan. *Beyond Suffrage: Women in the New Deal*. Harvard University Press, 1981.

Weathers, Betty Evans. *A Century to Celebrate: A History of the North Carolina Federation of Women's Clubs, 1902–1988, and GFWC of North Carolina, 1998–2002*. School of Graphic Arts, Masonic Home for Children, 2003.

Weindling, Paul. "German Eugenics and the Wider World: Beyond the Racial State." In *The Oxford Handbook of the History of Eugenics*, edited by Allison Bashford and Phillipa Levine. Oxford University Press, 2010.

Welborn, Eleanor Palmer. "Eugenical Sterilization in the United States, with Particular Attention to a Follow-Up Study of Non-Institutional Sterilization Cases in North Carolina, April 5, 1933 to January 1, 1939." Master's thesis, University of North Carolina at Chapel Hill, 1940.

Wells, Amy E. "Considering Her Influence: Sydnor H. Walker and Rockefeller Support for Social Work, Social Scientists, and Universities in the South." In *Women and Philanthropy in Education*, edited by Andrea Walton. Indiana University Press, 2004.

Wheeler, Marjorie Spruill. *New Women of the New South: The Leaders of the Woman Suffrage Movement in the Southern States*. Oxford University Press, 1993.

White, Deborah Gray. *Too Heavy a Load: Black Women in Defense of Themselves, 1894–1994*. W. W. Norton, 1998.

White, Ronald C., Jr., and C. Howard Hopkins, *The Social Gospel: Religion and Reform in Changing America*. Temple University Press, 1976.

Wiebe, Robert H. *The Search for Order, 1877–1920*. Hill and Wang, 1967.

Wilds, Sarah. "And the North Carolina Morons Lived | Happily Ever After: The Human Betterment League of North Carolina, 1947–1988." Master's thesis, University of North Carolina-Charlotte, 2019.

Wilkerson-Freeman, Sarah. "From Clubs to Parties: North Carolina Women in the Advancement of the New Deal." *North Carolina Historical Review* 68, no. 3 (July 1991): 320–39.

———. "Women and the Transformation of American Politics: North Carolina, 1898–1940." PhD dissertation, University of North Carolina at Chapel Hill, 1995.

Winling, LaDale C., and Todd M. Michley, "The Roots of Redlining: Academic, Governmental, and Professional Networks in the Making of the New Deal Lending Regime." *Journal of American History* 108, no. 1 (2021): 42–69.

Wisner, Elizabeth. *Social Welfare in the South: From Colonial Times to World War I*. Louisiana State University Press, 1970.

Woodside, Moya. *Sterilization in North Carolina: A Sociological and Psychological Study*. University of North Carolina Press, 1950.

Woodward, C. Vann. *Origins of the New South, 1877–1913*. Louisiana State University Press, 1951.

Wray, Matt. *Not Quite White: White Trash and the Boundaries of Whiteness*. Duke University Press, 2006.

Wright, David. "Mongols in Our Midst: John Langdon Down and the Ethnic

Classification of Idiocy, 1858–1924." In *Mental Retardation in America: A Historical Reader*, edited by Steven Noll and James W. Trent Jr. New York University Press, 2004.

Wyche, Mary Lewis. *The History of Nursing in North Carolina*. University of North Carolina Press, 1938.

Zelizer, Vivian. *Pricing the Priceless Child: The Changing Social Value of Children*. Basic Books, 1985.

Zenderland, Leila. *Measuring Minds: Henry Herbert Goddard and the Origins of American Intelligence Testing*. Cambridge University Press, 1998.

———. "The Parable of the Kallikak Family: Explaining the Meaning of Heredity in 1912." In *Mental Retardation in America: A Historical Reader*, edited by Steven Noll and James W. Trent Jr. New York University Press, 2003.

Zipf, Karin L. *Bad Girls at Samarcand: Sexuality and Sterilization in a Southern Juvenile Reformatory*. Louisiana State University Press, 2016.

Index

Italic page numbers refer to illustrations.

abortion ban, 219
Aid to Dependent Children (ADC), 190, 192, 195–96
Alabama, 73, 257n69
alcohol use, 44, 45, 63, 71, 121, 128, 133–34, 203
Alderman, John T., 155
American Association for the Study of the Feeble-Minded (AASFM), 129
American Breeders Association, 7
American Genetic Association, 7
American Psychological Association, 127
American Social Hygiene Association, 109
American Tobacco Company, 16
Anglo-Saxon identity and racial concept, 9, 62–63, 116–17, 227n20
apartheid, 34
arson: Caswell, 69, 82–85, 88, 133, 254n36; Samarcand, 165–70; court case, 165–70, 254n46
Associated Charities, 20, 160
Atlanta School of Social Work, 108
Aycock, Charles B., 35

Baggett, John R., 149, 252n25
Barr, Martin W., 83–84, 85, 142
BCPW Bulletin: on "bad heredity," 112–13; on family types, *113*, 114; on feeblemindedness, 111–12, *116*, *163*; on Mothers' Aid, *119*; on white boys, *117*. *See also* North Carolina Board of Charities and Public Welfare (BCPW)
Beasley, Roland, 97, 125, 156, 265n77
Beers, Clifford, 127

Being Well Born (Guyer), 195
benevolent societies, 78. *See also names of specific organizations*
Benson, J. McLean, 201, 203, 204, 205–6, 210, 287n1, 294n56, 294n64
"better babies" contests, 8, 63–64
Bickett, Thomas, 1, 36, 67, 79, 86, 95
Binet-Simon intelligence testing method, 48, 57, 275n43
Birth of a Nation, The (Dixon), 36
Bishop Tuttle Memorial Training School of Social Work, 108
Black Advisory Committee, 267n101
Black people: assumptions about inferiority of, 30, 33–34, 51, 62, 109, 114; "negro problem," 32, 33–34, 39, 107, 110, 235n71; reformatories and training schools for, 48, 97; welfare benefits for, 210–11; white reformers and eugenics strategies on, 8–9, 34; and women's reform work, 30–31, 78, 106–11, 189–90, 191–92, 231n32, 267n103. *See also* Black women; racial arguments; white people
Black Stork, The (film), 252n21
Black women: reform and social work of, 30–31, 78, 106–11, 189–90, 191–92, 231n32, 267n103; social clubs of, 26, 30; sterilization programs for, 15, 199, 211, 217. *See also* Black people; women
Blair, William A., 24
Blount, Marvin K., 155
Board of Charities and Public Welfare. *See* North Carolina Board of Charities and Public Welfare (BCPW)
Bold, Mark, 218

Bost, Annie Kizer: career of, 186–87, 288n8; at Conference for Social Service, 209; Eugenics Board membership of, 194; as head of BCPW, 191, 210, 258n5; on sterilization, 195, 197–98, 199, 206
Bradway, John S., 175–77, 180
Branson, Eugene Cunningham, 101
Braswell, James Cornelius, 150
Brewer, Margaret, 170, 172, 182
Brewer, Mary, 14, 158, 170–75, 177, 217
Brewer v. Valk, 14, 158, 170–78, 201, 285m45, 286n51
Brietz, Margaret, 130–31, 263n57
Brown, Julius, 87
Brown, R. Eugene, 160, 170, 181, 194, 195, 198, 291n34
Brown, Roy M., 274n42
Browning, Elizabeth, 30
Brummit, Dennis G., 85
Bryson, Edward, 179
Bryson, Sally, 84
Buck v. Bell, 14, 124, 150, 154, 158–59, 170, 181, 182, 286n52

"cacogenic" traits, 7, 55, 123, 131–41, 157, 181. *See also* feeblemindedness; fitness (term and concept); hereditary arguments about feeblemindedness
Cahn, Susan, 168–69
California, 8, 155
Carr, James O., 152, 153
cash assistance, 160, 189, 191, 192, 215. *See also* Aid to Dependent Children (ADC); Mothers' Aid; outdoor relief
castration, 73
Caswell Training School, 13, 52, 57–60; arson at, 69, 88, 133, 254n46; Crane's work at, 126–30, 144–46; establishment of, 42, 48, 76–77; expansion of, 87–89, 126; fires at, 70; funding of, 252n29; Johnson's work at, 97; mental testing at, 270n5; Parrott on, 66; reports on, 142, 144, 151–54, 255n54; sterilizations at, 198, 199. *See also* reformatories
Central Liberty Loan Committee, 94
Chamberlain-Kahn Act (1918), 79

Chambers, Mrs. Oscar, 184
Charity Organization Society of New York, 25
Charlotte Junior League, 207
Charlotte Observer, 79, 84
Chatham, Lucy Hodgins Hanes, 210
Cherokee, 6
Cherokee County, NC, 19–20
Chicago School of Civics and Philanthropy, 25
child labor, 3, 5, 12, 16, 17, 18, 32, 68
Chinese Exclusion Act, 10
Christ Church (Raleigh), 23
Christian ideologies: on charity services, 19, 21, 23, 25, 30, 33, 40, 46; eugenics and, 42, 61, 142. *See also* Progressive movement
Christian Law Institute, 218
church missionary societies, 30. *See also* female reformers and women's clubs
citizenship, 3, 10–12, 71, 228n26. *See also* voting rights
Civilian Conservation Corps, 190, 196
Civil Works Administration, 193
Clansman, The (Dixon), 36
Clark, William Grimes, 155
Commission on Interracial Cooperation, 110
Commission on Training Camp Activities, 79
Conference for Social Service. *See* North Carolina Conference for Social Service
Congress of Parents and Teachers, 134
constitutional rights, 10, 19, 287n66
Coon, Charles, 50
Cott, Nancy, 10
Cotten, Sallie Southall, 29–30, 37, 38
cotton industry, 17, 18, 41, 117, 184. *See also* industries
Country Life movement, 34
county homes, 19–20, 120
county-unit welfare system, 96
county welfare boards, 20
Craig, Locke, 32, 36
Crane, Harry W.: at Caswell, 126–31, 144–46; as director of Division of Mental Health and Hygiene, 124, 125; mental testing by, 90; speaking events of, 175; on

sterilization bills, 149, 170, 180; trainings and lectures by, 115, 123, 175
custodial institutions. *See names of specific institutions*

Daniels, Josephus, 32, 35
Daughters of the American Revolution, 54
Davenport, Charles, 53, 242n59
Davidson Book Lovers' Club, 38
Dean, Gordon, 179
Delaware, 155
delinquency, female, 76–84, 165–70, 254n39. *See also* Samarcand Manor; Stonewall Jackson Training School
Democratic Party, 4, 21, 35, 256n60
Denson, Claude, 22, 23, 46
Denson, Daisy: background of, 16; Board of Public Charities work by, 18, 21–26; Conference for Social Service and, 31; on feeblemindedness, 46; on Johnson's appointment, 97; legislative bills and, 240n32; on reformatory school, 50, 58; studies of eugenics by, 238n18. *See also* North Carolina Board of Public Charities (BPC)
Denson, Margaret Matilda Cowan, 22
Denson, Mary, 23
Depression. *See* Great Depression
deservingness, ideologies on poverty and, 2, 3, 9, 91, 185–86, 192, 193, 217. *See also* poverty
disabilities, 4, 7, 9, 43, 44, 48, 58–59, 76, 116, 252n21. *See also* feeblemindedness
disease: parasitic hookworm, 19; pellagra, 18–19; syphilis, 71, 133, 209, 250n9, 271n6; tuberculosis, 45, 60–61, 257n65; venereal, 6, 45, 71, 73, 79, 80, 87, 88, 131, 137, 167, 206–7, 251n14
Division of Field Social Work, BCPW, 190
Division of Mental Health and Hygiene, BCPW, 98, 124–31, 144, *145*, 193
Division of Public Assistance, BCPW, 190–91
Division of Work Among Negroes, BCPW, 110, 191, 192
Dix Hill mental hospital, 19, 88, 134, 147

Dixon, Thomas, Jr., 35–36
Dixon, W. H., 129, 144
Dosher, Lois, 165
Du Bois, W. E. B., 110
Duke Law School, 174, *179*
Duke Legal Aid Clinic, 174–77, *179*
Durham, NC, 16
Durham Crime Study Club, 175, 193–94

Eastern Band of Cherokee Indians, 6
Eastern Carolina Training School, 193
Eck, Lina Fehler, *139*
economic depressions, 12, 14, 15, 17, 121, 159–60, 184, 245n80. *See also* New Deal programs; poverty
Efland reformatory, 48, 78
Ehringhaus, John, 188, 289n13, 289n14
enslaved people, 6, 22
environmental cases of delinquency and feeblemindedness, 7, 44, 117, 130, 133, 203–4. *See also* feeblemindedness
epilepsy, 111, 244n72
Equal Suffrage Association, 38
Estabrook, Arthur, 8
Eugenical News, 56, 243n66
Eugenical Sterilization Act (1924), 150
eugenic family studies, 8, 43, *113*, 114, 123, 131–41, 195. *See also* North Carolina Board of Charities and Public Welfare (BCPW)
eugenics, 1–3, 6–15, 60–67, 158, 214–19; British roots of, 6; European programs for, 227n17; negative, 6, 7; positive, 6; public campaigns for, 8, 30, 63–65, 123, 141–46, 155, 157, 160–62, 231n31, 281n5. *See also* feeblemindedness; sterilization; sterilization laws
Eugenics Board of North Carolina, 158, 179–82, 194, 197–206
Eugenics Record Office (ERO), 7–8, 53, 113, 126, 128, 131, 154, 243n65
euthanasia, 13, 69, 70, 74–75, 252n21

factories, 4, 18
family studies, 8, 43, *113*, 114, 123, 131–41, 195. *See also* North Carolina Board of Charities and Public Welfare (BCPW)

Index 323

Farmers' Institutes, 28
fascism, 6
Federal Emergency Relief Administration (FERA), 188, 193, 289n13
feeblemindedness: "cacogenic" traits and, 7, 55, 123, 131–41, 157, 181; custodial institutions for, 13, 42, 48, 52, 57–60, 66; definition of, 1, 7, 236n7; delinquency and, 83–84; environmental causes of, 7, 44, 117, 130, 203–4; hereditary arguments about, 7, 41, 44, 55–56, 110, 111–13, 122, 130, 201–3, 212, 236n7; high-grade, 7; as "humanitarian cause," 48–54; low-grade, 7; as "menace," 43–48, 143; photographs claiming to depict, *116*, *163*; religious arguments about, 42–43, 45, 247n93; as "root of social problems," 2, 90–91, 111–12; segregation and, 41–43, 51, 65, 120, 240n39. *See also* disabilities; eugenics; poverty; sterilization
Fehler family, 134–41
female reformers and women's clubs, 21–31
First Baptist Church (Raleigh), 32
fitness (term and concept), 2, 8, 9, 11, 43, 70, 115–18, 199, 247n97
forced sterilization. *See* sterilization
Fourteenth Amendment, 10, 287n66
furniture industry, 11, 16, 171
FWC. *See* North Carolina Federation of Women's Clubs

Galloway, Thomas Coleman, 155
Gamble, Clarence, 210
Gardner, O. Max, 155, 159–60, 186, 187, 188, 189, 192
genealogical charts, *135*, *140*
Germany, 6, 256n61
Glenn, William Darby, 136–38, 275n43
Goddard, Henry H., 43, 48, 57, 236n7
Gosney, Ezra S., 182
Goudge, Mabel Ensworth, 126–27
Governor's Office of Relief (NC), 187
Gravely, Lloyd L., 155
Great Depression, 12, 14, 15, 159–60, 184, 191, 212, 215, 245n80. *See also* economic depressions; New Deal programs

Greensboro Record, 152
Groves, Ernest, 201, 209–10

Halbert, Leroy A., 95
Hanes, Frederic M., 207
Hanes, James, 210
Hardy, Hattie, 48
Hardy, Ira M., 13, 42, 48–54, 57, 60, 239n30
Hart, Hastings, 51, 97
hereditary arguments about feeblemindedness: at Caswell and other institutions, 41, 44; among medical doctors, 44; at national level, 236n7; studies of, 55–56, 130, 201–3; welfare officials and, 110, 111–13, 122, 212. *See also* "cacogenic" traits; feeblemindedness
Herndon, C. Nash, 210
Hester, Hanselle "Jerry," 173, 174, 177
Holmes, Oliver Wendell, 154
Hoover, Herbert, 121
Human Betterment Foundation, 175, 182
Human Betterment League of North Carolina, 210
Human Sterilization (Landman), 195
Hunter, Carey J., 24
Hunter, Helen, 210
Hutchins, Fred, 173, 177
Hutt, Mrs. W. N., 28
Hyatt, Henry Otis, 74
Hyatt, Sybil, 42, 54–57, 62, 74

Illinois Children's Home and Aid Society, 134
immigration: anti-immigrant sentiment, 56, 62; restrictions of, 6, 8
Indiana, 73
Indigenous groups, 6
industrialization, 4, 18
industries: cotton, 17, 18, 41, 117, 184; furniture, 11, 16, 171; railroads, 18; textile mills, 11, 16, 17, 172; tobacco, 11, 16, 17, 41, 117, 159, 171
inmates: mental defect arguments about, 25, 114; sterilization of, 84–85, 87; testing of, 272n18, 272n19. *See also names of specific institutions*

inspectors of state facilities, 20–21. *See also* North Carolina Board of Public Charities (BPC)
Institute for Research in the Social Sciences (University of North Carolina), 160, 263n64
institutional segregation. *See* segregation and feeblemindedness
intelligence testing, 48, 57, 81, 87, 90–91, 124, 130, 275n43
International Prison Congress, 24
involuntary sterilization. *See* sterilization
Iredell County, NC, 20
Ivey, Henry B., 155

James, Carmine, 130
John Locke Foundation, 217–18
Johnson, Alexander, 73, 251n17, 252n23
Johnson, Clarence A., 93
Johnson, Kate Burr, 93–98; on *Buck v. Bell*, 154; and hiring of Crane, 126, 127; on racial difference, 106–7; sterilization bill and, 154; on training workers, 101, 103; as welfare commissioner, 13, 90, 104, 107, 189
Johnson, Lester, 155
Joyner, James Yadkin, 31, 33
Jukes in 1915, The (Estabrook), 8, 123, 195

Kallikak Family, The (study), 43, 123, 195
Kentucky, 241n42
Kesler, M. L., 31
King's Daughters of North Carolina (organization), 23, 47, 78
Kinston, NC, 41, 52
Kinston Free Press, 49
Kitchin, William, 49

Larson, Edward, 236n3
Lassiter, William C., 179, *179*
Lathrop, Julia, 27, 35
Laughinghouse, Charles, 41, 43, 156
Laughlin, Harry, 55, 150
Laura Spelman Rockefeller Memorial, 104, 107, 111, 192, 266n82, 288n11
Lawrence, George H., 184, 201, 210
Lay, Lucy F., 143–44
League of Women Voters (NC), 91

Legal Aid Clinic (Duke University), 174–77, *179*
Lewis, Nell Battle, 123, 142, 167–68
Lingle, Clara Swift Souther, 37–38, 72, 97
Lingle, Thomas Wilson, 37–38
Lombardo, Paul, 218
Lost Cause ideology, 2, 22. *See also* white supremacy
Louisiana, 241n42
Lumbee, 6
Lynchburg State Colony (VA), 240n36, 257n69

MacLean, Angus W., 151
MacNaughton, Agnes, 80
marriage: education, 70; restrictions and laws, 6, 45, 69–73, 122, 134. *See also* miscegenation
Marshall, T. H., 228n26
McAlister, Alexander W., 39, 95, 120, 185
McBrayer, Louis Burgin, 31, 60–61, 63, 64
McCracken, J. R., 147
McDonald, William, 125–26
McGeachy, A. A., 78
McNairy, C. Banks, 57, 60, 273n28. *See also* Caswell Training School
McNaughton, Agnes, 166
Mental Health and Hygiene division, BCPW, 98, 124–31, 144, 193, 276n61
mental hygiene, 39, 115, 118, 125, 127, 141–42, 162, 193–97, 246n88
Mental Hygiene Association, 60, 71
Mental Hygiene Society, 175, 209
mental illness, 6, 7, 95, 114, 121, 127, 142, 157, 210. *See also* North Carolina State Hospital at Raleigh
mental testing. *See* intelligence testing
Michigan, 293n54
Miller, Justin, 175
Millner, Henry L., 154–55
miscegenation, 33–34, 72. *See also* marriage: restrictions and laws
Morganton asylum, 83
Morrison reformatory, 48
Mothers' Aid, 117–18, *119*, 163, 187–88, 189, 195–96, 201

National Association of Legal Aid Societies, 175
National Committee for Mental Hygiene, 88, 142
National Committee on Provision for the Feeble-Minded, 35
National Conference of Charities and Correction (NCCC), 24, 47, 73
National Conference on Social Work, 142
National Congress of Mothers, 34–35
National Industrial Recovery Act, 188
National Organization for Public Health Nursing, 35
National Youth Administration, 99
Nation's Health (newspaper), 144
natural selection, 247n94
"negro problem," 32, 33–34, 39, 107, 110, 235n71. *See also* Black people; white supremacy
Newbold, William, 129, 273n28
New Deal programs, 11, 14–15, 185, 186–92, 211–12. *See also* Great Depression; Social Security programs
New Hampshire, 293n54
New Jersey, 186
New Jersey State Home for Delinquent Girls, 186
News and Observer, 32, 35, 50, 155, 167, 207
New South, 3, 16, 21
New York School of Philanthropy, 16
New York School of Social Work, 97
North Carolina: economic and political climate of, 11–12, 14–15, 18, 226n11; eugenics program, 1, 8–10, 15, 158, 214–19; industries, 11, 16, 17, 41, 117, 159, 171, 184; rural population of, 17; social welfare system, 3, 9–10, 13, 18–21, 211–13, 259n20; state constitution, 19
North Carolina Board of Agriculture, 28
North Carolina Board of Charities and Public Welfare (BCPW): eugenic family studies by, 8, 43, *113*, 114, 123, 131–41; Field Social Work division, 190; funding of, 160, 187–88, 189, 190, 288n11, 290n17; Johnson's work at, 289n14; locations and districts of, 194–95; Mental Health and Hygiene division, 98, 124–31, 144, 193, 276n61; on mentally defective people, 197, 208; organization of, 95–99, 271n6, 271n10; post-1929 sterilization law and, 160–62; professional training by, 99–106, 185–86, 189–90, 194–95; Public Assistance division, 190–91; purpose of, 91; Social Security programs and, 212; Work Among Negroes division, 110, 191, 192. *See also BCPW Bulletin*
North Carolina Board of Health, 35
North Carolina Board of Public Charities (BPC), 18–29. *See also* Denson, Daisy
North Carolina Children's Home Society, 81
North Carolina Confederate Veterans' Association, 22
North Carolina Conference for Social Service, 12–13, 18, 31–40, 60, 70, 71, 144
North Carolina Emergency Relief Administration (NC ERA), 188–92
North Carolina Federation of Colored Women's Clubs, 30
North Carolina Federation of Women's Clubs, 26–28, 29–30, 37, 38, 60, 72, 78, 79, 94, 130
North Carolina Health Officers' Association, 87
North Carolina Hospital Commission, 48
North Carolina Medical Society, 49
North Carolina Salary and Wage Commission, 160
North Carolina School for the Feeble-Minded, 52
North Carolina State Hospital at Goldsboro, 83, 165, 188, 199, 293n53
North Carolina State Hospital at Raleigh, 19, 88, 134, 147

O'Berry, Annie Land, 188–89, 190, 290n20
Odum, Howard W., 102, 120
Old Age Assistance (OAA), 190
orphanages, 19, 20, 25, 31, 71, 97, 98, 118–20, 165
outdoor relief, 20, 215
ovariectomy, 279n90, 283n25. *See also* sterilization

Owen, Robert L., 32
Oxley, Lawrence, 106, 108, 109, 115, 191–92

parasitic hookworm, 19. *See also* disease
Parrott, Mattie, 66, 163
paternalism, 17, 20–21, 40, 42, 110
pellagra, 18–19. *See also* disease
Pennsylvania, 155
pensions, 21, 212
Pittsboro, NC, 16–17
plantation labor, 22
Poe, Clarence: as conference president, 31, 35, 36; as editor of *Progressive Farmer*, 31, 34
Poteat, William L., 32–33, 60, 61, 72, 151
poverty: county homes and, 19–20, 120; federal relief programs for, 11, 14–15, 185, 186–92; and ideologies of deservingness, 2, 3, 9, 91, 185–86, 192, 193, 217; new responses to, 21–26. See also *Brewer v. Valk*; economic depressions; feeblemindedness; welfare system
preventive social work, 193–97. *See also* social work
Priddy, Albert, 257n69
Problem South, 3–4
Progressive Farmer (magazine), 31, 34
Progressive movement, 5–6, 7, 11–12, 17–18, 21–22, 31–32, 229n6. *See also* Christian ideologies
public school education and teaching, 30
public welfare, 95–96. *See also* welfare system
Public Welfare Progress (bulletin), 142, 144, 145, 149, 154, 162, 165, 167, 281n7
Public Works Administration, 208

Quakers, 110, 175

race, construction of, 226n12
Race Betterment Foundation, 8
race suicide, 45, 62. *See also* Anglo-Saxon identity and racial concept; eugenics; immigration; white supremacy
racial arguments: and eugenics, 8–9; and feeblemindedness, 114–15, 120; in sterilization programs, 8, 15, 88, 124, 156, 217. *See also* Black people; segregation and feeblemindedness; white people; white supremacy
racial capitalism, 6, 11–12, 17. *See also* Black people; white people
Racial Integrity Act (1924; VA), 150, 278n74
racial uplift, 34, 109–10, 115, 267n95, 268n110
railroad industry, 18
Raleigh, NC, 16, 22
Raleigh Chamber of Commerce, 31
Raleigh Male Academy, 23
Raleigh Woman's Club, 21, 28, 93
Rankin, Watson Smith, 27, 31, 151–52
Rauschenbusch, Walter, 23
Reconstruction, 19
Reconstruction Finance Corporation (RFC), 187
Red Cross, 102, 261n35, 262n56, 263n63, 264n67
reformatories, 48. *See also* delinquency, female; Efland reformatory; Morrison reformatory; Samarcand Manor; Stonewall Jackson Training School
reform movements. *See* eugenics; female reformers and women's clubs; North Carolina Conference for Social Service; Progressive movement
religious arguments about feeblemindedness, 42–43, 45, 247n93
religious organizations, 26
Republicans, 19, 87, 217, 218, 256n60
Ring, Natalie, 3
Robson, Grace, 169, 209
Rockefeller Foundation, 121, 125, 207, 266n82
Rode, Nancy Fehler, 134–36
Roosevelt, Franklin Delano, 188. *See also* New Deal programs
Roosevelt, Theodore, 45
Royster, Hubert, 147–48, 162
Russell Sage Foundation, 97, 240n39

salpingectomy, 73. *See also* sterilization
Salvation Army, 81

Samarcand Manor: admittance to, 97; arson of, 165–70; Crane's study of, 276n55; establishment of, 78, 80, 253n35; funding of, 88, 253n33; sterilizations at, 198, 199, 283n25; studies of, 193
Sanders, Wiley Benton, 99–100, 101, 123
Scales, Alfred M., 78
School of Public Welfare (University of North Carolina), 101–2
Seaboard Medical Society, 49
segregation and feeblemindedness, 41–43, 51, 65, 120, 240n39. *See also* Caswell Training School.
sex education and hygiene, 65, 72
sharecropping, 17
Shivvers, Mandy, 130
Shotwell, Mary, 98–99
Simmons, Furnifold M., 35
social gospel, 23, 32, 38, 60, 61, 247n93. *See also* religious arguments about feeblemindedness
Social Security Act (1935), 190, 191
Social Security programs, 15, 190, 211, 290n25. *See also* New Deal programs
Social Service Quarterly (journal), 35, 39
social welfare programs. *See* welfare system
social work: by Black women, 30–31, 78, 106–11, 189–90, 191–92; caseworker profile, 104, 197, 265n80; gender dynamics of, 37–40, 216–17; on mental defects, 111–20; preventive, 193–97; training in, 99–106, 185–86, 189–90, 194–95, 196; by white women, 98–106. *See also* New Deal programs; North Carolina Board of Charities and Public Welfare (BCPW); welfare system
South Africa, 34
South Carolina, 79
South Dakota, 293n54
Southern problem, 3–4
Southern Progressivism. *See* Progressive movement
Southern Sociological Congress, 31
Spruill, Lydia, 13, 68, 69, 80–84, 88, 133, 254n46
St. Augustine's College, 108

Steiner, Jesse F., 102
sterilization, *148*; cost of, 294n64; of inmates, 84–85; institutional limits and, 84–88; McNairy on, 73–76, 85, 146; nineteenth-century debates on, 45–46; ovariectomy, 279n90, 283n25; in practice, 197–206, 283n25; public campaigns for, 8, 30, 63–65, 123, 141–46, 155, 157, 160–62, 281n5; public perceptions of, 206–11; statistics, 158–59, *164*, *200*, 225n2, 229n35; twentieth-century national debates on, 70. *See also* eugenics; feeblemindedness
Sterilization and Segregation (Goddard), 195
sterilization laws, 8, 146–51; 1919, 1, 13, 69, 85, 88, 124, 153; 1923 (proposed), 124, 149; 1924, discussion of, 149–50, 280n99; 1925 (proposed), 124, 150–51, 155, 278n75; 1929, 14, 124, 154–57, *161*, 279n90; 1933, 158, *176*, 179–82. See also *Brewer v. Valk*; *Buck v. Bell*
Stonewall Jackson Training School, 47, 77, 97, 99
strong-state liberalism, 3
suffrage, 3, 10, 30. *See also* citizenship
Summer School of Philanthropy (NY), 25
surgical operations. *See* sterilization
Survey (journal), 134
"Swamp Island" family, *132*, 141, 274n35
Swift, Wiley Hampton, 31
syphilis, 71, 133, 209, 250n9, 271n6. *See also* disease

taxes, ideology about, 5, 21, 107, 120, 207, 211, 215, 288n5
tenant farmers, 17
Tennessee, 31, 237n8
Texas, 237n8
textile mills, 11, 16, 17, 172. *See also* industries
Thompson, William A., 180, 239n30
Thornton, T. Spruill, 179
Tillis, Thom, 217
tobacco industry, 11, 16, 17, 41, 117, 159, 171. *See also* industries
Transylvania County, NC, 20
Trent, James, 43, 237n10, 238n19

tuberculosis, 45, 60–61, 257n65. *See also* disease
Tuttle, Emeth, 152, 261n43, 261n45

undeserving poor. *See* deservingness, ideologies on poverty and
United Daughters of the Confederacy, 22
US Army, 78
US Bureau of Education, 35
US Children's Bureau, 27, 35, 96
US Justice Department, 80

Valk, Arthur, 173
vasectomies, 73. *See also* sterilization
venereal disease, 6, 45, 71, 73, 79, 80, 87, 88, 131, 137, 167, 206–7, 251n14. *See also* disease
Vermont, 8, 293n54
Vineland Training School (NJ), 43, 51, 57
Virginia: eugenics program in, 8; mental institutions in, 237n8, 241n42; sterilization law of, 73, 149–50, 154, 257n69, 280n99, 287n62. See also *Buck v. Bell*
von KleinSmid, Rufus B., 175
voting rights, 10, 30. *See also* citizenship; suffrage

Waddill, Ella, 208–9
Wake County Memorial Association, 22
Wake family, 123, 133–34, *135*, 171, 194
Watauga Club, 35
Welborn, Eleanor, 201–3
welfare bulletin. See *BCPW Bulletin*
welfare law: 1917, 13, 95; 1919, 95–96
welfare system: Board of Public Charities involvement with, 28–29; development of, 3, 9–10, 13, 18–21, 94–97; federal policies and, 11, 14–15, 120–22, 185, 186–92, 211–12; female reformers and women's clubs' work with, 21–31; financial statistics on, 230n16. *See also* cash assistance; outdoor relief; poverty; social work; *and names of specific programs and organizations*
West Virginia, 237n8
Wettach, Robert, 170, 180
"What It Costs" (Hardy), 49
White House Conference on Child Health and Protection, 120
whiteness, 226n12. *See also* Anglo-Saxon identity and racial concept
white people: on degeneracy, 12, 62–63; elite class of, 4–5, 12–13; female delinquency, 76–84, 165–70; racial capitalism and, 6, 11–12, 17; reform networks and social work by, 21–31, 37–40, 189–90; as welfare officials, 98–106. *See also* Black people; racial arguments; racial capitalism
white supremacy, 4, 8–9, 22, 35, 116. *See also* Lost Cause ideology; racial arguments
Wilks, Fannie, 132
"Will You Help Find Out the Facts?" (Coon), 50
Wilmington, NC, 16
Wilson, Junius, 281n10
Wilson, William T., 173, 174
Wilson, Woodrow, 68
Winston, Ellen, 210
Winston-Salem Journal, 165
Wisconsin, 293n54
Woman's Club of Raleigh, 23, 78
Womble, Larry, 217
women: and gender dynamics of social work, 37–40, 216–17; reform networks and social clubs of, 21–31, 239n20; sterilization of (*see* sterilization); voting rights of, 3, 30
Women's Home Companion (magazine), 63
Works Progress Administration (WPA), 190, 210
World War I, 12, 22, 68
Wright, J. T., 273n28

Index   329

www.ingramcontent.com/pod-product-compliance
Lightning Source LLC
Chambersburg PA
CBHW020915220526
45357CB00035B/310